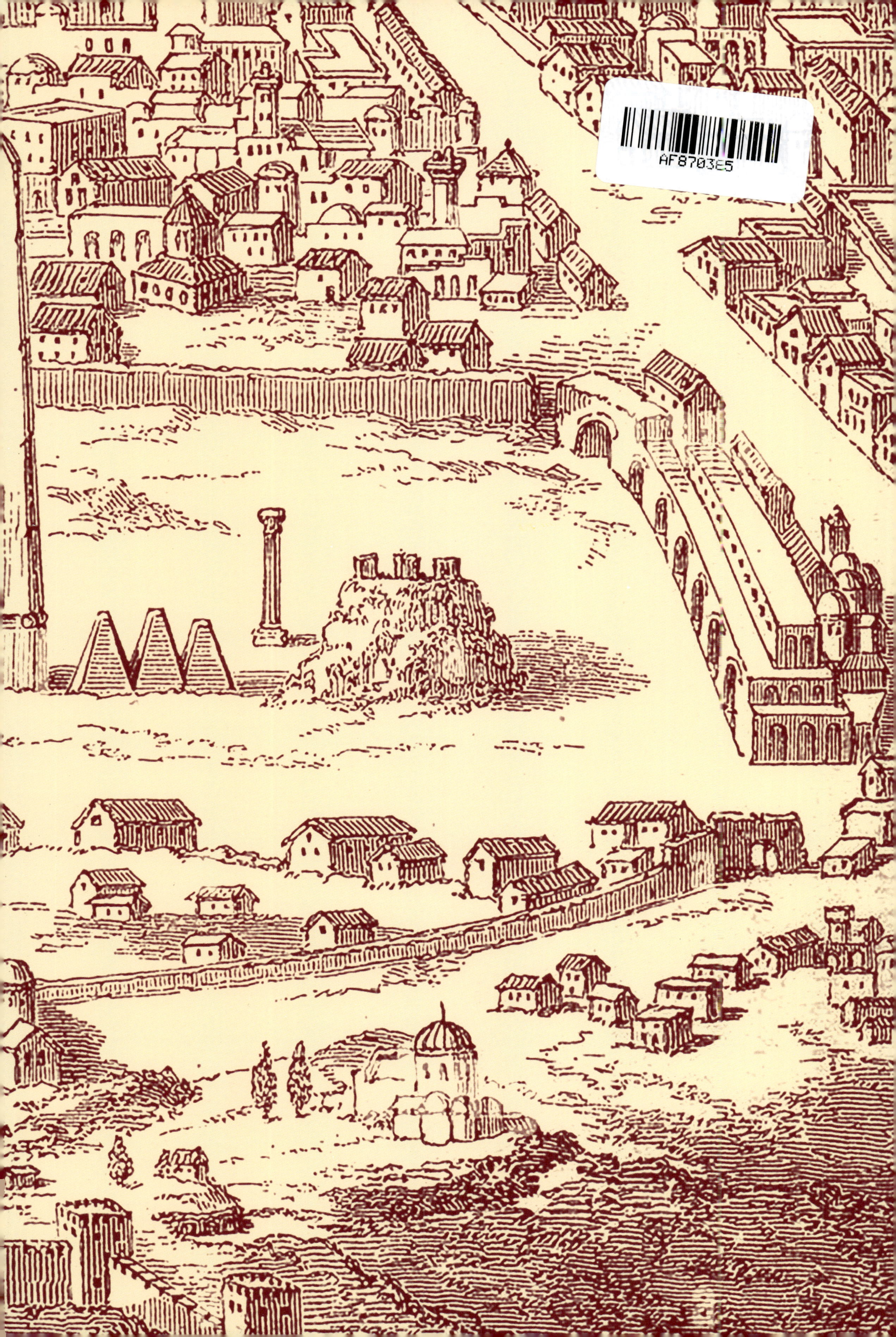

AF8703E5

Medicine and Hospitals in Byzantium

GEORGE C. PAPAGEORGIOU

Medicine and Hospitals in Byzantium

THROUGH THE LIFE OF A 12TH-CENTURY PHYSICIAN

Translated from Greek
Maxim Vasiljević

SEBASTIAN PRESS
LOS ANGELES

Published by
St. Sebastian Press

First Edition
Georgios C. Papageorgiou, *Η Ιατρική και τα Νοσοκομεία στο Βυζάντιο, Μέσα από τη ζωή ενός γιατρού του 12ου αιώνα*
(Athens: Hellenic Facsimile Editions – Ελληνικές Ομοιογραφικές Εκδόσεις, 2024)

Edited by
Bishop Maxim (Vasiljević)

Prepress for English Edition
Denis Vikić

Printing
Birograf COMP, Belgrade, Serbia

Contemporary Christian Thought Series, number 108

Copyright St. Sebastian Press & George C. Papageorgiou © 2025

Address all correspondence to:
Sebastian Press
1621 West Garvey Avenue • Alhambra, California 91803
E-mail: westsrbdio@gmail.com • Website: www.westsrbdio.org

Publishers Cataloging in Publication

Names:	Papageorgiou, George C. (George Constantine), 1945- author. | Vasiljević, Maksim, 1968- translator.
Title:	Medicine and hospitals in Byzantium through the life of a 12th-century physician / George C. Papageorgiou ; translated from the Greek, Maxim Vasiljević.
Other titles:	Η Ιατρική και τα Νοσοκομεία στο Βυζάντιο, Μέσα από τη ζωή ενός γιατρού του 12ου αιώνα. English
Description:	Los Angeles : Sebastian Press, [2025] | Series: Contemporary Christian thought series ; no. 108. | Translated from the Greek: Η Ιατρική και τα Νοσοκομεία στο Βυζάντιο, Μέσα από τη ζωή ενός γιατρού του 12ου αιώνα (εκδ. Ελληνικές Ομοιογραφικές Εκδόσεις, Αθήνα 2024). | Includes bibliographical references and index.
Identifiers:	ISBN: 9781964233222
Subjects:	LCSH: Physicians--Byzantine Empire--Fiction. | Hospitals--Byzantine Empire--Fiction. | Medical education--Byzantine Empire--Fiction. | Medical sciences--Byzantine Empire--Fiction. | Byzantine Empire—History--Fiction. | Istanbul (Turkey)—History--Fiction.
Classification:	LCC: PA5638.26.A617 M4313 2025 | DDC: 889.3--dc23

The Double-Headed Eagle of yours has flown afar,
Afar it soared, with all that's noble, all that's holy,
And its fourfold wings shall cast their mighty shadow
On other peoples, loftier peaks, and lands unknown.

Kostis Palamas

Contents

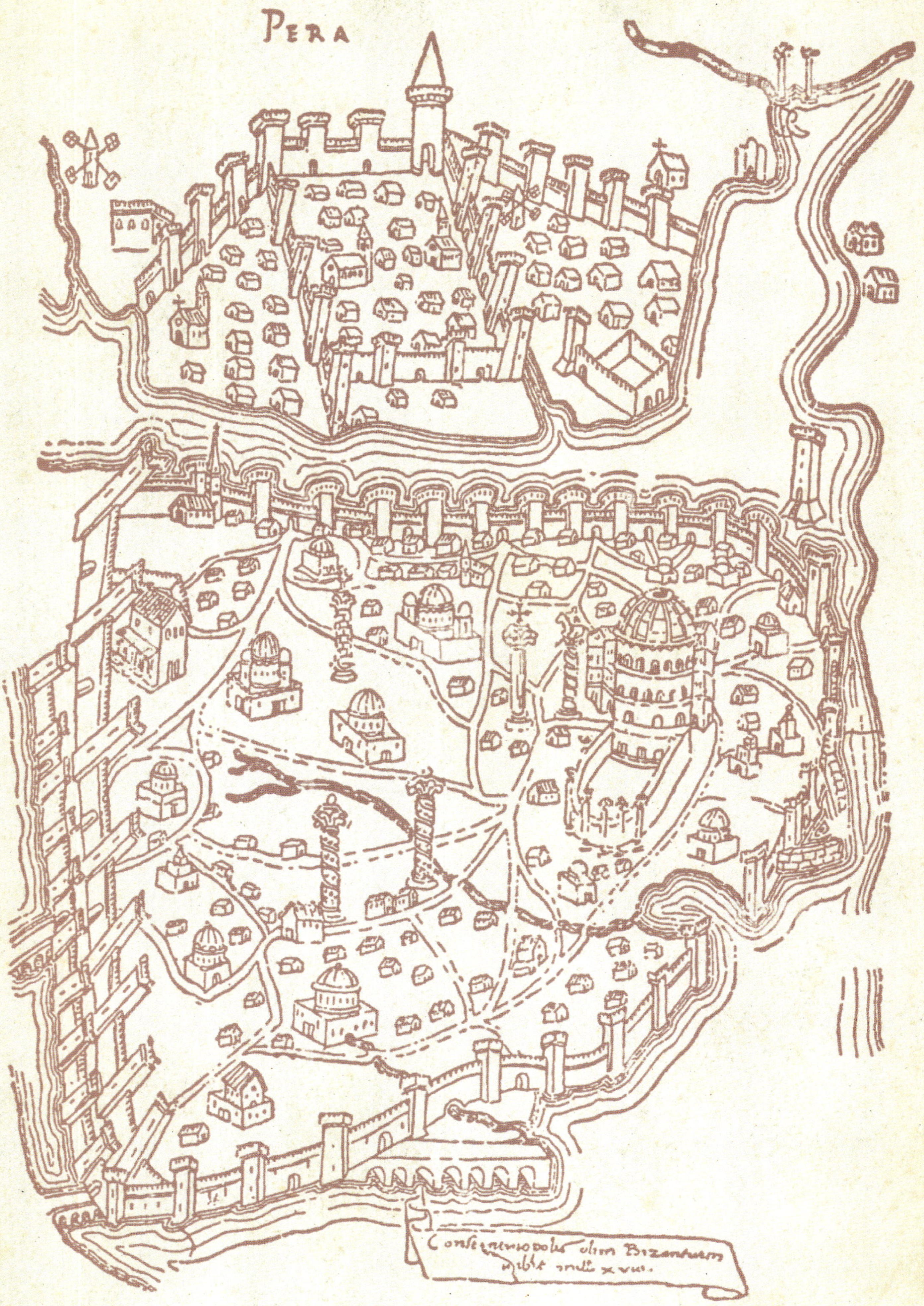

Map of Constantinople.

Christoforo Buondelmonti, Venice, 1422.

FOREWORD

During the 12th and 13th centuries, a decisive turning point occurred in the cultural and social landscape of Byzantium. In the 12th century, the dynasty of the Komnenoi Emperors ushered in the third and final great flourishing of the empire. The state was reorganized, strengthened both militarily and economically, and gained recognition from all the powers of the time. It came to be regarded as the most culturally and socially advanced state in Europe. Following the Komnenoi, a period of decline and disintegration set in during the twenty-year rule of the Angelos dynasty, culminating in the siege and fall of Constantinople to the Latins during the Fourth Crusade. The destruction of the City proved to be irreparable, and Byzantium never recovered its former power and glory. The dream of reclaiming the Queen of Cities lived on in the three Greek states founded after the fall: the Empire of Nicaea, the Empire of Trebizond, and the Despotate of Epirus. Among these, the first especially demonstrated remarkable military and cultural virtues, eventually recapturing Constantinople and reestablishing the Eastern Roman Empire—though as a mere shadow of its former grandeur.

During this period, Byzantine society stood among the most advanced in the Western world. The system of healthcare was remarkably developed for its time, as were the arts, the sciences, and the refinement of social life. Yet all these marvelous cultural and societal achievements of the "God-guarded" Empire remain unknown to most. It is a physician and philosopher of the era, Nikephoros Messenes, who undertakes to recount them for us, and his account is continued and completed by his student and successor, Nikolaos Melissenos.

Nikephoros Messenes is a fictional character. So is Melissenos. The historical figures and events described, however—as well as the intellectual, scientific, and cultural achievements of Byzantine society—are entirely real and carefully verified through the study of sources. Is Nikephoros, then, and are his friends imaginary? Yes—if by "imaginary" we mean a figure who gathers within himself the traits and experiences of several real people who truly lived. Yet in each of our lives, there are the events that actually occurred, and those we dreamed of, desired, or pursued. Our weaknesses, or the conditions of life, may have kept these from becoming reality. But are these aspirations and visions any less true than the things that happened? Certainly not. They mark our lives just the same. We might say, then, that Nikephoros and his companions are real persons—simply ones that no history book ever recorded.

The Byzantine Empire was never called by that name by its own subjects. It was always referred to as the Eastern (or Orient) Roman Empire, the "Christian Kingdom of the Romans," and later simply as "Romania." The term "Byzantium," derived from the ancient Greek city that preceded Constantinople on the same site, was coined in the 16th century by the German humanist Hieronymus Wolf, a student of Melanchthon. Though not historically accurate, the name Byzantium proved so elegant and effective that it prevailed internationally and is used in this text for the convenience of the modern reader. The same principle applies to the dating system. The Byzantines used the older Roman-Christian method of reckoning time "from the Creation of the world," according to which the birth of Christ occurred 5,508 years after the world's creation. Thus, the year 1150—the birth year of our narrator—would have been recorded as 6658 in his own calendar. To avoid confusing the modern reader, the dates have been adjusted to the current system.

The physician and philosopher of this brilliant Empire—which once shone in power and culture, and now, humbled, is literally gathering its fragments in Nicaea, in Pontus, and in Epirus—invites us on a fascinating journey through time, where we shall encounter the significant figures and the radiant civilization of an era too often wronged by oblivion. Above all, he will reveal to us the marvelous achievements of Byzantium in the field of medicine and public health, incomparably more advanced than those of other states of the same period. Let us follow him...

The Early Years

My name is Nikephoros Messenes. I was born in Patras in the year 6658 from the Creation of the world, according to the traditional reckoning of the Roman Empire—or in 1150 Anno Domini, as the Western dating has come to prevail, and which we too are gradually beginning to adopt. Patras, the great city of the Peloponnese, had known great glory throughout its long history, stretching back to antiquity. In the time of the Macedonian emperors, about two hundred years before my birth, it was the most important city of the Empire after the Queen of Cities (Constantinople) and Thessaloniki. It was a major commercial hub, the principal port to the West, and held strong trade and cultural ties with Southern Italy—especially Sicily—regions that had been Greek since ancient times. Many scholars and merchants had come from there. In Sicily, there were still many Greeks, and perhaps my father's surname bears witness to some ancestral origin from the city of Messene.

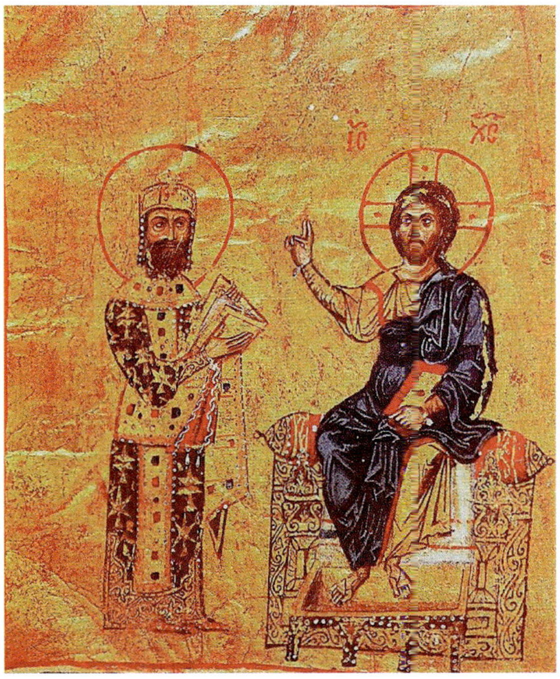

Alexios I Komnenos

Miniature illustration, Zonaras (Zigabenos), Dogmatic Panoply, 12th century, Vatican Library, Rome.

When I was born, our Empire was in a state of brilliant flourishing—its last—under the reign of the Komnenoi dynasty. The Emperor was Manuel I, a prudent man and a fearless warrior. He reigned for thirty-seven years, from 1143 to 1180, continuing the great work of his grandfather, Alexios I, and his father, John II, known as Kaloiōannēs—"Good John."

The first three Komnenos emperors ruled the Empire for a hundred years (1081–1180) and succeeded in healing the wounds inflicted by the Seljuk Turks in the East and the Normans in the West through their invasions—the former in Asia Minor, the latter in Italy and Sicily. They skillfully managed the forces of the Crusaders during the first three Crusades and, with their help, succeeded in reclaiming many lost provinces and expanding the Empire's reach in Asia Minor and Italy. Most importantly, they secured internal stability and prosperity, which led to the flourishing of commerce, literature, and the arts.

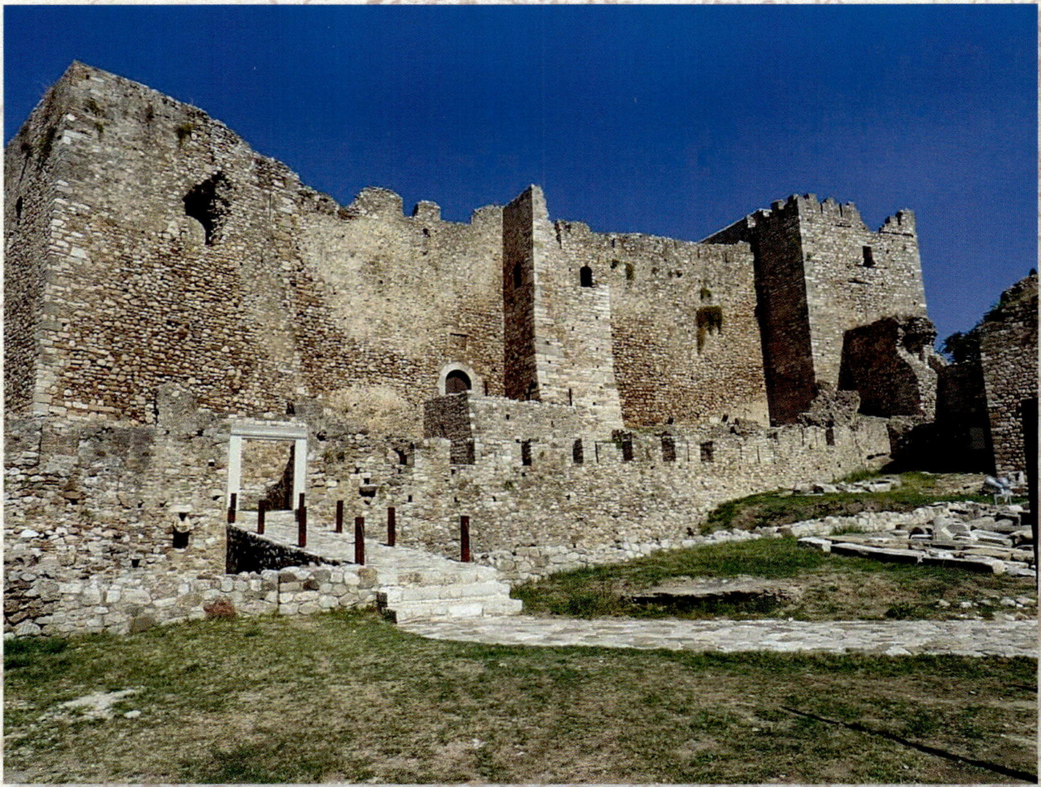

The Fortress of Patras.

Patras is distinguished by its large harbor, where ships dock from all parts of the East—but primarily from the West. The city itself, however, is built about a kilometer and a half inland, on a natural rise surrounding the fortress constructed by our great Emperor Justinian, atop the ruins of the ancient acropolis and the temple of Poseidon, which had stood there since antiquity. At the port, one finds only the warehouses for goods and the homes of fishermen and port officials. The region has long suffered from raids by barbarian peoples—first the Goths and the Heruli, and more recently the Slavs, Saracens, and Normans—but the city was well fortified and withstood many sieges. Its greatest flourishing came in the 9th and 10th centuries, thanks to the silk and purple dye trade, as well as carpet weaving, which was taught to us by Persian craftsmen who arrived in the 7th century. Most of the fertile plain and hills surrounding the city were covered with mulberry trees for the breeding of silkworms. The processing of purple dye was a long-standing tradition in Patras—the finest purple silk fabrics in the Mediterranean were produced here. Legend surrounds the story of Lady Danielis, a noblewoman who lived here about two hundred years ago. She owned vast stretches of land and operated specialized workshops for silk and purple dye. With her immense wealth and noble bearing, she captivated the imperial inspector Basil, who had been sent to oversee production and taxation. A few years later, Basil was proclaimed emperor as Basil I the Macedonian. Countless tales circulated in Patras about Danielis and her possible love affair with the emperor. My grandmother used to tell me that she had visited him in Constantinople, where he honored her with titles and high offices. What is certain is that in the end, she left her immense fortune to his son, the next emperor, Leo the Wise.

My father was also involved in the trade of silks and purple-dyed fabrics. Our family was not wealthy, but we were well enough off that my father agreed to have me pursue an education, rather than oblige me to follow him into the trade. Fortunately, my older brother John was interested in our father's profession and even had many ideas for improving it. This greatly eased my father's decision to honor my own wish. He ensured that we received a good education at school, where we studied according to the ancient model: Greek language, mathematics, and philosophy. The study of the Greek language was especially important, because all scholarly writings—as well as imperial decrees and laws—were composed in ancient or highly archaic Greek, and it was essential that we could understand them. The spoken language had diverged somewhat from ancient Greek, especially in its syntax and everyday vocabulary. Although most of the people did not have the opportunity to pursue formal studies, education was held in the highest esteem in our society. It was regarded as the "art of arts and science of sciences." People praised those with a cultivated mind and broad knowledge, while they mocked the ignorant and the uncouth. Education was referred to as "paideia" (formation),

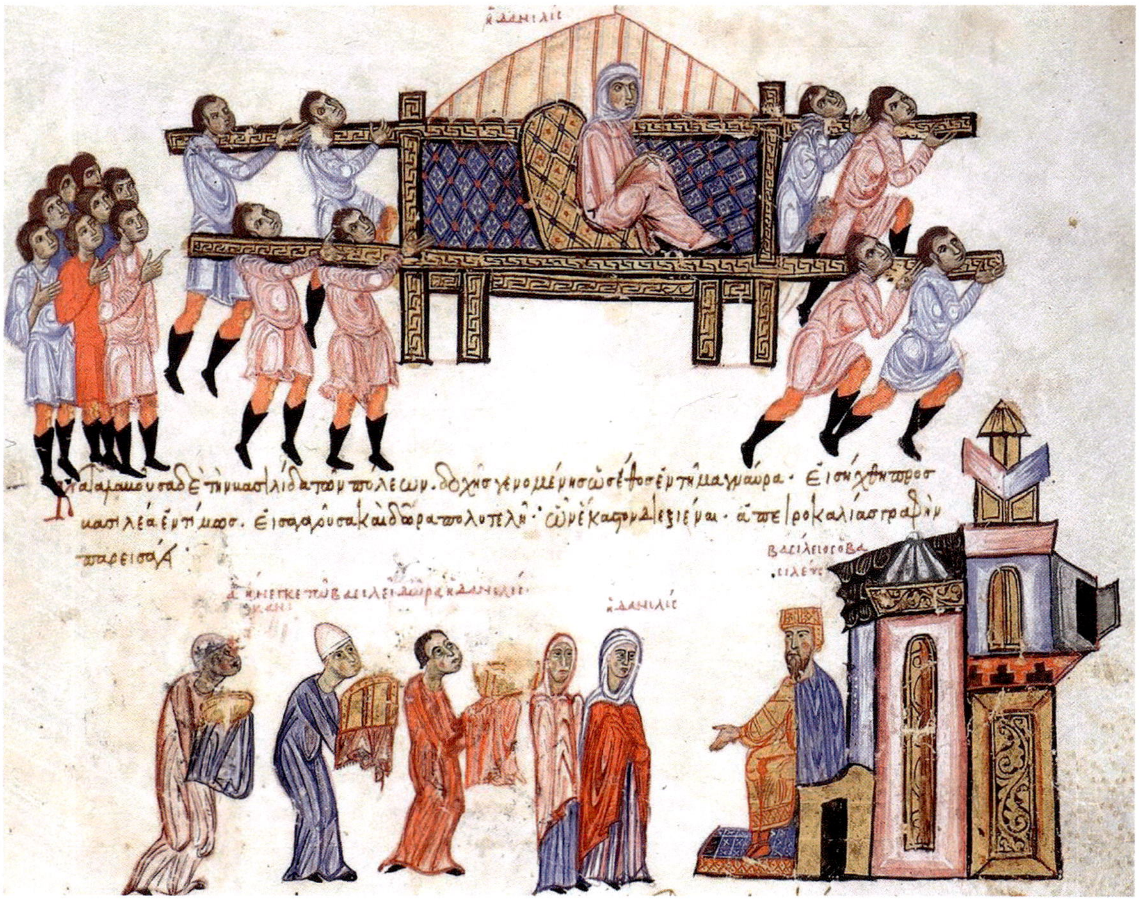

Danielis Travels to Constantinople.
Miniature, Skylitzes, 12th century National Library of Spain, Madrid

and one who was uneducated was called "apaideutos" (unformed or uncultivated).

Nevertheless, only a few were able to acquire a truly substantial education, since schools were private and a certain level of financial comfort was necessary for a child to study. There were, of course, quite a few people who could read and write. But the truly educated were few, and even fewer were those who could earn a living through the learning and knowledge they had acquired in school—such as palace officials, high-ranking clergy, tax collectors, physicians, notaries, and teachers.

So, when I turned six years old, I began school, where the first thing we learned was the "holy letters"—also called "propaideia" (preliminary education). There were quite a few propaideia schools in Patras, usually simple rooms near churches or monasteries, where the teachers—whom we called *grammatistes*—were most often monks or priests. I went to school with great joy. My school was next to the Church of the Pantocrator, a large church built about 150 years earlier, upon the ruins of the ancient Temple of Olympian Zeus, which had once stood in the center of the ancient agora. There, our teacher was Father Porphyrios, a kind and gentle monk who served at the church and taught us reading, writing, arithmetic, and grammar.

My school was one of the best in the city, and I was fortunate that it was located close to our home, so I didn't have to walk far like other children who

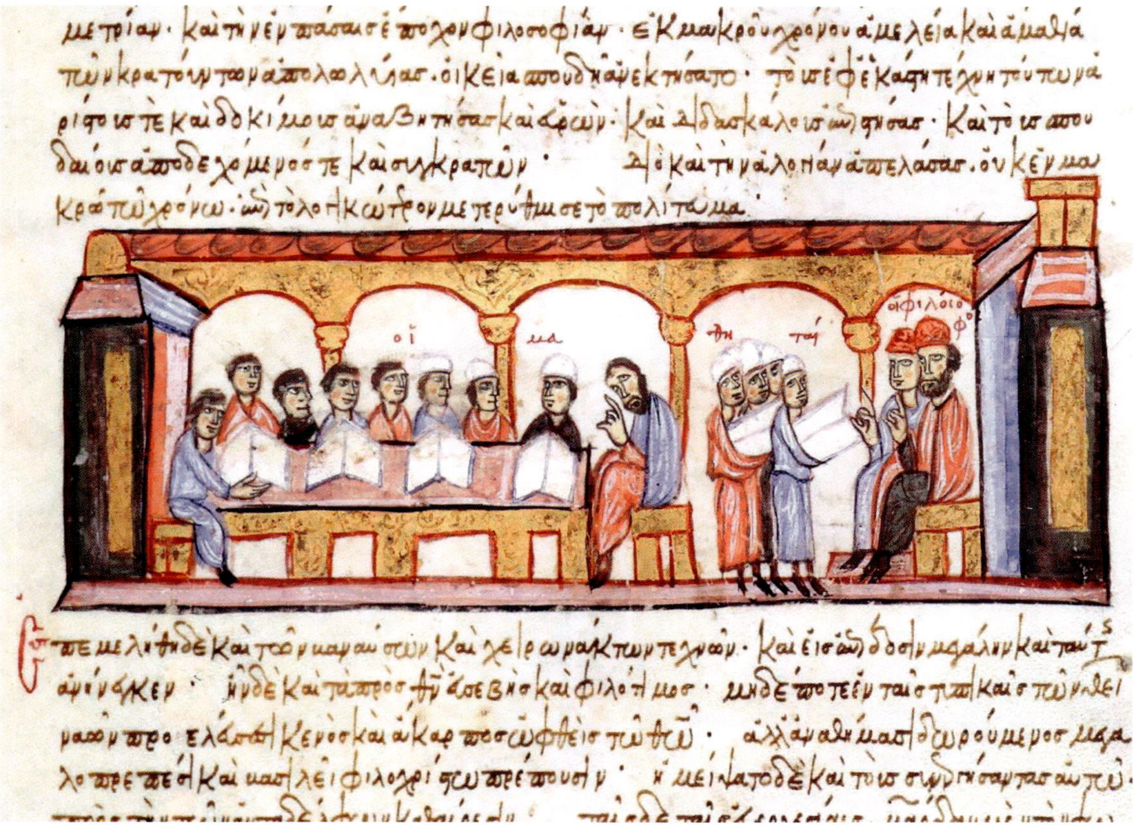

Students and Philosophers.

Miniature, Skylitzes, 12th century National Library of Spain, Madrid.

lived in distant neighborhoods or the suburbs. The classroom was spacious and bright, with seating for all the students: the *anaváthres*, tall wooden chairs, and the *skímbodes*, low stools. Whoever arrived early would secure a good seat, so I always made sure to rise early in order to sit in one of the front anaváthres. Later, however, once the teacher had formed an opinion of each student's diligence and performance, he would assign seats himself, placing the best students on the tall chairs. At the front of the room stood the teacher's throne, a raised chair where Father Porphyrios sat, and in front of him was the lectern, where we placed our books. Books were a precious commodity, and the teacher guarded them with reverence. Our school had a fair number of books. On the right-hand wall, as we faced the teacher, was the inscription: "Fear God," and on the opposite wall: "Honor your parents." Our school, like most in the Empire, was private, and the cost of tuition was burdensome for most families. Thus, education remained a privilege of the financially well-off. Emperor Alexios Komnenos had founded a school in Constantinople where poor or orphaned children could

The Church of the Pantocrator in Patras.

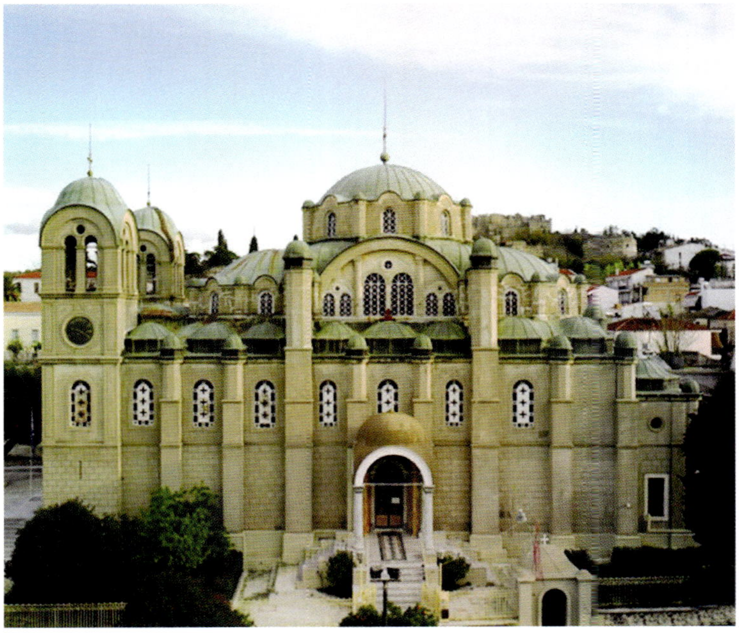

study for free, but this did not resolve the broader issue. Still, in the schools there was no discrimination of race or ethnicity—all citizens of our multiethnic Empire had equal rights. Distinctions were made only between diligent and careless students. At the same time, the bishoprics had also established and maintained strictly ecclesiastical schools, where the primary focus was religious education.

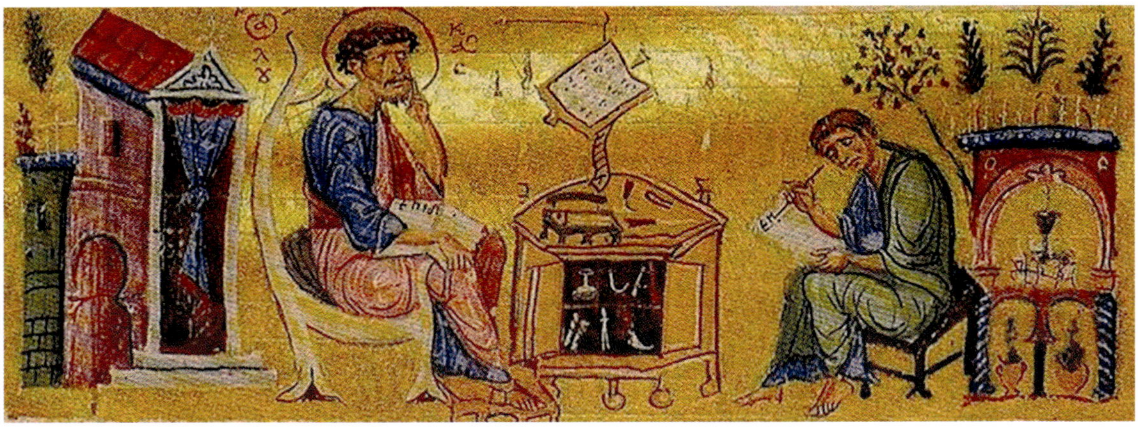

The Evangelist Luke Dictating the "Acts"

Miniature, 11th century, Monastery of Pantocrator, Mount Athos.

Lessons lasted from morning until afternoon every day. In between, we took short breaks, and at midday there was a pause for a meal. The food that Father Porphyrios gave us he called a "blessing," and it usually consisted of bread and cheese, though we often had salted fish as well. Naturally, the lunch break was the most pleasant part of the day. Father Porphyrios was a kind man and treated us with love, but he was determined to teach us, and so he was very strict when it came to laziness and indifference. Punishments were administered with a rod, and they were quite frequent. But the harshest punishment, reserved for more serious offenses, was being denied food. This was the educational mindset of the time; in fact, there was a saying: "He who is not beaten, is not educated" ("Ho mē dareis ou paideuetai"), meaning, "Whoever doesn't get a beating, doesn't learn his letters." Sometimes, particularly unruly children were even expelled. These punishments had the full approval of our parents, who regarded the teacher with deep respect and a sense of obligation. In the afternoons, we returned home—except for a few children who had come from nearby villages to study, and whom our teacher hosted at the school.

The main textbooks we used were the Psalter and Homer. Father Porphyrios taught us reading and writing by training us to syllabify texts slowly, to memorize them, and to write them "asphaltí"—that is, without mistakes. He referred to grammar as "to Hellenize the tongue" ("τὸ ἑλληνίζειν τὴν γλῶσσαν") and considered it of great importance. He was very patient, requiring us to engage in endless repetition. He was also highly methodical, guiding us from the easier material to the more difficult, only after ensuring we had mastered the basics. He welcomed every question about things we did not understand and never tired of repeating explanations. We memorized large portions of the Psalms, and to a lesser extent, passages from the Iliad. We could understand the Psalms to some extent, but Homer's language was very difficult. Nevertheless, we learned with great enjoyment the captivating stories of the battles fought by the heroes of Troy, which our esteemed *grammatistes* (teacher) explained to us with vivid clarity. For most of the students, his lessons were a genuine delight.

We went to school in our everyday clothes, without any kind of uniform or identifying mark. We carried with us the *mársipos*, a leather or cloth satchel, in which we kept the *schedárion* and the stylos, or *grapheion*. The schedárion was a wooden tablet coated with wax, on which we inscribed letters using the stylos—a pointed stylus with a sharp tip. The flat end of the stylos was used to smooth out the wax and erase the markings. It was a simple and inexpensive way to learn writing, allowing us to correct our many mistakes.

Much later, in the second level of education, we began to write using a reed pen (*kálamos*) and ink on small pieces of parchment or paper, which we had recently begun importing from China. In earlier times, papyrus had also been used, but by then it had fallen out of use. The *kálamos* was literally a reed, specially sharpened, which we dipped into black ink. Manuscripts were rolled into scrolls. Needless to say, paper and parchment were precious, and only the most careful students were permitted to write on them, usually by copying Homer or sacred texts. Now, as I write these lines, seventy years later, our Empire produces its own paper, and no longer depends on imports from China. And so, I have the luxury of writing down my memories.

Father Porphyrios taught us the newer minuscule script, which was more artistic than the majuscule, or capital-letter script, used by the ancient Greeks and Romans up until the 8th century. Minuscule writing had the advantage of incorporating accents and breathings, and, above all, it occupied less space, making books smaller and easier to read. In Arithmetic, we learned "to count" (*psēphízein*), meaning to calculate using our fingers or small pebbles that we would collect and carry in our *mársipon*. Our teacher taught us the four operations: *epísoureusis* (addition), *aphaíresis* (subtraction), *pollaplasiasmós* (multiplication), and *epimerismós* (division). I loved my lessons deeply—I thirsted for learning, especially the astonishing stories of the Iliad and the Odyssey. At home, I would study and review the material and retell the stories to my sister. As a result, I became one of the best students, and the teacher assigned me to sit in one of the front *anaváthres*.

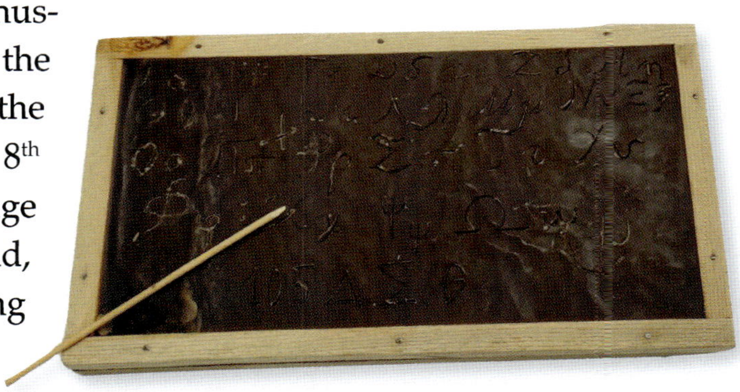

Wax Tablet

I had the great fortune of growing up in a loving family. My father, whom we held in deep respect, was just and kind, though—due to the mindset of the time—he was obliged to appear strict. He would leave very early each day for work, and his return home was always an important event. My mother, who essentially ruled the household, cared for him with affection, and we all showed him our respect. She had a strong and sociable character and made sure that we lacked nothing. She was strict with us, but behind that strictness we could clearly see her deep love and concern for us. We were only three siblings: Ioannis, myself, and our younger sister, Iphigenia. Ioannis had what one might call a business mind. He loved our father's trade and had helped him in the shop from a young age. Like me, he studied preparatory education so that he could learn language and arithmetic, and he also took private lessons to improve his Greek. That was sufficient for a life in commerce. He worked alongside our father and helped him adapt to the new conditions of trade, especially later on when we relocated to Constantinople. I owe him a great deal, for by taking over our father's business, he gave me the freedom to pursue my studies, and he also supported me financially during my early years. Although, as a practical-minded person, he considered my devotion to endless studies—without clear financial return—a kind of futile endeavor, deep down he was proud of his brother. He was a serious and quiet boy, knew what he wanted, and was truly our father's main support.

My sister was a gifted young woman—beautiful, intelligent, and full of spirit. She, too, loved learning, but at that time, the fate of girls was different. There were no schools for women, and only a few girls from wealthy families received an education at home through private tutors. Our family had no such means. Although there was no formal prohibition against women holding public office or pursuing studies, the opportunity simply did not exist. There are examples of women who became empresses, such as Irene of Athens, Zoe the Macedonian, and Theodora, as well as distinguished intellectuals like Pulcheria and Athenais-Eudokia in the time of Theodosius II, the poetess Kassiani, and more recently Anna Komnene, daughter of Emperor Alexios, who wrote a major historical work, the *Alexiad*. In it, she describes the history of her era—a precious monument of our civilization. Anna, in fact, possessed profound knowledge of medicine. But these are

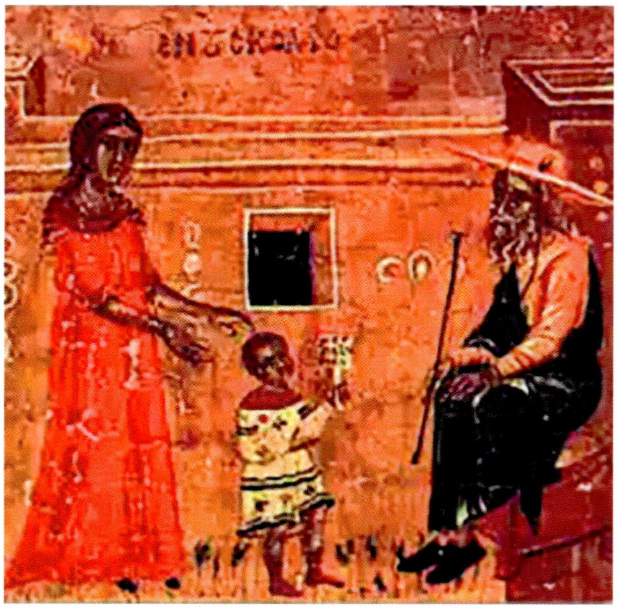

A Mother Brings Her Child to the Teacher.

Detail from a portable icon of Saint Nicholas, Patmos Monastery.

exceptions, gifted women who also had the good fortune to be wealthy. For most girls, the best prospect in life was a successful marriage. However, there was one field in which women participated equally with men—that of charitable institutions and hospitals. There, women could serve as deaconesses, midwives, medical assistants, and even as female physicians. I learned this later when I worked as a doctor in the Queen of Cities, and I will elaborate on it further on. Iphigenia, just a year younger than me, had a great love for learning, and—being influenced by me—she too wanted to pursue an education, but that was impossible. Yet every afternoon when I returned home from school, I would sit with her and recount everything I had learned that day. It was also the best way for me to reinforce my own knowledge, and it made me one of the top students. My sister would absorb knowledge eagerly, memorizing texts and repeating what I told her. My mother, pleased with her love of learning, did not insist that she devote herself solely to household chores, but allowed her to study with me. Thus, she mastered the language beautifully, learned to speak correctly, to read and write, and acquired a solid grounding in basic arithmetic.

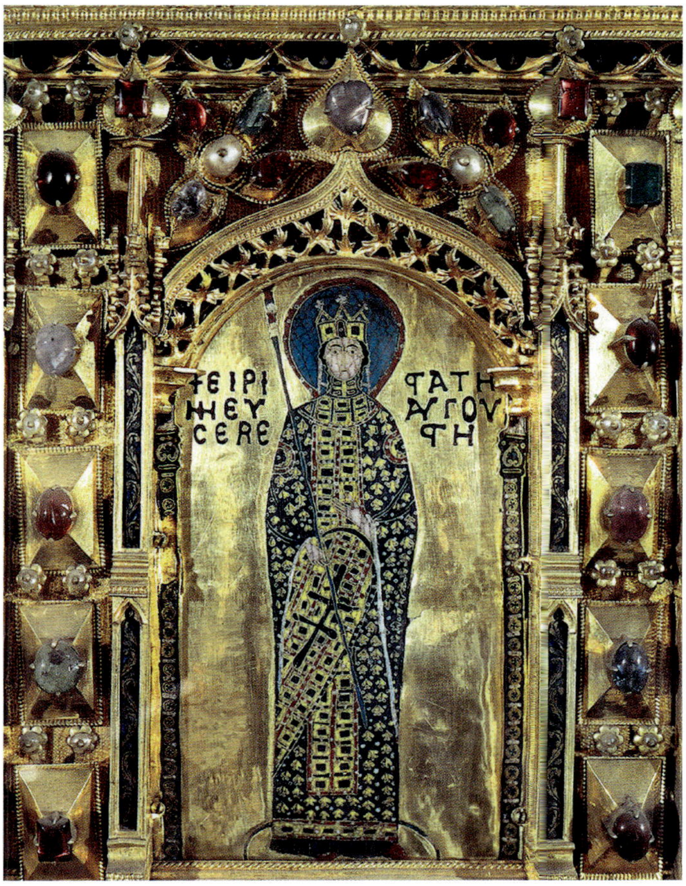

Irene of Athens.

Enamel on the ornate golden altar screen (Pala d'Oro) of Saint Mark's, 12th century, Venice.

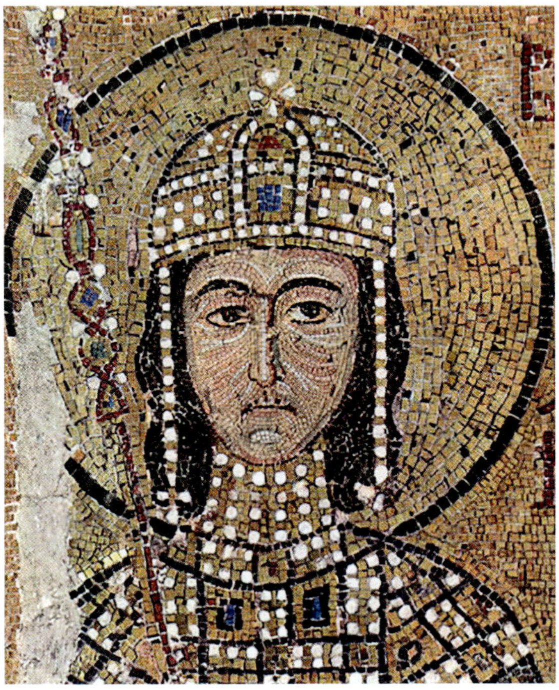

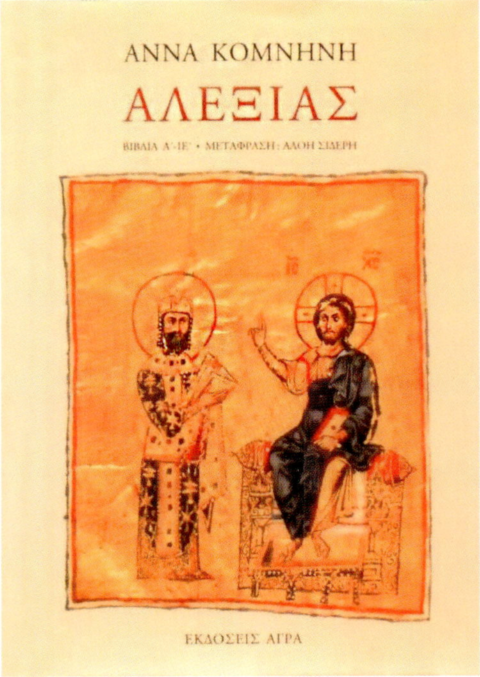

Left:
Anna Komnene.

Mosaic, 12th century, Hagia Sophia.

Right:
The Alexiad by Anna Komnene.

Agra Publications, 2005

The four years of basic education passed quickly, and I was to continue with the second stage of my studies, the so-called "encyclical education." This too lasted four years and was held in different schools, which were again private. The teachers, who were also the owners of the schools, were no longer clergy but were called *grammatikoi*. They were better trained and better paid than those who taught in elementary education. There were very few such schools in Patras, and naturally, the number of students was much smaller. I parted from Father Porphyrios with sadness. He held great affection for me, appreciating the diligence I showed and the effort I put into my studies. In fact, as I was leaving, he gave me a small wooden icon of the Theotokos, which I always kept in my *mársipos* as a student, and later carried with me through every stage of my life.

My new school was located in the area of the ancient city, at some distance from the fortress, from where—like from a balcony—one could see the sea and the mountains across the water in Central Greece: the three-peaked Chalkeia and the gentle Taphiasos, which the people called Paliovouna. In the afternoons, as I left school, I would look westward, past the mountains of Aetolia toward the Ionian Islands, and behold the sunset, which the people of Patras say is one of the most beautiful in the inhabited world. At the edge of the large square facing the sea were the ruins of the ancient wall, beneath which lay the old artificial harbor, the *skaptos limēn*, which had once been connected to the open sea by a canal. It was there that Antony and Cleopatra disembarked before the great naval battle of Actium. Later, Augustus also disembarked there, and he became a benefactor of the city. Still later, Nero visited our city—the same year as the Apostle Andrew, our patron saint. My teacher was named Euthymios Tornikes, and although he was young, he possessed great learning. He had a passion for ancient Greek literature and the Greek language. Through my diligence and growing knowledge, I gained his trust and confidence.

Encyclical education was divided into two stages. The first included three main subjects, known as the *Trivium*: Grammar, Rhetoric, and Poetry. The second stage consisted of four subjects: Arithmetic, Geometry, Astronomy, and Music—collectively known as the *Quadrivium*. This educational structure was a direct continuation of the system of Classical Greece. These seven disciplines are mentioned by the sophist Hippias, who lived in the late 5th century before the birth of our Savior. Plato, in his *Republic*, even states that the subjects of the *tetraktys* are essential qualifications for the *guardians of the City*.

Books were a luxury in those days, just as they are now. Tornikes was an admirer and disciple of the great intellectual Arethas, who had been born and had lived in our city two hundred years earlier. He left behind a significant body of work in philosophy and theology. Known as Arethas of Patras, he had been a student of the great Photios, and left a rich collection of books in

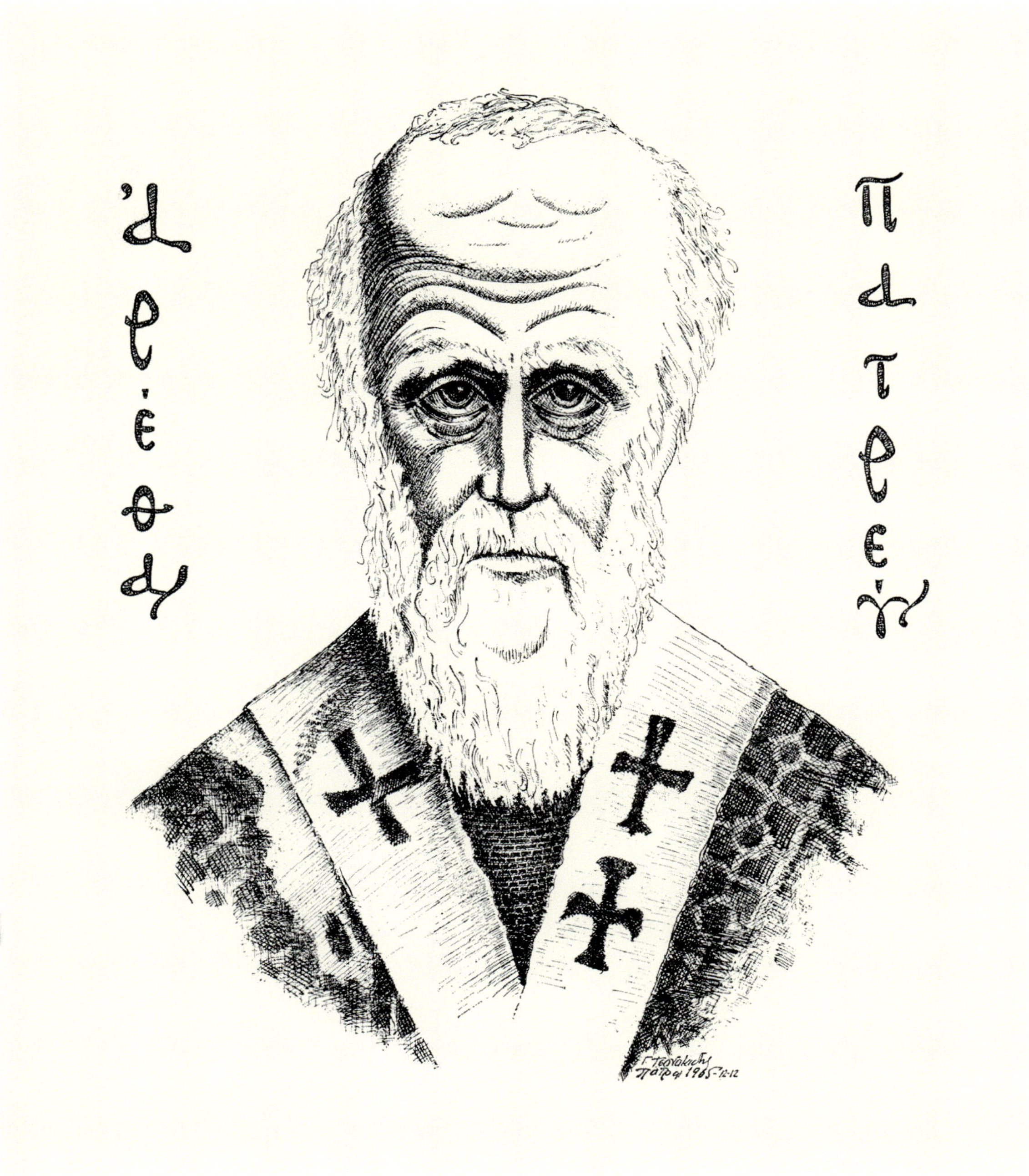

Arethas of Patras.

Engraving by Georgios Tsonakidis, Municipal Library of Patras.

Patras. Books could also be found in many monasteries, which, following the teachings of Saint Basil, not only founded libraries and scriptoria, but also supported learned monks who studied the texts in the monastic libraries and taught them to others. Tornikes, too, possessed a respectable personal library, and his school was considered one of the finest in the city.

In antiquity and during the early centuries of the Empire, manuscripts were rolled into scrolls, which were called *tomoi*. However, storing and reading them was inconvenient. Thus, a more practical format was invented: the *biblion*, or book. The earliest books were called codices, and they consisted of several folded sheets. When the number of folded sheets was three or six, they were called notebooks (*tetradia*). By stitching together many such tetradia, a full book was formed. For covers, they usually used wooden boards or leath-

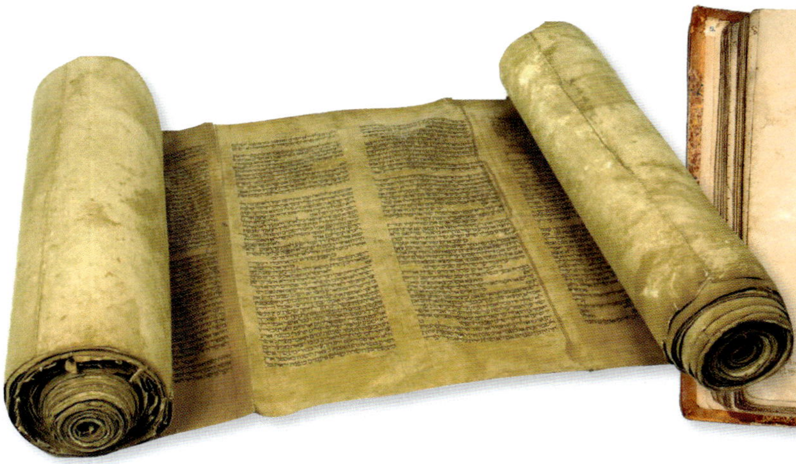

Papyrus.
Illustrated Bible.

Ink on leather,
15th century, Spain.

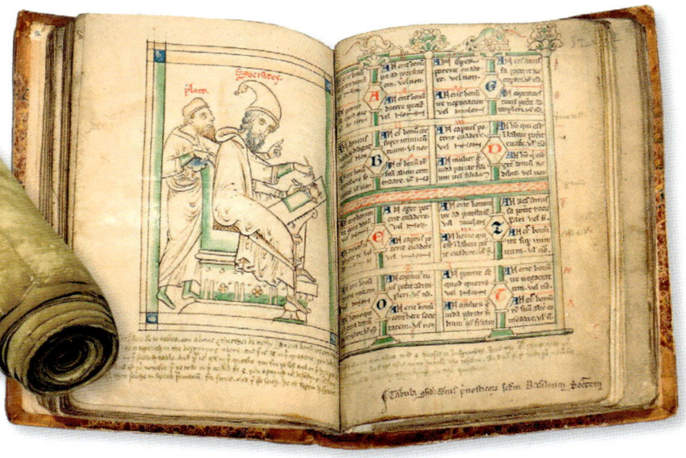

Old Book.

Unknown author, 13th century
Bodleian Library, Oxford.

er. But when a book was intended for liturgical use in a church, or commissioned by a wealthy patron, its exterior would be made of precious materials, such as ivory, gold, or silver. Books were—and still are—very expensive. A medium-sized book could cost as much as half the annual income of a well-paid public official. As a result, most scholars throughout their entire lives were unable to acquire more than twenty books. For this reason, it was customary then—as it still is now—for them to regularly borrow books from one another. Only a few intellectuals or court officials, through great sacrifice, managed to build large personal libraries. Among them were Patriarch Photios, Arethas of Patras, and Theodora Kantakouzene.

Grammar was the principal subject, and great emphasis was placed on it, as it was the key to speaking Greek correctly. The method of studying and teaching it was based on ancient texts by our Greek forebears. The most important textbook was the *Art and Grammar* (*Téchnē kai Grammatikē*) by Dionysius Thrax, who lived in the 2nd century before the birth of the Savior. His work was founded on the grammatical studies of the Stoic philosophers. Tornikes owned a copy of this book and taught us the details of declensions, the tenses of verbs and nouns, irregular verbs, and much more that we had to memorize perfectly ("farsí", by heart and with precision).

Rhetoric was another subject to which great attention was given. Tornikes taught us the proper structure of speech and the skilled and refined use of language. He used to tell us that mastery of language is a passport into society, and the key to success in any profession: for example, the politician or diplomat, who must persuade in negotiations; the lawyer, who must convince the judges; or the clergyman, who must preach effectively from the pulpit. He emphasized that, as written in the Acts of the Apostles, chapter 21, verse 37, the Apostle Paul escaped torture and execution simply because he spoke Greek to the Roman commander—proving himself a cultivated man, not an uncivilized bandit.

Finally, the crowning achievement of our education was Philosophy. Our teacher taught us Logic, Ethics, Dogmatics, and Metaphysics with great passion, based on the writings of the great Aristotle. *Mathematical science* was also considered part of Philosophy, though it was taught in the next stage of our studies.

The first cycle of my studies lasted two years. I continued to share my knowledge with Iphigenia, but now things had become more difficult. It required a great deal of time, and my sister had grown older and needed to help with household duties, which would prepare her to become a good "oikokyra"—a housekeeper or homemaker. Thus, our collaboration became less frequent, but during that period, Iphigenia learned to handle the Greek language exceptionally well.

In the second cycle of studies, during the third and fourth year, we were taught the Tetraktys: Arithmetic, Geometry, Astronomy, and Music. The teaching of Mathematics was based on the Arithmetic of Pythagoras and Diophantus, as well as the Geometry of Euclid. Tornikes was enraptured by the harmony of numbers, the symbolism of Pythagoras, the equations of Diophantus, and the theorems of Euclid. Such was his passion that he transmitted to us

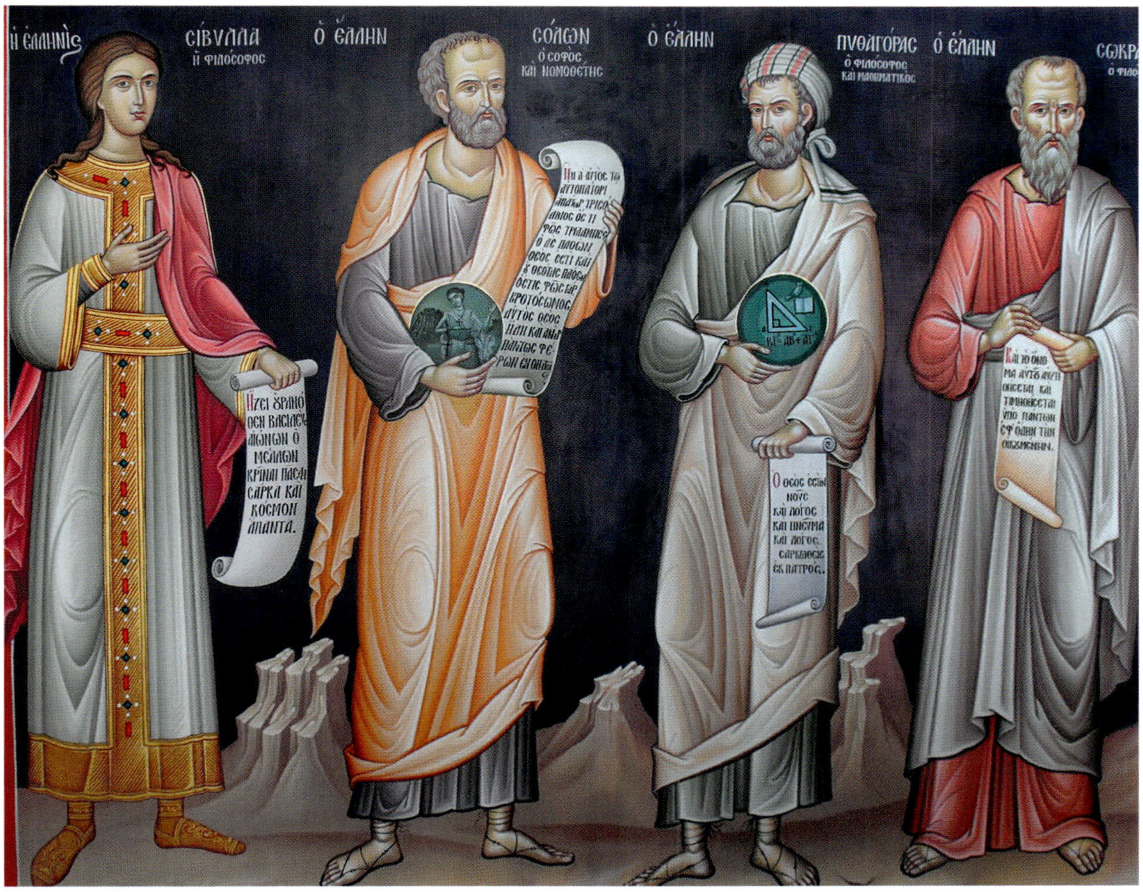

Ancient Greek Philosophers. The Sibyl, Solon, Pythagoras, and Socrates.

Monastery of Great Meteoron.

his enthusiasm and love for these subjects. Astronomy was another deeply engaging discipline. He taught us from the *Phaenomena*, a poem by Aratus, which describes the constellations, the phases of the moon, and even weather prediction. Music, finally, was the chanting of our ecclesiastical hymns, especially the masterpieces of Romanos the Melodist.

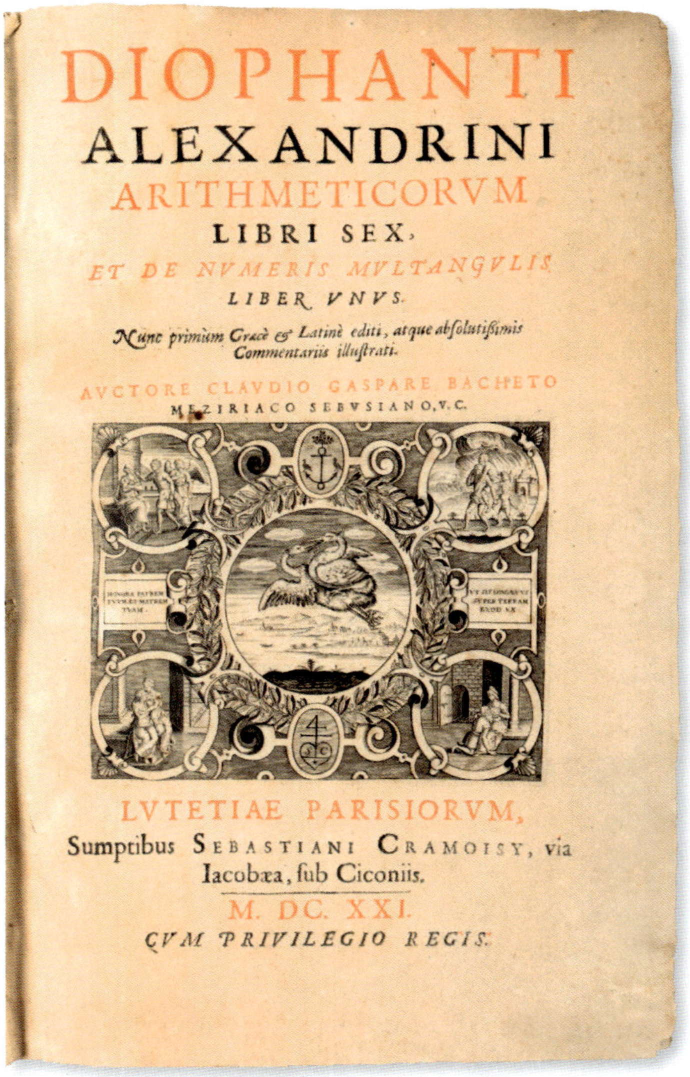
DIOPHANTI
ALEXANDRINI
ARITHMETICORVM
LIBRI SEX,
ET DE NVMERIS MVLTANGVLIS
LIBER VNVS.
Nunc primùm Græcè & Latinè editi, atque absolutissimis Commentariis illustrati.
AVCTORE CLAVDIO GASPARE BACHETO
MEZIRIACO SEBVSIANO, V.C.
LVTETIAE PARISIORVM,
Sumptibus SEBASTIANI CRAMOISY, via Iacobæa, sub Ciconiis.
M. DC. XXI.
CVM PRIVILEGIO REGIS.

Latin Translation of Diophantus.

Ed. Bachet, Paris, 1621.

From the ancient texts, we studied both the Iliad and, in parallel, the Bible. Homer, according to Saint Basil the Great, was the great *teacher of the virtues*. We also studied other poets, but far more briefly than Homer. In addition, we were taught nine classical tragedies by the great tragedians: The Persians, Prometheus Bound, and Seven Against Thebes by Aeschylus; Ajax, Electra, and Oedipus Tyrannus by Sophocles; Hecuba, Orestes, and The Phoenician Women by Euripides. These tragedies were taught in all the schools of the Empire for centuries, and for this reason, they came to be known as "Byzantine tragedies." In addition, we studied three comedies by Aristophanes: Plutus, The Clouds, and The Frogs, as well as excerpts from other ancient Greek authors. Naturally, we studied the entire Bible, both Old and New Testaments. We would memorize entire passages, and Tornikes would dictate various texts that we were required to copy *asphaltí*—that is, without error. Religious education was integrated into the general curriculum, but specific instruction in dogmatics and church order was given to us by a hieromonk who would come expressly for that purpose.

My encounter with the writings of the ancient authors was truly fascinating. I quite literally devoured the books of these great thinkers who illuminated the world, and whom we, as Greek-speaking Romans, citizens of the Eastern Roman Empire, rightfully feel to be our natural heirs. Fortunately, my city gave me access—at least—to the essential works of antiquity. I was able to borrow books and read them at the school, even after class hours, since students were not permitted to take books home, for obvious reasons. My deepest interest lay in philosophy and mathematics—which, after all, is not so different from philosophy. So, alongside Homer, Aristotle, and the tragic poets,

I was captivated by arithmetic, with the harmony of its reasoning, and geometry, with the clarity and precision of its theorems and proofs. Tornikes would speak to us about Archimedes, who, with his levers and pulleys, managed to lift and sink the Roman ships that besieged Syracuse; about Eratosthenes in Alexandria, who calculated the circumference of the Earth; and about Aristarchus of Samos, who estimated the distances of the sun and moon and proposed that the Earth revolves around the sun, not the other way around. All of this awakened within me a longing for knowledge—a desire that would lead me to truth, beyond the foolish superstitions and the ignorance that prevailed among the common people. I resolved to pursue higher learning at the most esteemed intellectual institutions, at any cost. I yearned to learn as much as possible, and I had no desire whatsoever to engage in commerce in order to make money or become wealthy. The horizons of Patras felt too narrow for me. I longed to travel, to discover the world, but above all, to reach our great Queen of Cities, Constantinople, the center of the world. But how could I make that happen?

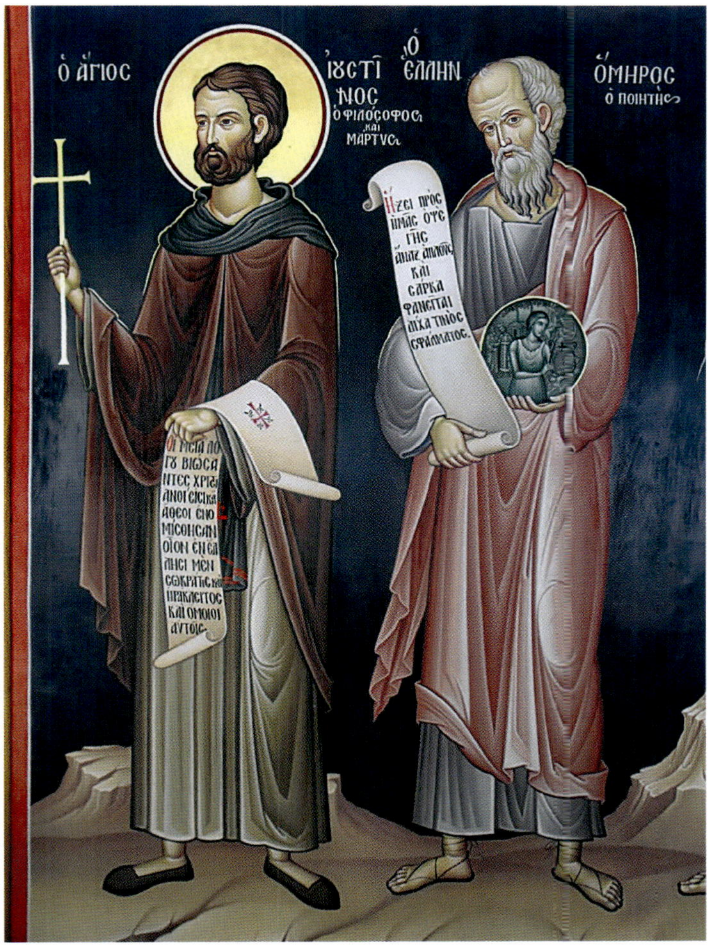

Saint Justin and Homer.
Monastery of Great Meteoron.

When I completed my encyclical education, I was nearly fifteen years old. Tornikes awarded me my graduation certificates, with distinction. In fact, because I was skilled in calligraphy, he entrusted me with copying certain texts for him on precious paper, which we still imported from China at the time. I felt great anxiety about my future. There was no university in Patras. For higher studies, one had to go to the Capital, or to one of the great traditional cities of the Empire. Since antiquity, these included Athens, Antioch, Berytus (Beirut), Edessa, and Gaza in Palestine. By now, however, Athens had fallen into sad decline, and all the other cities I mentioned had been conquered by the Arabs since the 7th century—that curse upon the Romans—which deprived the Empire of its richest and most cultured provinces, Egypt and Syria. From that time onward, our state lost its universal territorial character, but in turn, it gained greater homogeneity, having been reduced primarily to Asia Minor and the Balkans—regions that were now almost exclusively Greek-speaking.

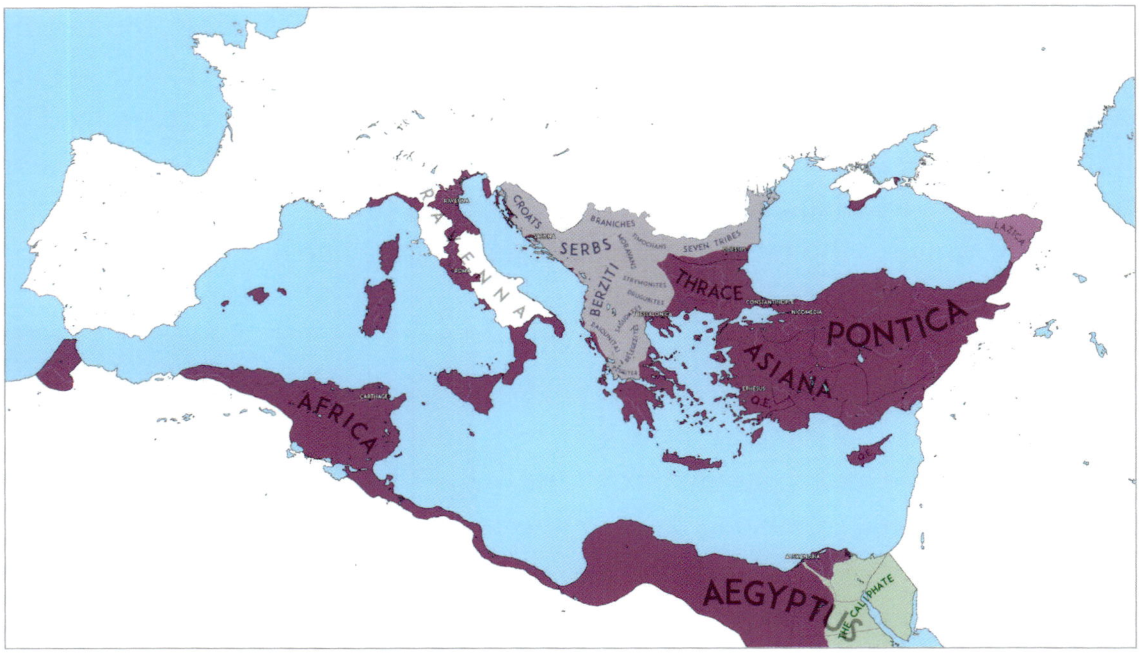

The Empire after the death of Heraclius.

The martyred Emperor Heraclius, who decisively defeated the Persians, recovered the Holy Places and the eastern provinces of the Empire as far as Mesopotamia, and triumphantly brought the True Cross back to the City, lived to see all these victories lost in the face of the unstoppable surge of Islam. Heraclius reigned from 610 to 641 after the birth of the Savior. Through superhuman efforts, he modernized the administrative system, reorganized the Empire, which his incompetent predecessors had brought to ruin, and—fighting on the front lines alongside his soldiers—pushed the Empire's borders to Mesopotamia and Libya. He humbled the most powerful state in the region—the Sassanid Persian Empire. It was he who established the Greek language as the official language of the state, recognizing the universal legacy of Greek civilization. He also replaced in official documents and coinage the Latin title "Imperator Caesar Augustus" with the Greek "Basileus", following the example of Alexander the Great.

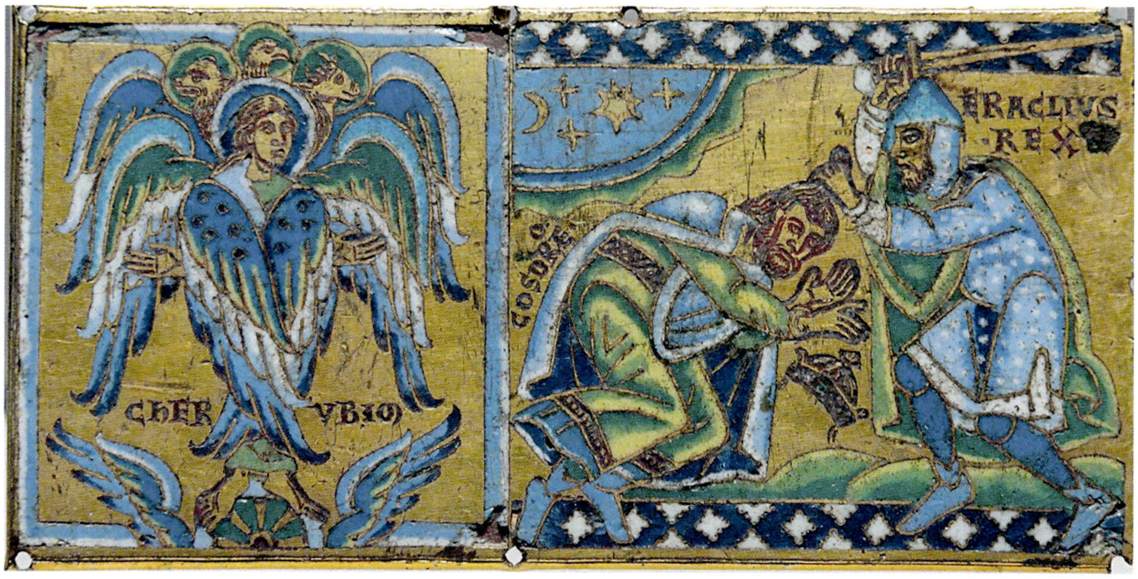

Heraclius defeats the Persian King Khosrow.

Enamel, 12th century, Louvre Museum, Paris.

Together with the progressive Patriarch Sergius, the author of the *Akathist Hymn,* he (Heraclius) attempted to bridge the gap between the Orthodox and the Monophysites of the eastern provinces by proposing a middle way, known as Monothelitism. But the religious leaders of the time did not accept it. The inhabitants of the eastern provinces continued to feel alienated from the central administration. The end of this great leader was tragic. A sudden force of desert tribesmen, armed with the fanaticism of a new religion—which we initially mistook for a Christian heresy of the Monophysites—swept into the wealthy provinces of Egypt and Syria. These were the Arabs, and the religion was that of Muhammad. Our armies met theirs in battle in the year 636, at the river Hieromyax—called Yarmouk by the barbarians—a tributary of the Jordan River in Palestine.

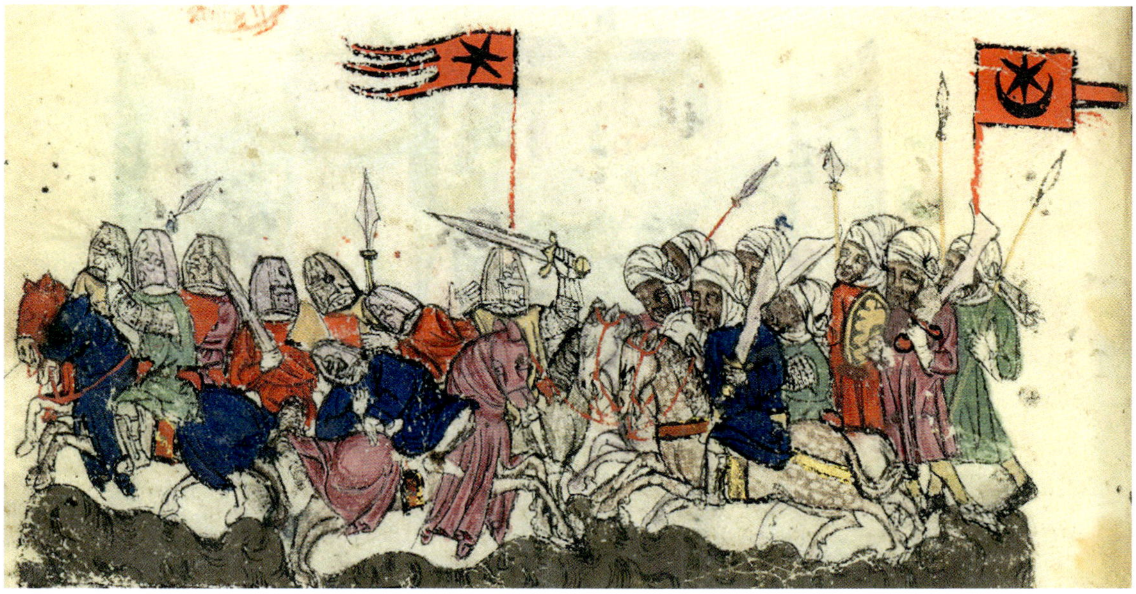

The Battle of Hieromyax (Yarmuk).

By an anonymous Catalan artist, 12th century, National Library of France, Paris.

At that time, the Roman army was the most disciplined and battle-hardened force in the world. Our cataphract cavalry and dense, heavily armed infantry were considered invincible. The general was the Emperor's brother, Theodoros Trithourios. Victory seemed assured. And then the unthinkable happened. Our unbeaten army, though exhausted from the endless battles against the Persians, was defeated by a horde of wild demons, who charged screaming on their swift horses, striking from all directions against the phalanxes of our soldiers. It was the heaviest defeat we had ever suffered. Our army was utterly annihilated. The provinces of Egypt, Syria, and Palestine fell permanently into the hands of the Arabs. The Hellenized populations of those regions—whom the uncompromising policies of the Patriarchate had already alienated spiritually, because they had adhered to Monophysitism—soon came to be Islamized in religion and Arabized in language, under the threat of the Arab sword. These provinces were lost forever to the Roman State and to Hellenism. Heraclius could not endure the blow. The achievements of a titan-

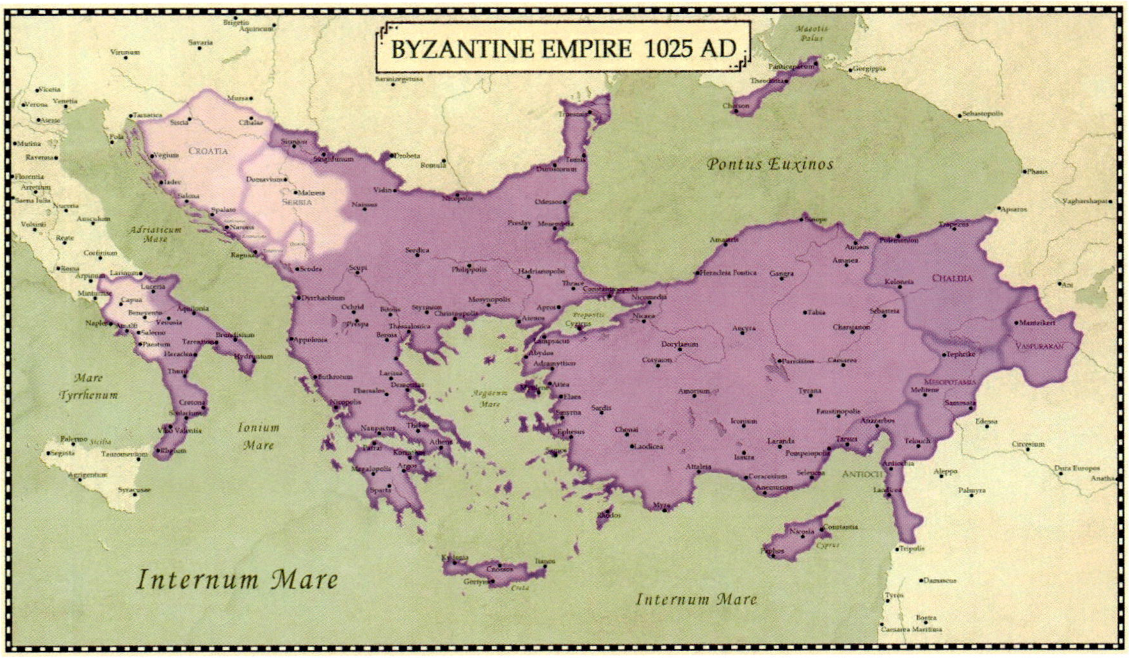

The Empire under Basil the Bulgar-Slayer in 1025.

ic twenty-year effort were swept away in a single day. He fell into deep depression, withdrew into his palace, and never recovered. He died a few years later, consumed by grief. Yet the Empire remained one of the strongest powers in Europe, and the most culturally advanced. It passed through difficult times, but during the Macedonian dynasty, which lasted nearly two centuries, and reached its height under Basil II the Bulgar-Slayer in 1025, it once again became the most powerful state in Europe, possessing an unrivaled navy, thanks to its use of Greek fire. Our Empire extended across all of Asia Minor to Armenia, the entire Balkan Peninsula up to the Danube, and Southern Italy, from Naples southward. But even this glory did not last long.

From the depths of the East came a new calamity: the Seljuk Turks. With their lightning-fast cavalry, they began conducting raids and pillaging across Asia Minor, bringing great devastation to the most vital region of the Empire. The brave Emperor Romanos IV Diogenes resolved in 1071 to strike them with a decisive blow and rid Anatolia of their presence once and for all. He set out with a large army, composed of heavy infantry and cavalry, and met the Seljuks at Manzikert, deep in Armenia.

Romanos fought on the front lines, just like Heraclius once did. The battle was fierce and lasted all day. At the critical moment, betrayal played its disastrous role. Andronikos Doukas, who commanded a large portion of the army and coveted the throne, spread the false rumor that the Emperor had been killed, and withdrew with his troops. The remaining soldiers panicked, broke their formation, and were slaughtered by the Turks. Romanos was captured while fighting, grievously wounded, but still alive. When they brought him before the Seljuk sultan Alp Arslan, the latter, admiring his bravery, asked him: "If you were in my place, how would you treat me?" The valiant Roma-

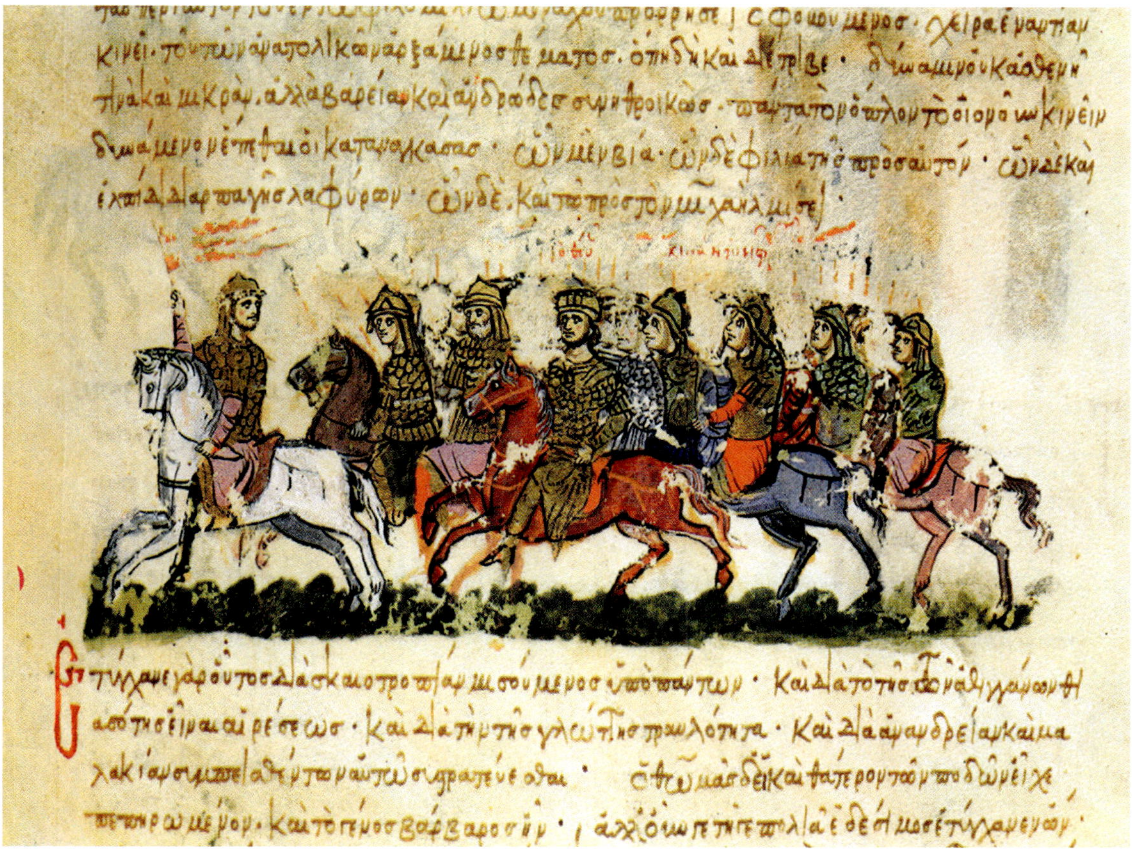

The Battle of Manzikert.

Miniature from Skylitzes, 12th century, National Library of Spain, Madrid.

nos replied without hesitation: "I would kill you." Let us not forget—this was the Emperor of the Romans addressing a barbarian invader, whom he naturally regarded as a rebel and usurper. "And how do you want me to treat you?" asked the Muslim ruler. "As you would a king," answered the proud captive. The noble Seljuk indeed treated him as a king, and—after receiving a large ransom—returned him to the Romans. This was the second devastating defeat of our army, one that shattered the international prestige of the Empire. The greater part of Asia Minor, which was the richest and most populous region—the very backbone of the State—was lost to Hellenism. The Turks settled there permanently, leaving to Byzantium only a portion of the western and northern coast. In the last century, under the prudent administration of the Komnenoi emperors, the State recovered many of the lost territories in Asia Minor and in Italy, yet it never again attained its former glory.

Constantinople, the Queen of Cities, was—and remains—the cultural center of the world, home to the earliest "Universities" in Europe, such as the *Pandidakterion*, founded in the year 425 by Emperor Theodosius II. At the Pandidakterion, subjects taught included Philology, Rhetoric, Roman Law, Grammar, Philosophy, and Medicine. A major advancement in Higher Education was introduced by Caesar Vardas, who in 849 established this Pandidakterion within the Magnaura Palace, where Philosophy, Geometry, Astronomy, and Grammar were taught—what was then referred to as "external wisdom" or "education from without" (*exō sophia* or *thyrathen paideia*). It was from this in-

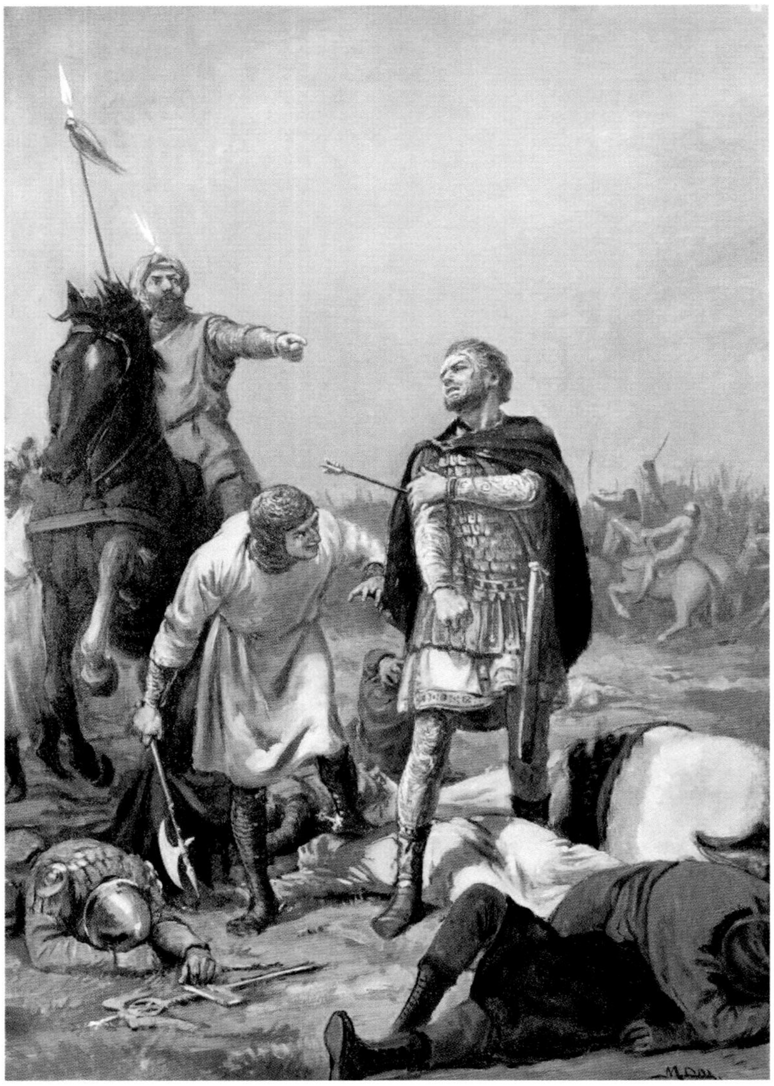

Romanos Diogenes is captured at Manzikert.

Lithograph based on a painting by Margaret Dovaston, London, 1915.

novation that the institution took its name. In 1045, under Emperor Constantine IX Monomachos, the Pandidakterion was restructured and became a proper university. Two major schools were founded: the *Didaskaleion ton nomon*, meaning the School of Law, and the *Gymnasion*, or the School of Philosophy. At the first school, the science of Law was taught for the formation of fully qualified jurists, judges, and state officials. At the School of Philosophy, all other sciences were taught. Today, particularly in the field of Medicine, the University does not confine itself to the theoretical education of students but aims primarily at the acquisition of practical medical knowledge and experience. This is achieved through training in hospitals—known as *Xenones*—which house rich medical libraries. Practical training is an official part of the academic program and is validated by the granting of a Medical Diploma. For higher theological studies, there is the Patriarchal School or Academy, founded in the 7th century and directly under the jurisdiction of the Ecumenical Patriarchate. All this information had captivated me and stirred my imagination. My dream was to study in the capital.

When I completed my general education, I faced a great dilemma: how would I fulfill this dream of mine? Unlike the secondary schools, attendance at the "University" was free of charge—but how could I support myself in the Capital?

My family simply could not afford the cost, nor could I demand such an expense from my father. We had no relatives or friends in the City who could host me. One possible path was to become a monk in a monastery that supported learning, and, with the knowledge I had already acquired, ask to be sent to study in the City and later serve the Monastery's mission. But despite my deep faith in God—instilled in me by my mother and my first teacher, Father Porphyrios—I felt no calling whatsoever toward the monastic life. Torni-

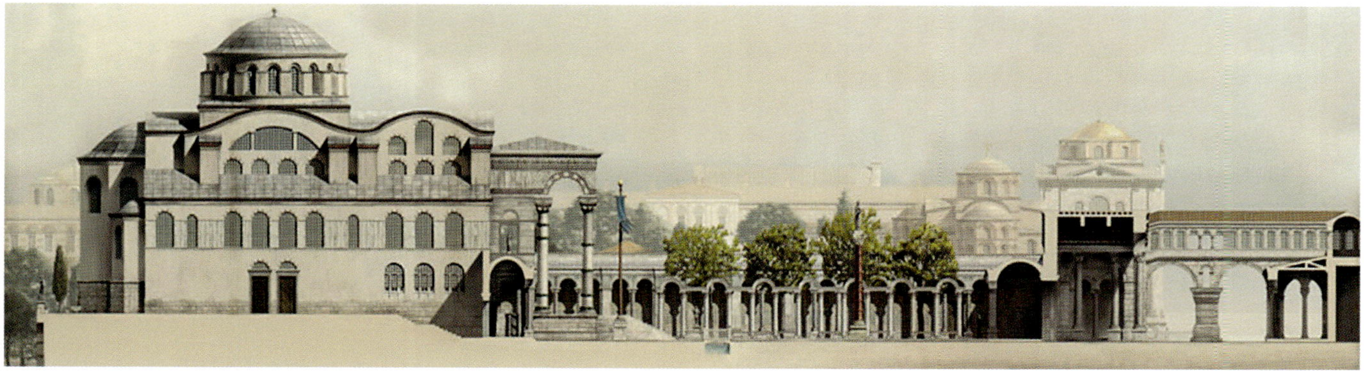

The Pardidakterion of the Magnaura. *Reconstruction by Antoine Helbert, 1870.*

kes, who was fond of me, offered real support in my predicament. He agreed to let me continue at his school as his assistant—without pay, of course. And so, I remained a "grammar assistant" for about two years. During that time, I would go to the school and examine the students to ensure they had studied, organize the books, and supervise those who were writing so they wouldn't ruin the precious paper. But most importantly, I had access to the teacher's library—and not only that. I was also able to borrow books from others in his name, which they gladly allowed, since Tornikes was held in high esteem and trusted by all in the city. During this period, certain events occurred that marked my life deeply and gave decisive momentum to my plans and aspirations.

A close friend and classmate of mine during our elementary studies was Nikolaos Kalavros, the son of a general goods merchant. As his name suggests, his ancestors likely came from Italy, and his father maintained commercial relations with Brindisi. Nikolaos lived relatively near us, and our mothers were acquainted. However, his father was peculiar and antisocial. Nikolaos, having inherited his mother's good nature, was an honest and modest man who loved knowledge. He had a brilliant mind but was not at all arrogant, unlike most top-performing students at the time, who formed a select minority among the other children. We had formed a close friendship, and like all teenagers, we explored the world together, held endless conversations after school, and shared our dreams for life. Despite being well-off, Nikolaos' father was firmly opposed to the idea of him continuing his studies. He considered the preparatory education more than sufficient and wanted to keep him in the family business. The teachers, seeing the potential of the boy, pressured his father to allow him to pursue his elementary education, but it was in vain. He finally agreed only after Tornikes, who greatly admired Nikolaos, persuaded him that an educated man would bring much more prestige—and therefore profit—to the business. Tornikes also promised to accept his son with reduced tuition fees. We completed our studies with nearly equal grades, and our teacher had praised us both for our achievements. My friend began working in his father's business—but not for long. One winter day in 1166, he suddenly fell ill. He developed chills, a high fever, and a dry cough. The women in the

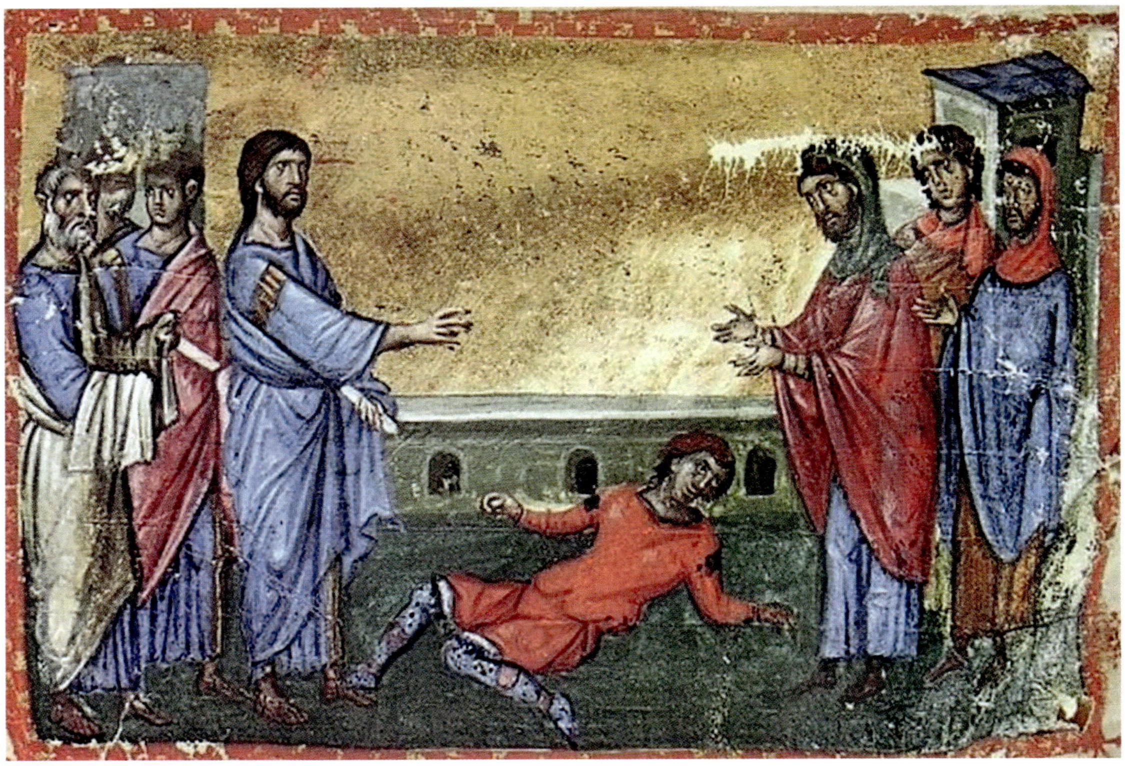

Christ Healing the Sick.

Miniature, 15th century, Iviron Monastery, Mount Athos.

household applied the folk remedies of the time—warm compresses and poultices—but to no effect. Within two days, he also experienced shortness of breath and extreme fatigue. They called for a practical doctor, who administered some medicine and diagnosed a severe case of pneumonia. He warned that if the fever didn't subside, Nikolaos would need to be taken to the hospital. But it was too late. The next day, he began to deliriously ramble, gasping for breath. By evening, he passed away. I was at his home and witnessed his final moments. I saw the unspeakable grief of his mother—and of his father too, who lost the pride of his heart, "the greatest of hopes," as an ancient epigram says.

This event shook me to the core. The pain of losing my friend so unjustly made all my desires and plans seem futile. What meaning can there be in spending one's life in philosophical and intellectual pursuits, when a life in full bloom can so easily be snuffed out? What thought, what lofty concept, can ever replace the presence of a beloved person? It was the first time I came so close to pain and death. I realized that the world suffers from illnesses that destroy lives and bring sorrow to defenseless people. I came to understand that my choices should not be guided by pleasure or ambition, but by a desire to offer help to those who suffer, to ease their pain as much as possible. I resolved to study medicine—to explore the wisdom humanity has gathered in this sacred field, to understand the mysteries of health, illness, life, and death, and to wage battle against disease, which I came to see as the greatest injustice a person can face.

My teacher, Euthymios Tornikes, was also deeply saddened by the unjust death of Nikolaos. He held him in high regard and had great expectations for him. He was moved by my decision to pursue medicine and wholeheartedly agreed with my choice. He did his best to support me in every possible way. There were many so-called practical doctors, but most of them were mere quacks, not held in high esteem by the people. Their knowledge was rudimentary, often mixed with charms and incantations—a legacy of antiquity. The truly learned and competent physicians were few, and to become one of them, I would have to go to Constantinople. There, I would need to study first the writings of the ancient masters and then those of the more recent great physicians of our Roman Empire, all of which were composed in the Greek language. And, of course, I would have to engage in hands-on training at one of the great hospitals of the City, more commonly referred to as xenones[—hospices that served as both places of healing and of learning.]

The beginning would be made with the study of Hippocrates. In his library, my teacher had several treatises by the great father of the Art of Medicine. He told me he could borrow others if needed. I devoted myself to their study. This great healer was the first to separate medicine from magic and superstition, applying instead careful observation and the methodical study of patients, along with systematic descriptions of symptoms and the course of each illness. He always assessed symptoms in conjunction with the patient's personality, thoroughly questioning them about past ailments, their parents, and their family situation—what we now call a case history. *He treated each case as unique and taught us that we should not investigate disease in general, but the specific patient.* In his time, as in ours in the 12th century, it was commonly believed that illnesses were punishments from God. This mistaken view branded the unfortunate sufferer as a sinner, adding guilt to the pain of sickness, implying that either the patient or someone close to them was responsible for causing it. Hippocrates boldly declared: *"God is the cause of nothing"* (*ouk estin ho*

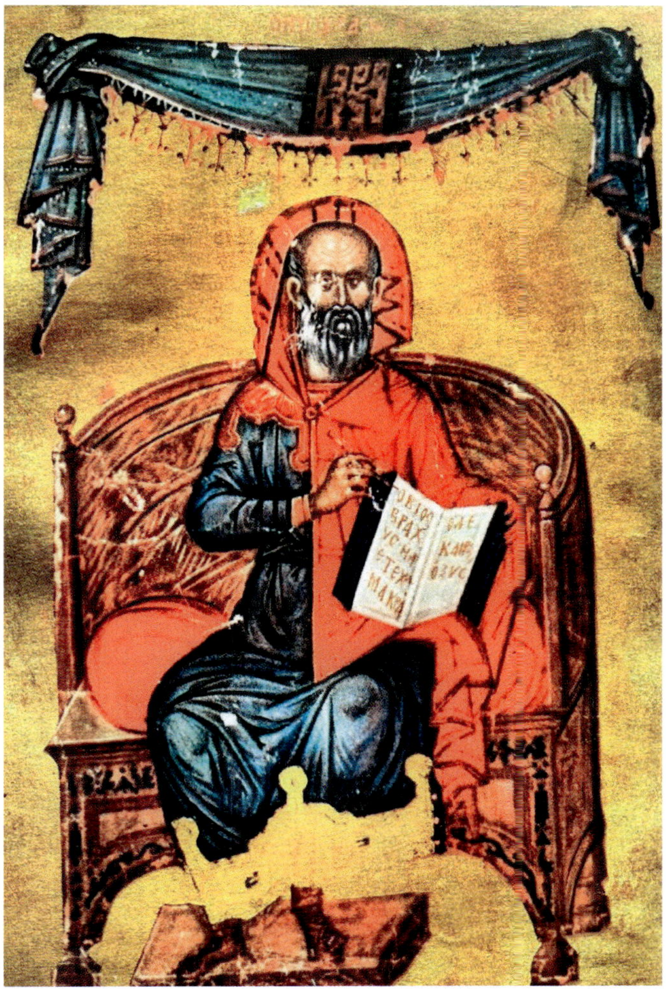

Hippocrates Depicted as a Bishop.

Miniature, 14th century
National Library of France, Paris.

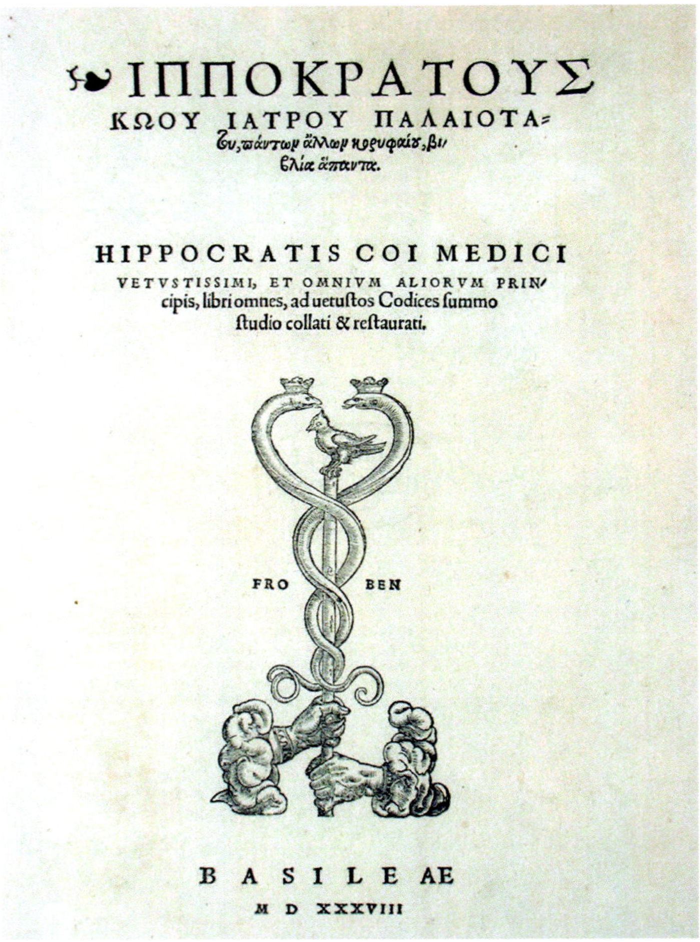
ΙΠΠΟΚΡΑΤΟΥΣ
ΚΩΟΥ ΙΑΤΡΟΥ ΠΑΛΑΙΟΤΑ-
του, πάντων ἄλλων κορυφαίου, βι-
βλία ἅπαντα.

HIPPOCRATIS COI MEDICI
VETVSTISSIMI, ET OMNIVM ALIORVM PRIN-
cipis, libri omnes, ad uetustos Codices summo
studio collati & restaurati.

BASILEAE
M D XXXVIII

Complete Works of Hippocrates.
Basel, 1808.

Theos aitios oudenos) and taught that illness results from human or natural causes, which can be investigated and treated.

Lacking at the time a basic knowledge of anatomy, I was unable to fully grasp the descriptions of various treatments—especially surgical ones, such as abscess drainage or fracture reduction. However, I held fast to his famous maxim: "What medicines do not heal, iron heals" (*okosa pharmaka ouk iētai, sidēros iētai*)—by which he meant the surgeon's knife and cautery. For this reason, I began by reading his general works: the *Oath*, the *Law*, On the *Physician*, *On the Art*, and the *Aphorisms*. In these texts, the Great Teacher sets forth the principles that must guide the physician in the practice of his profession. The guiding principle, he said, must be "To benefit, or at least do no harm" (*ofelein, ē mē blaptein*): that is, the physician must seek to help the patient—or, at the very least, avoid causing him harm. He also describes how a physician ought to behave, his obligations, but also his privileges within society. And I began to realize how profound it is for one to assume such a role in life. Two years passed in study and waiting. I enriched my knowledge in Philosophy and Medicine, all the while hoping and preparing. The historical events that took place during that time were generally distressing—but for me, they opened the door to the opportunity of a lifetime.

Hippocrates' Aphorisms

Life is short, the Art long, opportunity fleeting, experience treacherous, judgment difficult

It is preferable to prevent than to cure

It is preferable to benefit than not to harm

Those diseases which medicines do not cure, iron (*surgery*) cures. Those which iron cannot cure, fire (*cauterization*) cures. And those which fire cannot cure, are to be reckoned wholly incurable

Both sleep and insomnolency, when immoderate are bad.

Persons who are naturally very fat are apt to die earlier than those who are slender.

Those things which one has been accustomed to for a long time, although worse than things which one is not accustomed to, usually give less disturbance; but a change must sometimes be made to things one is not accustomed to.

For extreme diseases, extreme methods of cure, as to restriction, are most suitable

Neither repletion, nor fasting, nor everything else is good when more than natural

We cannot know medicine if we do not know what man is

Hippocratic Oath

I swear by ... all the gods and goddesses, making them my witnesses, that I will fulfill according to my ability and judgment this oath…:

To hold him who has taught me this art as equal to my parents and to live my life in partnership with him…

To regard his offspring as equal to my brothers ... and to teach them this art—if they desire to learn it—without fee and covenant…

I will apply dietetic measures for the benefit of the sick according to my ability and judgment; I will keep them from harm and injustice.

I will neither give a deadly drug to anybody who asked for it, nor will I make a suggestion to this effect.

I will not give to a woman an abortive remedy. In purity and holiness, I will guard my life and my art.

Whatever houses I may visit, I will come for the benefit of the sick, remaining free of all intentional injustice, of all mischief and in particular of sexual relations with both female and male persons, be they free or slaves.

What I may see or hear ... in regard to the life of men ... I will keep to myself, holding such things shameful to be spoken about.

If I fulfill this oath and do not violate it, may it be granted to me to enjoy life and art, being honored with fame among all men…

if I transgress it and swear falsely, may the opposite of all this be my lot.

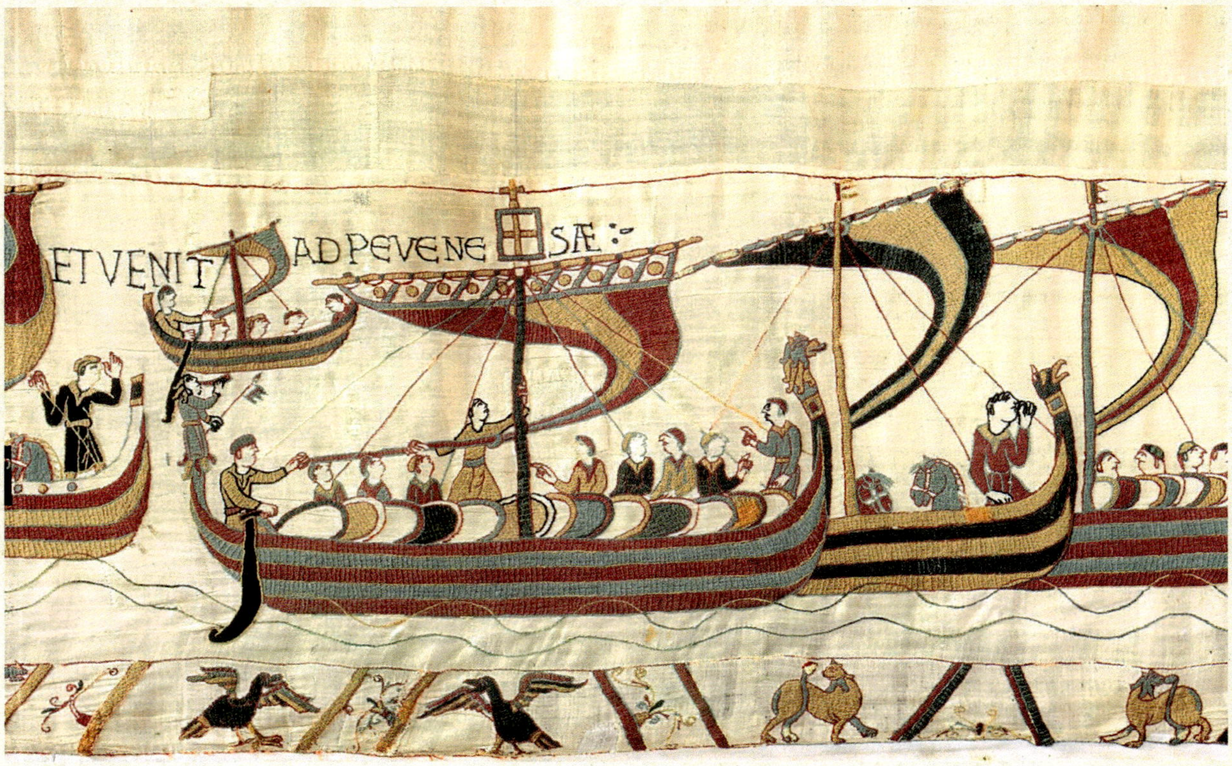

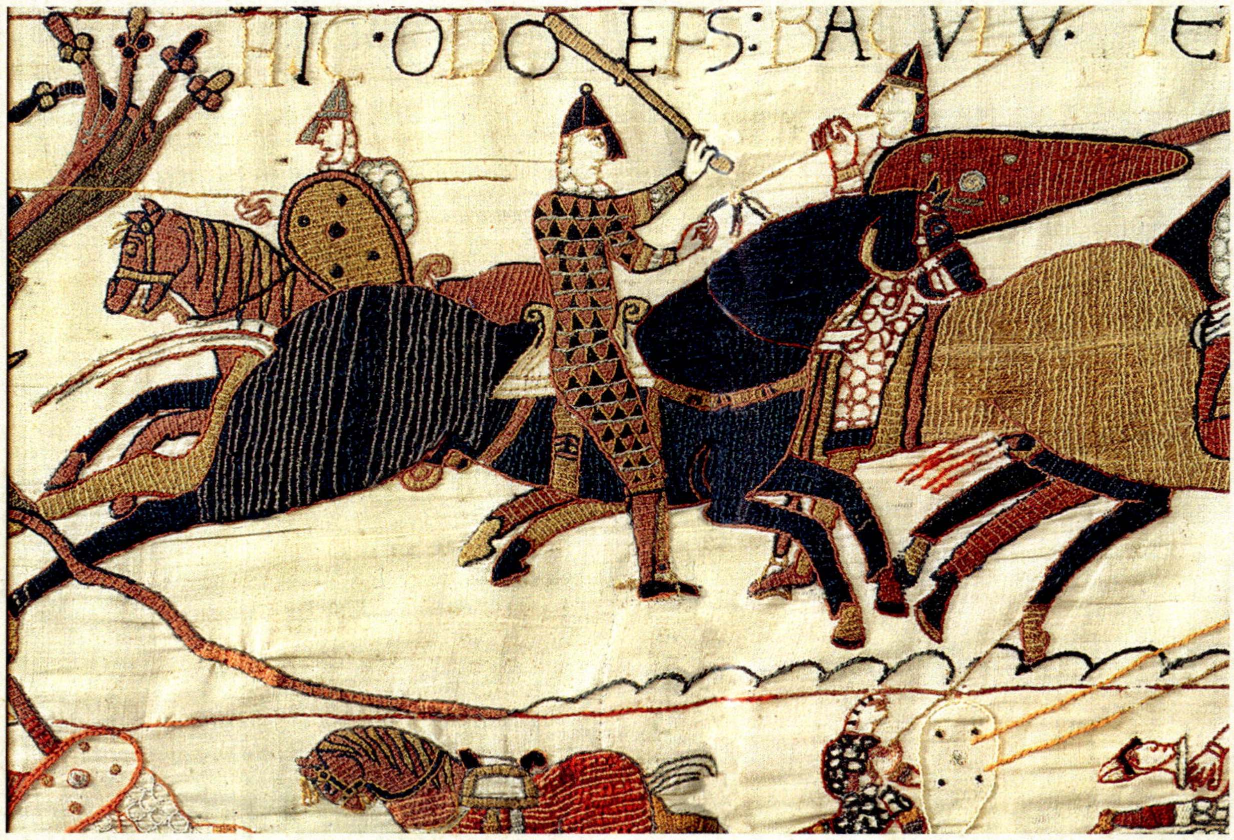

Norman ships and cavalry.

Embroidered Bayeux Tapestry, 11th century, Bayeux, France.

As I have said, the most glorious period of our later Empire came to an end in 1071 with the calamitous defeat at Manzikert and the definitive loss of the greater part of Asia Minor. Yet that disaster alone did not suffice. Though we had secured ourselves from the north—through the crushing of the Bulgarians and the Christianization and reconciliation with the barbarian Rus of Kiev—a new threat arose from the West: the Normans. They are a tribe that originated in the lands of Scandinavia, as their name indicates (men of the North). Being skilled seafarers and fierce warriors, they launched raids across Northern Europe, where they overcame the Franks and settled in a large region of France that took its name from them—Normandy. They quickly adopted the French language, and Normandy became an independent duchy within the Kingdom of France. In 1066, just a few years before the disaster at Manzikert, the Duke of Normandy, William, claiming the inheritance of the English throne as a relative of the last king, Edward, landed with a great fleet at Hastings. There he defeated the English and Harold, the local claimant to the throne, and was crowned King of England, while still retaining dominion over the Duchy of Normandy. William, who came to be known as "the Conqueror," transferred the capital of the realm to London and entrusted the administration of the country mainly to his fellow Normans. The Norman houses have ruled England ever since, and the English aristocracy speaks the French language.

Another large group of Normans, with their agile ships, passed through Gibraltar and arrived in Southern Italy, where they initially served as mercenaries for us, assisting General George Maniakes in his attempt to recapture Sicily from the Saracens. Within a few years, their capable leader, Robert Guiscard—whose name means "the cunning"—took advantage of the poor governance by the incompetent successors of Basil the Bulgar-Slayer and established an independent duchy in Calabria, which until then had belonged to our Roman Empire. The Normans defeated our weakened forces and gradually seized all of our possessions in the region. In that same fateful year of 1071, when the Seljuks overran Asia Minor, the Normans seized our last stronghold, Bari, and completely expelled the Byzantine Romans from Italy. But they did not stop there. Sixty years later, in 1130, Robert's nephew, Roger II, conquered Sicily from the Arabs and united it with Southern Italy into a great Norman Kingdom, in which he was proclaimed "King" (Rex).

From 1080, when the Komnenoi dynasty took the helm of Byzantium, the Empire began to recover both militarily and economically. Letters and the arts flourished, and some of the lost provinces were retaken. However, the threats from both East and West remained grave. Our people first came into close contact with the peoples of Western Europe—whom we collectively called Franks or Latins—during the First Crusade, which took place from 1096 to 1099. The Franks, under the pretext of liberating the Holy Places, were in truth seeking new lands to rule and easy wealth to plunder. Our capable Emperor Alexios I skillfully managed to handle them, allowing them to pass through the Empire's territory and even using their help to recover large regions of Asia Minor. They, in turn, conquered vast lands in Syria and Palestine and established the Kingdom of Jerusalem along with various Principalities and Counties, where they imposed their rule. This first encounter with the Christians of the West proved unsuccessful. Our people quickly realized the great difference in mentality, and conflict became inevitable.

But the bitter experience came with the Second Crusade, which took place three years before my birth, in 1147, and lasted for three years. Our Emperor, kyr Manuel, had to face the arrogance and rudeness of the Germans and the French, who passed through our territories without any respect for our people. Still, he managed the situation well and gained significant territorial benefits. To that end, he formed an alliance with the King of Germany, Conrad III. However, the Germans were at war with the Normans of Sicily. Thus, Roger II took this alliance as a pretext to plunder the lands of Romania. His fleet, under the command of the admiral (amirales) George of Antioch—a Greek Sicilian—captured Corfu and plundered the Peloponnese, Athens, Thebes, and Corinth.

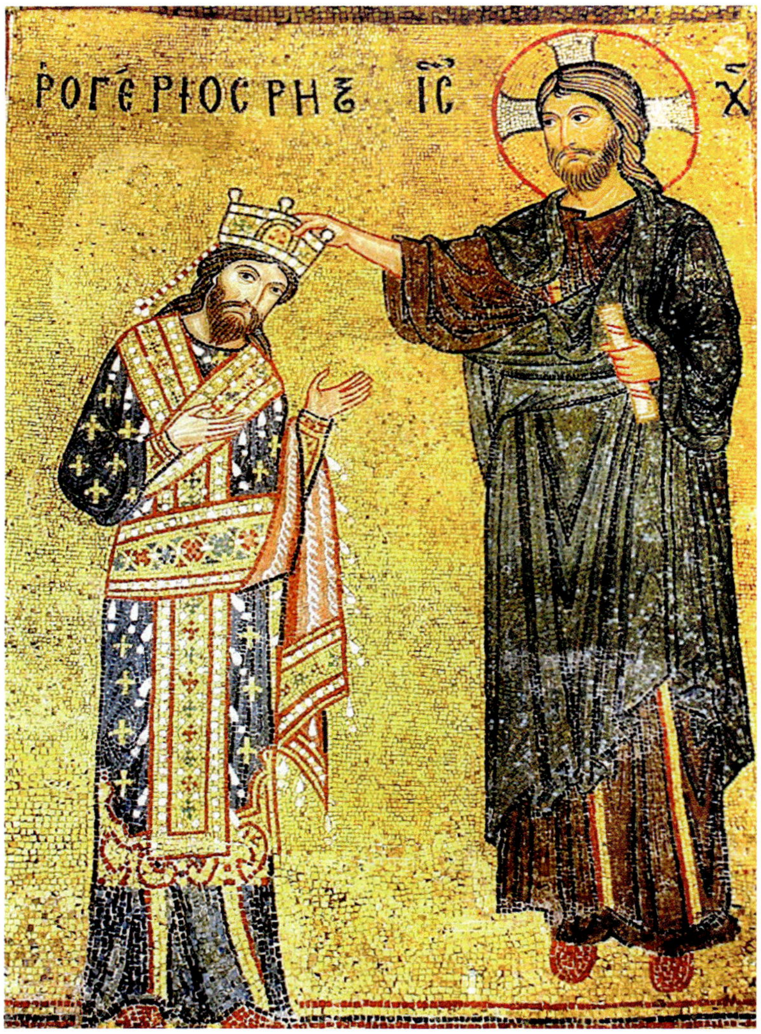

Roger II is crowned King by Christ.
Mosaic, 12th century, Church of Martorana, Palermo.

We were gripped by great fear in Patras, for we did not know whether they would attack us as well. People began hiding their goods in fear of a raid and prepared to take refuge in the fortress. I remember my father's anguish, as he stood to lose all his merchandise. Fortunately, the Normans did not besiege Patras. However, they transported thousands of captives to Sicily, who then taught them the arts of commerce and the processing of silk and purple dye—skills that had once been the near-exclusive domain of old Hellas. Here I must confess that Roger, though hated by us, was a very capable ruler. He promoted learning and the arts, making use of Greek artisans and scholars, as well as Saracen merchants in Sicily, without distinction of race or religion. When I was seven years old, the Normans once again plundered Euboea and Almyros. The Norman threat was a constant shadow, ever returning. On the other hand, a new naval power with a formidable fleet began to rise in the Adriatic—Venice. The stability of the western coasts of Greece began to be seriously threatened. Rumors circulated about a Third Crusade, this time to be launched with Venetian ships, which would conquer Western Greece and the Peloponnese. The future of trade with the West became entirely unpredictable, and an economic catastrophe seemed increasingly likely. Thus, in the year 1168, my father made a momentous decision: we would leave Patras and move his business to the safety of Constantinople.

This news was for me like a gospel of joy. Not only would I come to know and live in the jewel of the civilized world—the City of cities, the legendary Constantinople—but I would also be able to fulfill my dream of studying medicine. With deep emotion, I bid farewell to my teacher, Euthymios Tornikes, to whom I owe so much and whom I will never forget. I also said goodbye to my friends and to the beloved city where I grew up. Yet such was the joy of my expectations that I felt no sorrow at all; on the contrary, I could hardly wait for us to depart.

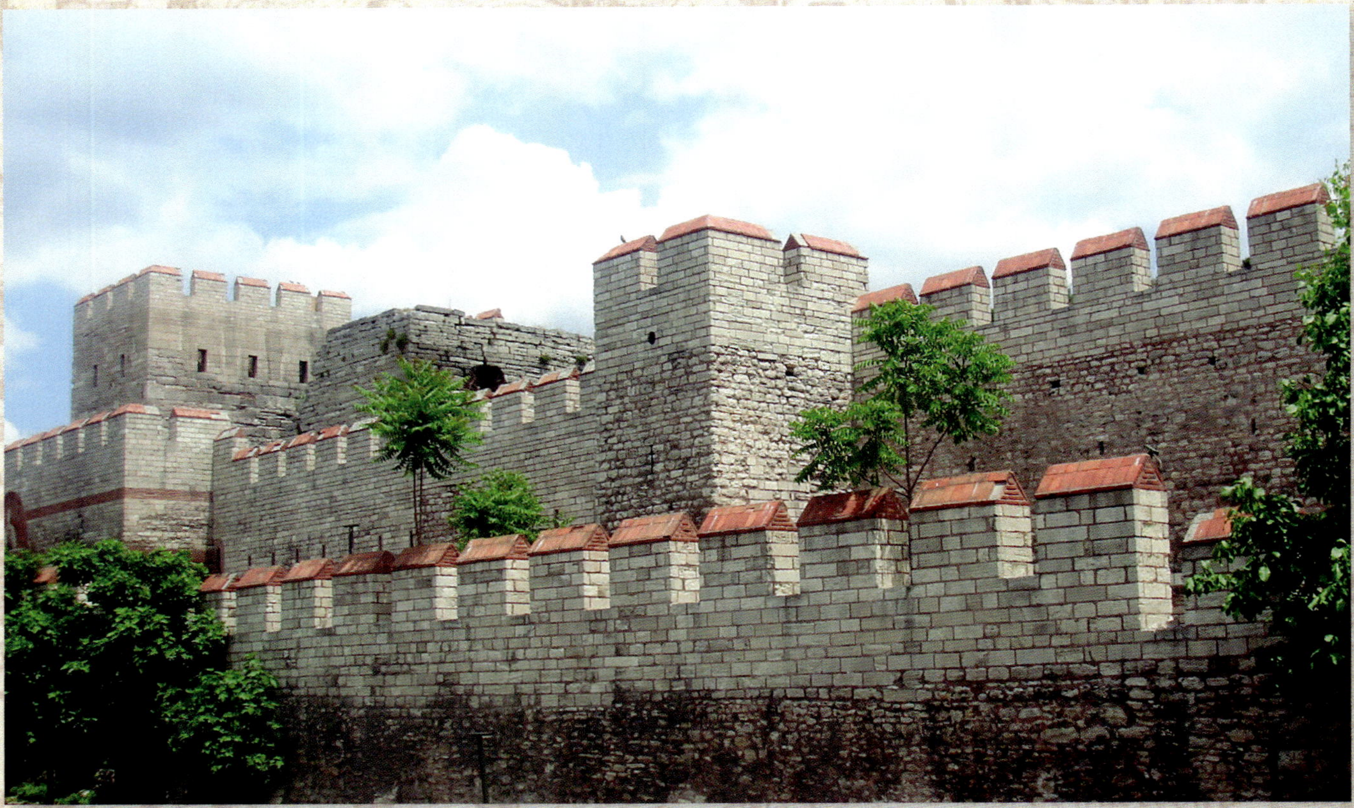

The land wall. *Photo by Bigdaddy1204, 2006.*

IN CONSTANTINOPLE

The journey to the City could only be made by sea, as proper roads did not exist and overland travel was wholly unsafe. We followed the same route our trade caravans used when transporting silk and purple-dyed cloth to the capital. We loaded our belongings and as much merchandise as my father could secure onto wagons. Our departure was deeply moving—neighbors and friends came to bid us farewell with mixed emotions: some with sadness at our leaving, others with the natural envy felt toward those setting out for the fabled Capital. Together with a group of fellow merchants and escorted by a few armed guards, we set out for Corinth. The journey was exhausting, through clouds of dust raised by the wagons and horses, and always under the threat of bandits. It took three full days of continuous travel along a rugged wagon trail, yet through magnificent countryside: we delighted in the lush greenery, the countless mulberry trees of the Achaean plain, and the view of the sea framed by the mountains across the way—first the nearby Tafiasos, then the sharp peak of the Aselinos mountain, which the people called Giona, and finally the majestic, snow-capped summits of Mount Parnassus.

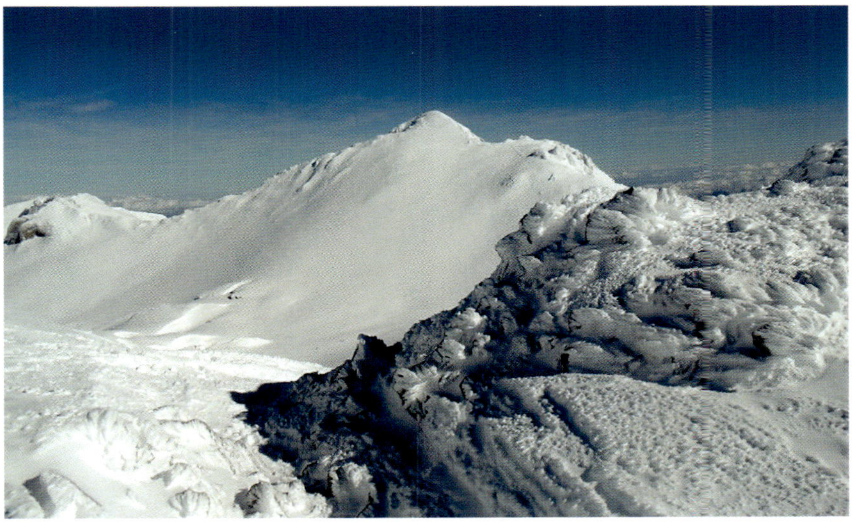

Top: Mount Parnassus, the mountain of the Muses.

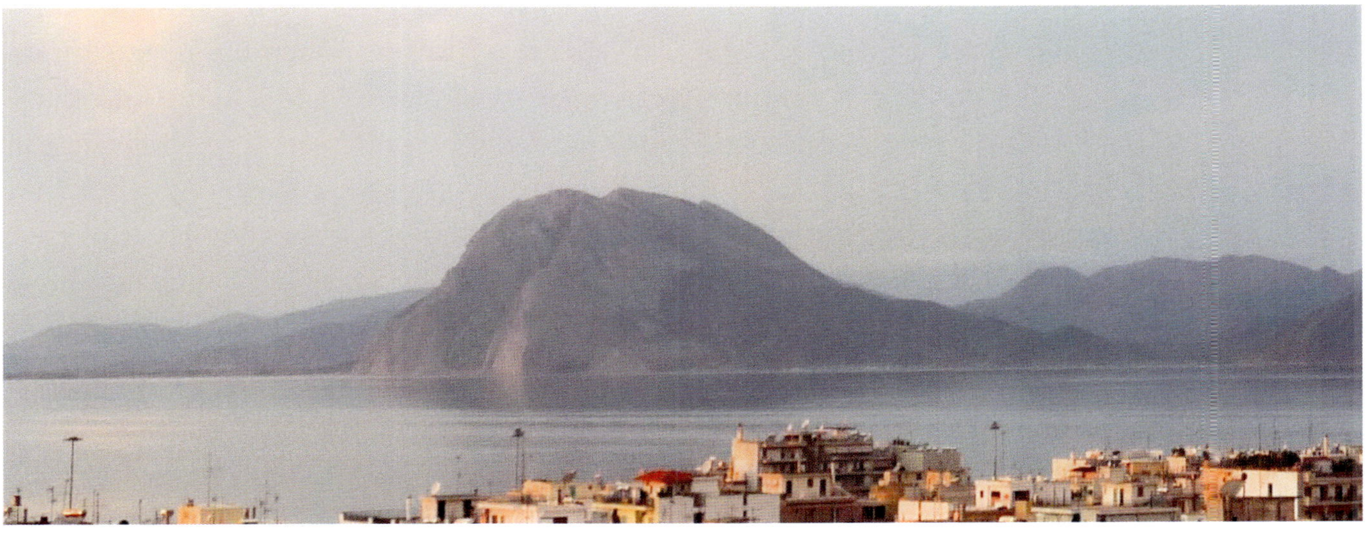

Bottom: Mount Tafiasos (Paliovouna), view from Patras.

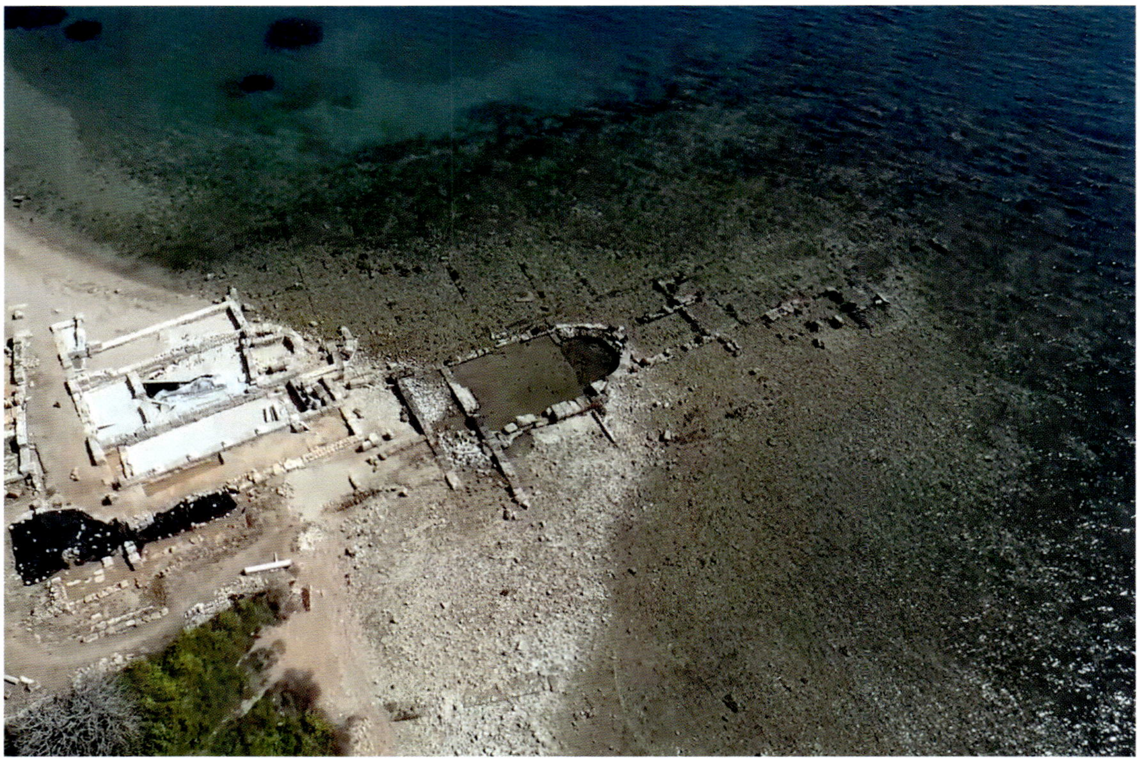

The ancient harbor of Kenchreai in Corinth.

Photo: Loutraki365, 2020.

We passed Cape Rion, the narrowest point between the Peloponnese and the mainland, where the Gulf of Patras ends and the Gulf of Corinth begins. By afternoon, we reached Vostitsa—ancient Aigion—a city that once knew great glory but had long since fallen into decline, ever since the Slavic raiders devastated it in the 9th century and imposed a new name, which, nevertheless, prevailed. We spent the night in roadside inns, taking many precautions for our safety. We had completed the first 27 miles. Over the following two days, we covered the remaining 60 miles to Corinth, journeying through a landscape of breathtaking greenery. We first arrived at Lechaion, its port, where we stopped briefly before continuing on to the safety of the city, where we settled temporarily.

Corinth at that time was experiencing commercial prosperity similar to that of Patras. Built beneath its impregnable fortress, the Acrocorinth, it possessed two port towns: Lechaion on the Corinthian Gulf and Kenchreai on the Saronic Gulf. After a three-day stay in Kenchreai, during which the necessary arrangements and preparations were made, we boarded a merchant ship transporting fabrics and grain to the City, and we set out to sail across the Aegean

Our merchant ships were relatively small compared to warships, but they were wide and hollow—just as Homer described—thus allowing for great cargo capacity. They were moved solely by the wind, as oars were no longer necessary after the invention of the triangular sail, which made it possible to sail even with side winds or slightly opposing ones. The single rudder at the stern, which had replaced the two steering oars previously used until the 10th century, made the ships faster and more maneuverable—an essential feature for avoiding pirates. The elimination of the need for rowers made voyages more economical and, consequently, more frequent. This gave a great boost to trade and, more broadly, to communication between regions of the Empire as well as with our neighbors across the Mediterranean and the Black Sea.

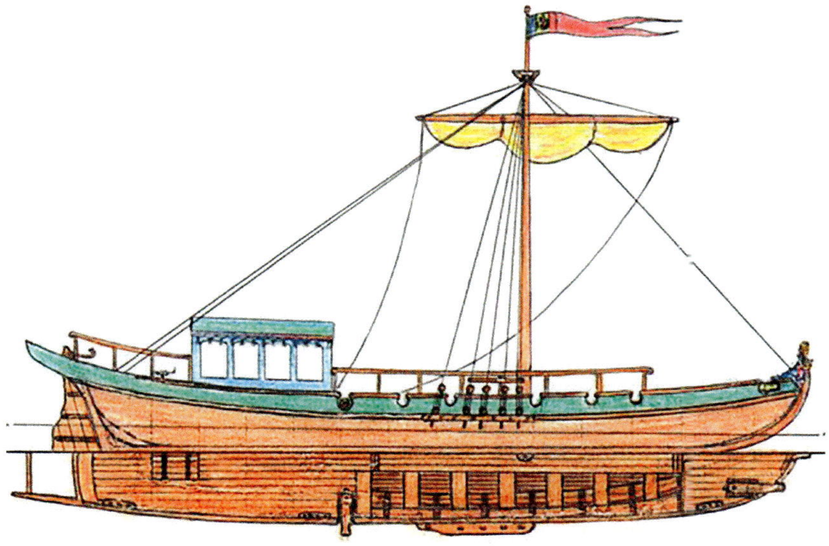

Ship similar to a Byzantine merchant vessel of the era.

We set out on a beautiful morning, with fair weather and a gentle Zephyr that carried our ship over the blue waters of the Saronic Gulf. We passed to the north of Aegina and sailed along the cape of Sounion, where I could see the marbles of the temple of Poseidon gleaming in the sunlight, towering above the rock. Then we sailed through the strait of Caphereus, between Euboea and Andros, and entered fully into the Aegean Sea. The strait of Caphereus is always swept by strong winds and currents, and passing through it is rather difficult. We were thoroughly shaken. After Caphereus, we set a course northeast and sailed near the western shores of Lesbos, until we drew near the coast of Asia Minor at the mouth of the Hellespont.

The Aegean archipelago, full of islands, is marked by the instability of its winds, which often change direction and intensity—unlike the Ionian Sea, where the winds are steady. Thus, Aegean captains are considered particularly skillful and capable. Our journey lasted several days, giving me the opportunity to get to know the captain and speak with him. He was a sharp-witted sea wolf from the Cyclades, full of curiosity about the process of dyeing with purple. He asked me many questions, and I answered as best I could—though not going into too much detail, for I didn't know them thoroughly myself. In turn, he explained to me the ways sailors navigate. He showed me the astrolabe, with which he measured the height of the sun during the day, thereby determining the point of midday. Thus, he could orient himself by knowing the cardinal points of the horizon. At night, he explained his navigation by showing me the stars—the Great and Little Bear, and the Pleiades. The last star of the Little Bear was the so-called Pole Star, which steadily pointed north, and the entire celestial dome seemed to revolve around it. My knowledge of astronomy helped me understand what he was saying and also to impress him with my questions. He also showed me the famous *periplous*—a kind of map that depicted landmarks, ports, and coastlines for the entire Aegean. It was an indispensable aid, although he, by now, after so many voyages, knew it all by heart. He told me that such maps also existed for the Ionian Sea, the Black Sea, the Cretan Sea, and other waters of the Mediterranean. This journey taught me much about the seafaring traditions of the Empire. The captain,

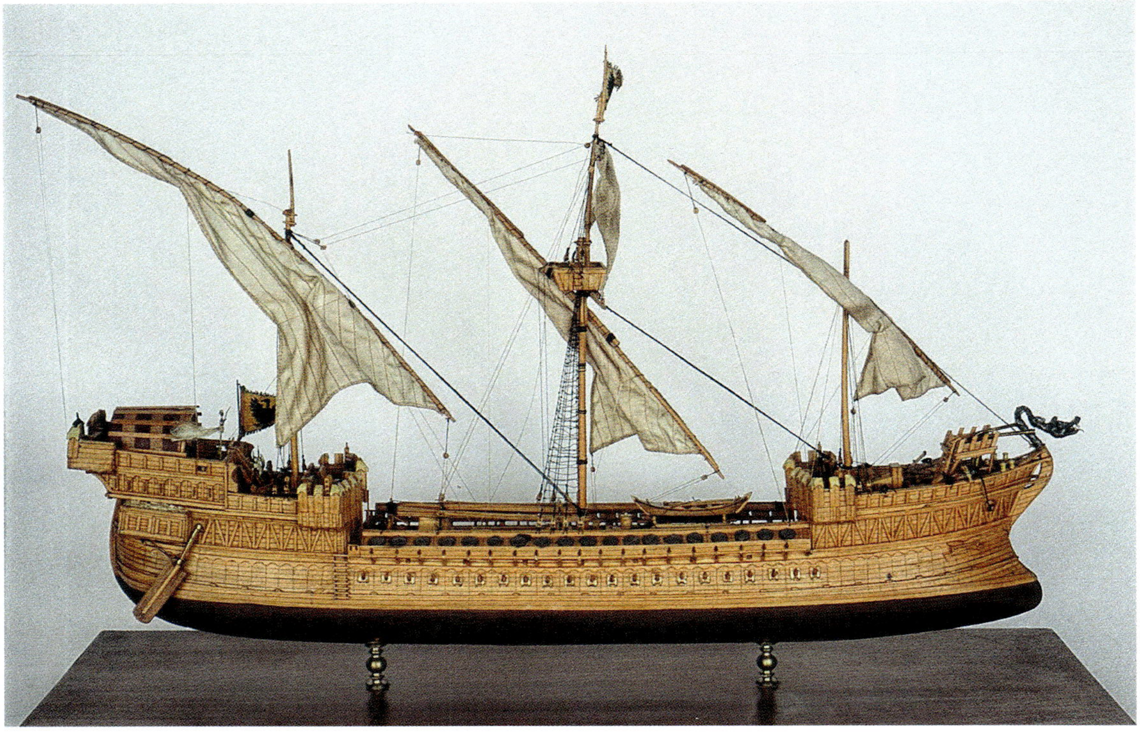

Byzantine *dromon*.
Hellenic Maritime Museum, Piraeus.

an old sea dog, had also fought in our navy. Seeing my interest, he would tell me many things about our Imperial Navy as well.

Our warships, known as *dromōnes* or *chelandia,* were larger than merchant vessels and were equipped with sails as well, but their main source of propulsion came from rows of oars, arranged in two tiers. Until about a hundred years ago, our fleet held dominance over the Mediterranean, and the naval power of the Empire was considered unbeatable. The *dromōnes* had a large siphon mounted at the prow, which projected *Greek fire* onto enemy ships, and at the base of the main mast there was a wooden structure, the *xylokastron,* from which marines, protected behind its walls, would launch projectiles and arrows at the enemy. Unfortunately, after the glorious Macedonian dynasty, the incapable Emperors who followed neglected the fleet, while at the same time new naval powers appeared in our seas—the Normans, the Venetians, the Genoese, and others—who gradually took control of trade. What was worse, we began to entrust them with the naval defense of the Empire, hiring their ships as mercenaries. Yet even so, the Aegean was still a Roman sea, and our Navy remained a formidable force.

Our ship passed through the Hellespont and entered the Propontis—the famed Sea of Marmara. To our right, we encountered an island, Prokonnesos, and continued toward the Bosporus, along the northern shore of the Propontis. My anticipation had reached its peak. Soon, the shores and the walls of the City came into view, gleaming in the sunlight. The sea walls were built right up to the edge of the coast, leaving no space for enemy landings. They stood 10 to 13 meters high and 3 to 4 meters thick, and every so often, towering watchtowers rose from their line. Seeing the walls, I understood the discouragement of the barbarians who came intending to besiege the City—many of whom departed empty-handed without even attempting it. Yet the awe I felt before the sea walls was nothing compared to the overwhelming impression I had upon beholding the land walls, which guarded the City from the mainland. Constantinople, built upon seven hills, forms a triangle—the base being its western, landward side. The other two sides are washed by the Propontis to the south and the Golden Horn to the north. The apex of the triangle lies at the mouth of the Bosporus. The two coastal sides are protected by sea walls, while the landward base is fortified by the legendary land walls, which stretch for 5,600 meters. The land walls are double-layered, with their height—including the battlements—reaching approximately 8 and 13 meters, respectively. Every 50 meters, towering watchtowers alternate along both lines of fortification. In front of them lies a deep moat, 20 meters wide. The sight is awe-inspiring. Both the land and sea walls are pierced with numerous gates. Among the most prominent are the Golden Gate, the Gate of Saint Romanos, the Gate of Selymbria, the Gate of Adrianople, the Xylokerkos Gate, the Gate of Rhegion, and the Gate of Charisius, among others.

We disembarked at the *Port of Theodosius*, the main commercial harbor along the shores of the Propontis. The City boasts many harbors, both on the Propontis and along the Golden Horn. The impression the port made on me was entirely new—I had never seen anything like it. The harbor in Patras, by comparison, now seemed quite small. Here, a bustling and colorful crowd, clad in strange and varied garments, moved constantly to and fro. Ships from every corner of the Mediterranean and the Black Sea docked at this port. Besides the Roman merchants, sailors, customs officers, and guards, one could see haughty Franks and Venetians, barbarian Russians and Bulgarians, cunning Saracens, and all sorts of peoples—Jews, Armenians, Turks—who came to the City for business, dressed in their distinct and peculiar garments and speaking their incomprehensible tongues. Naturally, in order to communicate with the authorities, they had to speak Greek. So you would hear every kind of sound and noise, and Greek spoken with heavy or singsong accents—

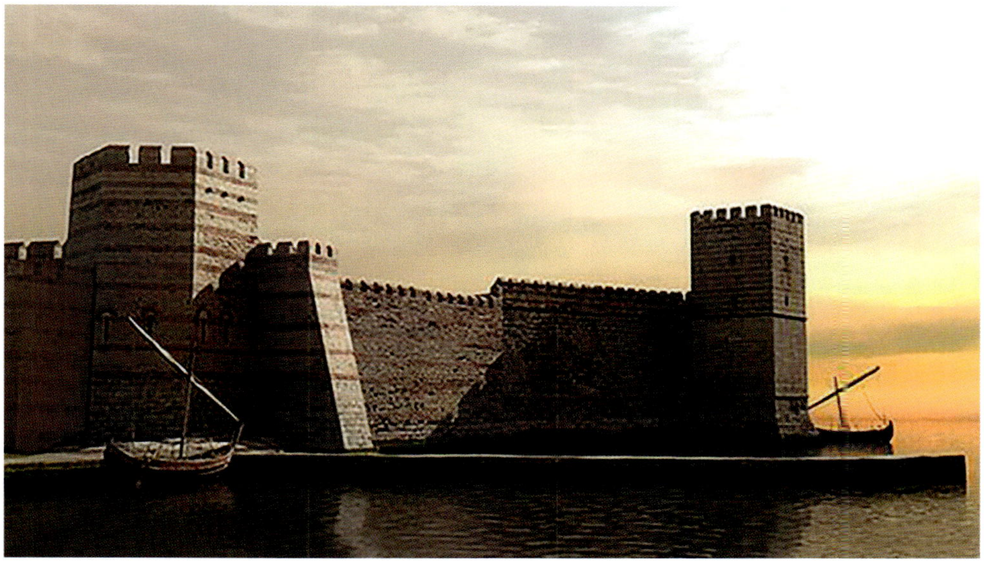

The Sea Walls: *Reconstruction from Byzantium 1200.com*

full, of course, of mistakes. As someone aptly put it, in the ports there is a jumble of "Greeks, Hellenizers, Hellenized, and those merely mimicking Greekness."

My father had made arrangements with a merchant from the capital, Theodoros Vlemmides, with whom he had been collaborating for years. Vlemmides had kindly taken care of finding us a place to live—a difficult task in the City. He would now work together with my father, who had connections with the markets of Italy, Sicily, and generally the lands of the West, while Vlemmides would contribute his own experience with the markets of the East, the Black Sea, and the northern Balkans to their joint enterprise. Vlemmides, who was quite well-off, welcomed us at the port accompanied by two servants. He had instructed us to meet him at the Gate of Aemilianus—one of the two gates (the other being the Gate of the Jews) through which one could enter the City from

Constantinople in the 12th century.

R. Janin, Paris, 1950.

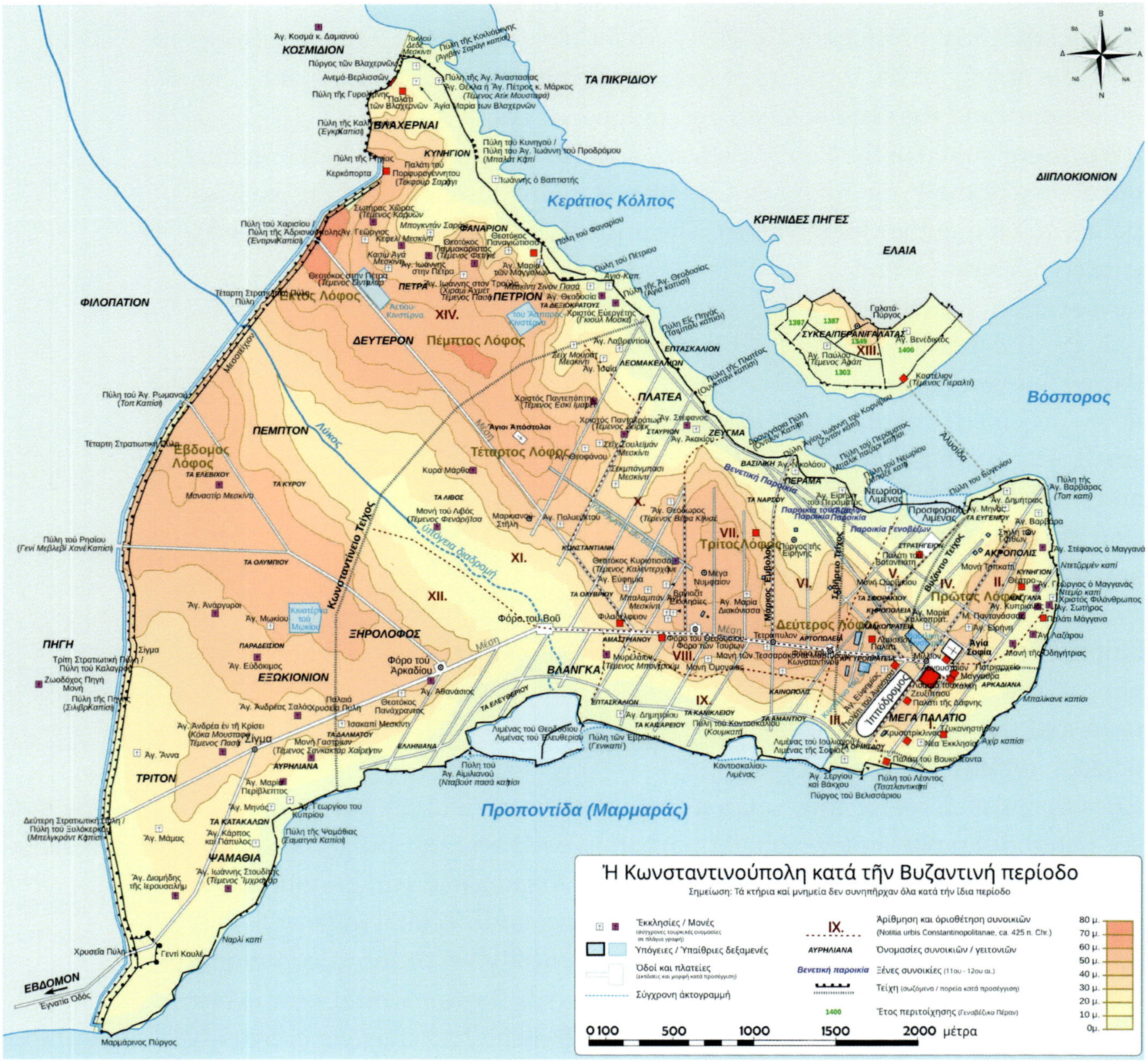

the harbor. He was easily recognizable by his simple yet dignified attire and his well-groomed beard, now beginning to turn grey. He greeted us warmly; after embracing my father, he respectfully greeted my mother and then us children, showing particular tenderness toward young Iphigenia. Our belongings were loaded onto a large wagon, and we set off for our home, which was quite a distance away, in the district of Petra, in the northwestern part of the City.

Petra was near the Palace of Vlachernae and the renowned Monastery of Chora. We first took a rather narrow road heading north, which led us to the famous Mese, or Imperial Avenue—the main thoroughfare of the Queen of Cities—stretching in two branches across the City like a slanted "Y." It begins at the Hippodrome and runs westward all the way to the land walls. This boulevard is broad and straight, lined with elegant homes—some of the most expensive in the city—and adorned on both sides with beautiful arcaded galleries, where countless shops offer anything one might desire. Taking a turn, one branch of the road leads to the southern part of the Wall, to the Golden Gate. From a point on the road near the great Forum of Theodosius, the northern branch begins, reaching as far as the Gate of Adrianople and the Palace of Vlachernae, in the northern section of the Land Wall. This is the route we followed. Along the way, I gazed in wonder at the houses, the squares, the countless churches, and the grand public buildings. What I saw surpassed even my wildest imagination. The journey felt endless—I had never imagined a city could be so vast. The house that Vlemmides had secured on our behalf was very beautiful, and Petra proved to be a well-to-do, urban neighborhood. We settled in with great joy, deeply impressed by the layout of the house. It was two-storied. On the ground floor there was a central hall, which would serve as the reception area for guests and for my father's merchant associates. There was also a room with a large hearth for heating, along with the icon room, the kitchen, the bath, and the laundry area. On the upper floor were four bedrooms. I was especially happy to have a room of my own, where I could keep my books and spend quiet hours reading and dreaming, making plans for the future. Our neighborhood was very desirable, for it was adjacent to the area where the emperors had built a second palace as early as the 6th century, named after the Church of the Theotokos of Vlachernae that stood nearby.

Traditionally, the Emperors resided in the Sacred Palace, next to the Hippodrome and Hagia Sophia, which were located at the other end of the City. But Alexios I Komnenos found it more convenient to settle permanently in the Vlachernae district, which lay next to the land walls—and his successors did the same. In fact, the current Emperor, Lord Manuel, fortified it, added new halls, and named it the *New Palace.*

The Komnenoi were great emperors, yet they made a grave mistake—one that proved fatal in the long run. They placed the entire weight of the Em-

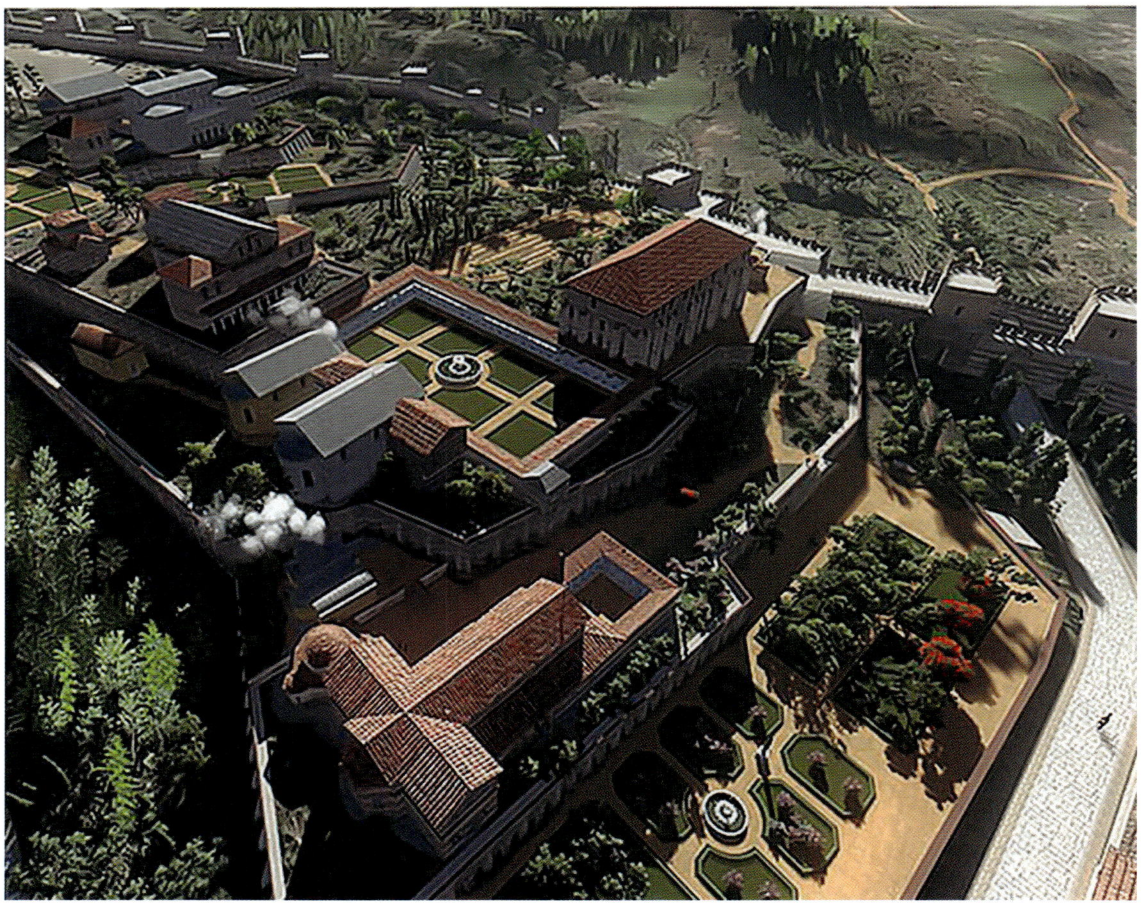

The Palace of Vlachernae.
Reconstruction by Byzantium 1200.com

pire's defense on the land forces of the army. Underestimating the power and greed of the Latins, instead of strengthening our war fleet—which previous emperors had unfortunately neglected—they deemed it more advantageous to rely on the naval might of Venice, granting it, in return, extensive commercial privileges and customs exemptions. The Venetians settled in the northern part of the City overlooking the Golden Horn and established an entire colony. Local merchants began to suffer, losing their livelihoods. In an attempt to counterbalance the exclusive dominance of the Venetians, Lord Manuel granted similar privileges to the Genoese, the Pisans, and the Amalfitans, who in turn settled along the northern coast of the City, beside the Venetians. But this was not the right solution. The Latin colony in the City grew large, and the fierce competition between them led to armed clashes and mutual massacres, to such an extent that the Emperor was eventually forced to intervene and expel many of them. At the time of our arrival in Constantinople, there were around 60,000 Latins living among a population of 450,000. Vlemmides explained to my father the problems that the competition from the Italians was causing for the local merchants, as well as the hostile sentiments that had developed between the two communities—sentiments that had, regrettably, taken on a national and religious character, framing the tension as a conflict between Orthodox Greeks (Romans) and Roman Catholic Latins.

These problems affected my enthusiasm very little. I could think of nothing else but the grandeur of the greatest and most beautiful city in the world, and the prospects of my studies. In regard to the latter, I was fortunate. Theodoros Vlemmides, although a merchant, belonged to a prominent family of intellectuals and had many connections within the intellectual circles of the Capital. My first concern was to get to know the City—to walk its streets, to admire its magnificent monuments, to delight in it, to take it all in until my heart was full. I was eighteen years old, with the courage and curiosity of youth—and legs of iron. For days on end, I walked from morning till night, wandering through the vast City. I wanted to know every part of it, to touch it, to feel it. Vlemmides had a son my age, Manuel, who helped me by giving me advice on what to see and what to pay attention to. I would wake up at dawn, alongside my father and brother who left for their work, and I would set out, walking the City all day long to explore it. I began with the *Neon Palation* of the Vlachernae, which was nearby. Of course, I could only admire the majestic building from a distance—its vaulted arcades, battlements, and large windows left a deep impression on me. Through those windows, I hoped I might catch a glimpse of the Empress herself—the famed Maria of Antioch and Poitiers—whom Lord Manuel had married a few years earlier in his second marriage. They said she was the most beautiful woman in the world. She was twenty-three at the time. Of course, I did not see her, though I lingered near the palace gate for quite some time, until a guard eventually sent me away. Just a little farther from our house stood the most beautiful church in the city—after Hagia Sophia, of course. The Monastery of Chora, or of the Karyai, left one utterly speechless with its magnificent mosaics. I don't even know how long I stood there gazing at them. Then I followed the Mese—the Middle Road—to-

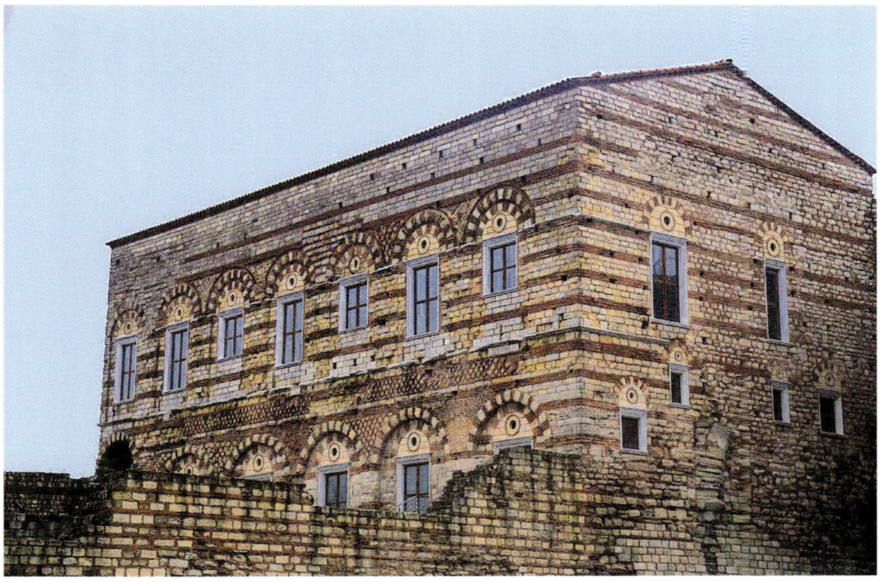

The Palace of Vlachernae.

Restoration, 2015.

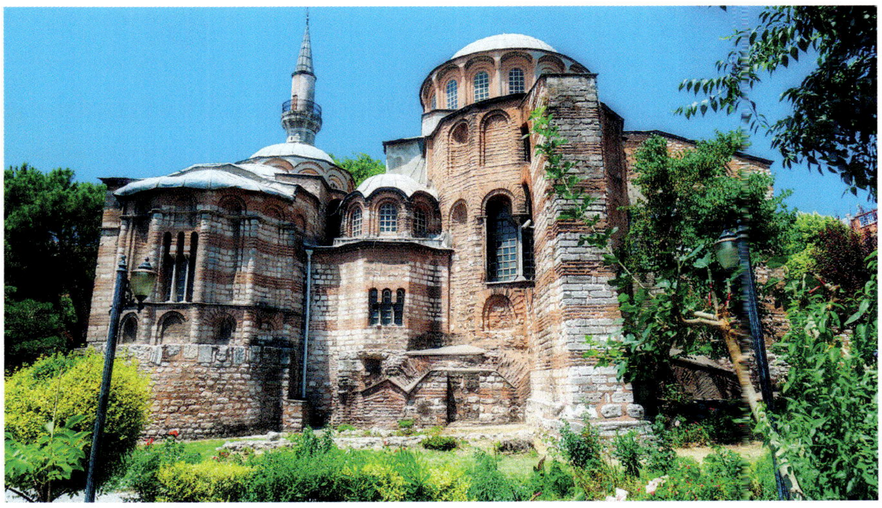

The Monastery of Chora.

Photo: Darwinek, 2009.

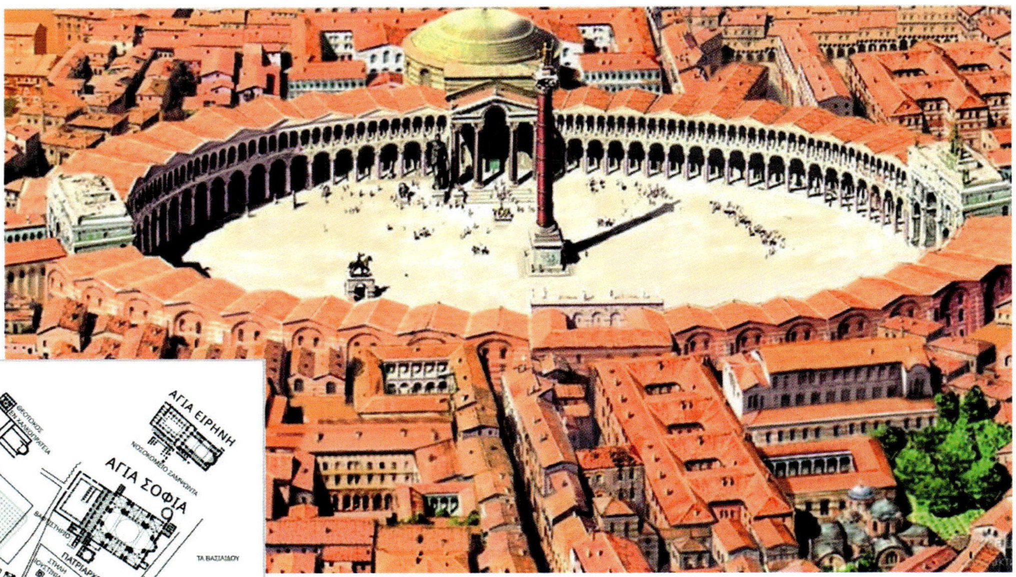

Column of Constantine the Great.

Reconstruction by Antoine Helbert, 1870.

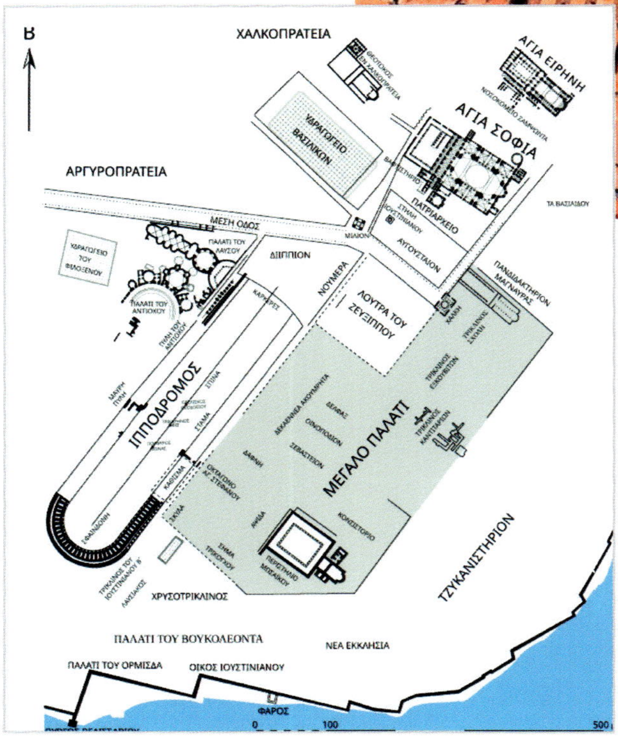

The Center of Byzantine Constantinople.
The Chalke Gate District (Chalkoprateia).

ward the city center. Every part of it pulsed with life. People coming and going, merchants calling out their goods, groups of friends chatting in the street. Every so often, I would step off into the side alleys, where I encountered the humble homes of the working classes. One thing that truly impressed me was the great care given to the water supply of the City. It is filled with cisterns—covered water reservoirs—I counted at least seven myself. I later learned that there were around 100 large public cisterns and many smaller private ones, which together stored nearly a million tons of water within the city. The water was channeled through underground pipes to fountains scattered throughout various parts of the city. The magnificent, towering aqueduct of Valens, which carries water from the forests of Thrace to supply the city's cisterns, dominates the skyline and imparts a sense of grandeur and security. Along the *Mese Odos*, the city's grand avenue, lie the largest plazas, known to the locals as phoroi, a name derived from the Latin *forum*, meaning marketplace or public square. Indeed, these were the places where the finest shops could be found. I strolled and marveled at the Forum of Arcadius, the Forum of the Ox, the Forum of Theodosius, and finally arrived at the awe-inspiring, vast, circular plaza—the Forum of Constantine the Great. The *Mese Odos* meets the great plaza on both its eastern and western sides through two magnificent arched gates. A circular colonnaded portico encloses the entire square, and on its northern side stands the imposing Senate House—the *Megalē Synklētos*. At the center of the plaza once stood a marble column crowned by a statue of Constantine the Great, the city's illustrious founder. Alas, just eighteen years ago, in 1150, a violent storm brought the statue crashing down, shattering it to pieces. In its place, Emperor *Kyr-Manouēl* erected a grand cross.

After passing the Forum of Constantine and heading eastward, I reached the heart of the city, where the Hippodrome lies, the legendary Church of Hagia Sophia, and the Sacred Palace—the traditional seat of the emperors.

I admired Hagia Sophia from the outside—we would visit it later during the Divine Liturgy. I simply had not imagined it to be so immense. On its southern side lies the vast square of the Augusteion, where the great market of the city is held. From there begins the Mese Odos, and one finds a column, the Milion—or Stadiometron—where the distances from the Capital to the major cities of the Empire are inscribed. Next to it stand the Baths of Zeuxippus, the Palace of Daphne, endless arcades, the Oinopodion, and many other smaller palaces and halls, gardens and terraces, which together form the complex of the Sacred Palace—not a single building, but a collection of splendid structures, colonnades, and magnificent gardens. Everywhere one sees ancient statues and decorative columns. Further down lie other palaces as well—the Boukoleon Palace, the Palace of Antiochos, and other grand edifices beyond what my mind could fully grasp.

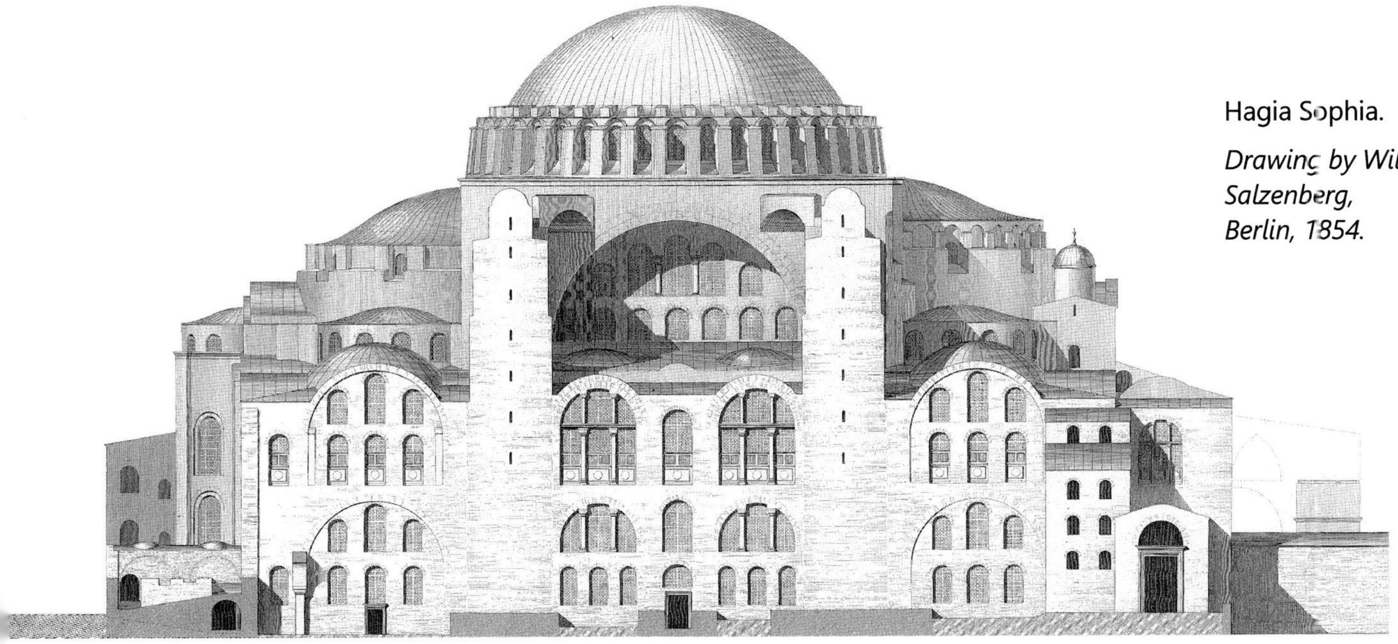

Hagia Sophia.

Drawing by Wilhelm Salzenberg, Berlin, 1854.

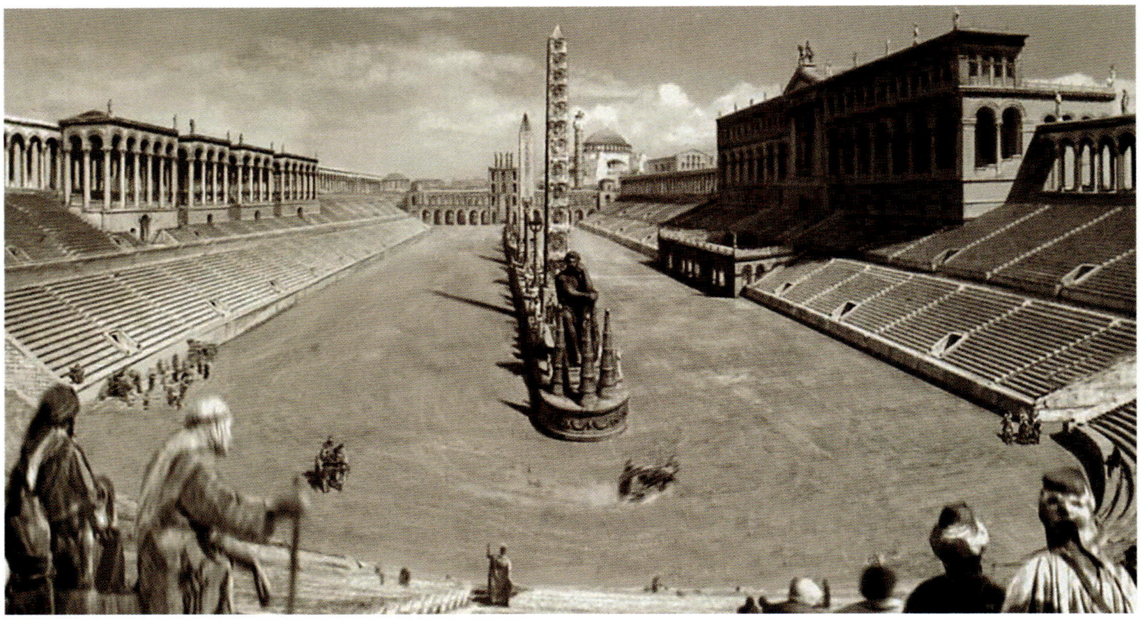

The Hippodrome of Constantinople. *Reconstruction by Antoine Helbert, 1870.*

Next to the Palace lies the vast Hippodrome, which fortunately was open and I was able to enter. Passing through a large courtyard, one first encounters the stables, now empty. Opposite them stands a tower crowned by four magnificent bronze horses—works of the ancient sculptor Lysippus—that looked almost alive. Through the tower's gate, one enters the interior of the Hippodrome. The arena is about 450 meters long and 80 meters wide, divided in the middle by a platform. Surrounding it are forty rows of marble tiers for the spectators. The space is adorned with numerous votive offerings and statues; the most striking are the Obelisk of Theodosius, brought from Egypt, and the Serpent Column, brought from Delphi, whose top once held the tripod of the Pythia. I didn't linger long in the Hippodrome, despite the grandeur and awe it inspired in me as I imagined it packed with crowds and the chariots racing through the elliptical track. I was eager to reach the place of my dreams—the temple of learning.

Indeed, toward the eastern end of the Sacred Palace complex stood the Palace of Magnaura, which housed the *Pandidakterion*. I stood in silence before that magnificent edifice. For hours I marveled at its grand domes, its elegant columns, the statues of ancient philosophers adorning the entrance, and the great mosaic of Christ above the lintel. The *Pandidakterion* was closed—it was still summer. Classes would begin in October, one month after the start of the Indiction. I hoped that by then I would have managed to arrange my registration and see it from the inside as well. On the northern side of the Sacred Palace complex stood the Palace of the Mangana, which housed the famous Imperial hospice of the same name—that is, the hospital where medical studies were conducted.

To complete my impressions of Constantinople, I must recount the experience of the Divine Liturgy we attended at Hagia Sophia—that architectural marvel achieved by the engineers of the 6th century, perfected by the artisans of ornamentation with their elegant designs and peerless mosaics. We had been told that the church's construction was such that light itself creates unbelievable impressions. A few days later, our whole family went together, before dawn, to give thanks to God.

Inside, the vast church was gently illuminated by the light of chandeliers and candles. Matins had already begun. The choirs of chanters sang the troparia in harmony, creating an atmosphere of profound reverence. I marveled at the immense dome, the spherical triangles at its base, the ornate columns, the mosaics adorning the entire church, softly glowing in the half-light.

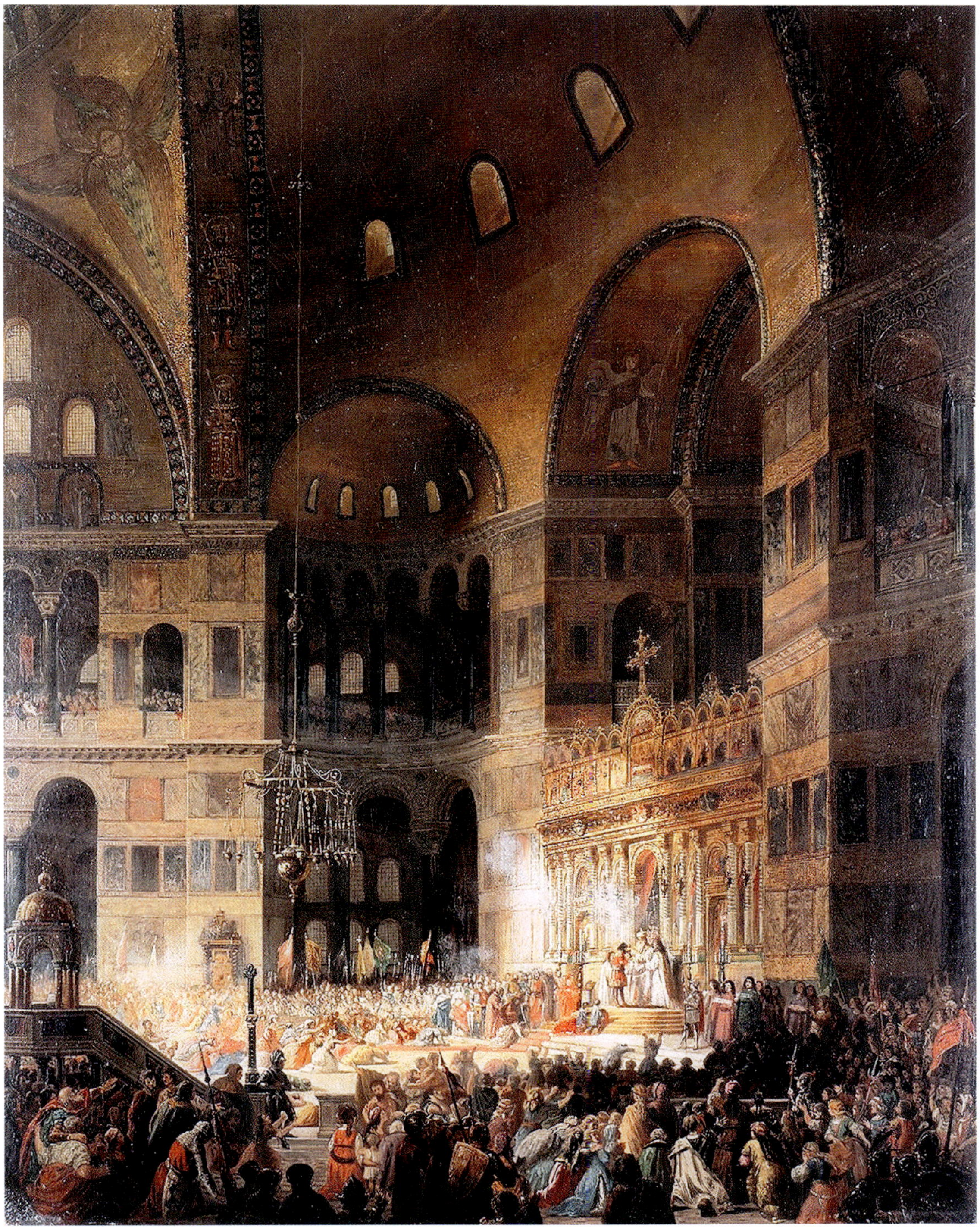

Hagia Sophia.

Painting by Gaspare Fossati, 1849. Swiss National Museum, Zurich.

Slowly, dawn broke. The Psalms of Praise (*Aínoi*) had begun, the voices of the chanters swelled, and the rhythm quickened. The sun rose brilliantly into the clear summer sky. I do not know how they achieved such perfect synchronization. The Doxology followed, and the voices of the chanters became thunderous while the bells rang out joyfully, their peals echoing with celebration. Church attendants, using long rods, began to swing the great chandeliers so that even the inanimate danced in glorification of the Creator. And then something unexpected happened. Through the many windows of the sanctuary, the triumphant light of the newly risen sun poured in. The walls and colonnades were suddenly illuminated. The golden mosaics came to life, gleaming as they reflected the light. The faces of the saints on the walls, as well as those of the worshippers, were bathed in radiance—everyone gazing heavenward in awe, as if witnessing a miracle. The slanting rays of the sun, entering through the countless windows at the base of the dome, created a dazzling plane of brilliance and light. The dome itself appeared to detach from its base and hover, weightless, above the light. The bells rang out joyfully, and the people turned this way and that to take in the transcendent sight. The entire congregation chanted with emotion: "Glory to Thee, who hast shown us the light." It was then that I understood why the barbarian Rus', who had come about two hundred years earlier as envoys of their prince Vladimir to determine which faith their people should follow, upon witnessing the Divine Liturgy in Hagia Sophia, said: "We knew not whether we were on earth or in heaven." The service ended without our even realizing it. We returned home utterly enchanted—proud that our nation had created such masterpieces, and grateful to God that we had been deemed worthy to live in this city.

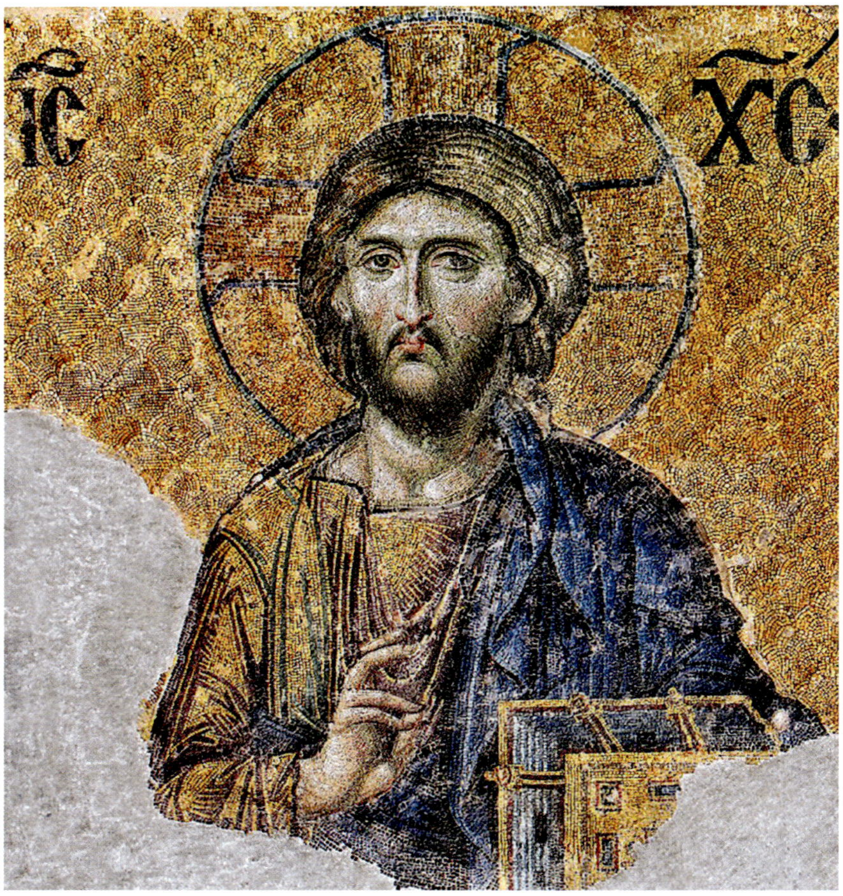

Christ Pantocrator.
Mosaic, 10th–11th century, Hagia Sophia.

My father's business partner, Theodoros Vlemmides, was a respectable and honorable man. He had a fine family—three sons and a daughter named Antigone. His two eldest sons followed in their father's footsteps, and together with our parents and my own brother Ioannis, they formed a fine trading team, working creatively, with mutual understanding and trust. Their house was near ours, and we met often. I became close friends with the youngest of the Vlemmides children, Manuel, who was almost a year younger than I. Like me, he had no interest in commerce and longed to pursue his studies. His interests, however, leaned more toward philosophy and theology, and he had not ruled out the possibility of becoming a clergyman. He was deeply cultivated, with a profound education, and despite being a native of the capital while I was a naïve provincial newcomer, he treated me with great courtesy and sincerity. We had endless conversations—about philosophy, literature, medicine, and the aims and values of life—as we wandered through the streets and squares of the city. Manuel showed me all the notable places and introduced me to his circle of friends, other young men who were also preparing to study at the *Pandidakterion*. Deep within, I felt grateful to my teacher, Euthymios Tornikes, for the education he had given me, for I realized I was in no way inferior to them—neither in knowledge nor in the refined use of the Greek language. Not for a moment did I feel at a disadvantage, and I must emphasize that the society of Constantinople, and of the Roman Empire more broadly, was very tolerant at that time, as it had long been. There was no prejudice based on origin, background, or ethnicity. Nobility was not determined by bloodline but by merit. Even the humblest villager from the remotest province could rise to high office—even become emperor—provided he was capable. The only essential requirements were adherence to the Orthodox Christian faith and knowledge of the Greek language. Most emperors of the past were of humble origin. There was no aristocracy of blood in the Roman Empire. Of course, social classes existed, as did differences in wealth, influence, and education—but these were not predetermined by birth. Everyone had the chance to strive and shape their own destiny. The aristocracy of blood—the *noblesse,* as the Franks called it—was a novel fruit, a recent import from the West. There, a feudal system had developed from the very beginning, when the Germanic tribes who conquered the Western Roman Empire shattered it into various "kingdoms." These invaders established a system of governance centered on semi-independent local lords, who divided the land

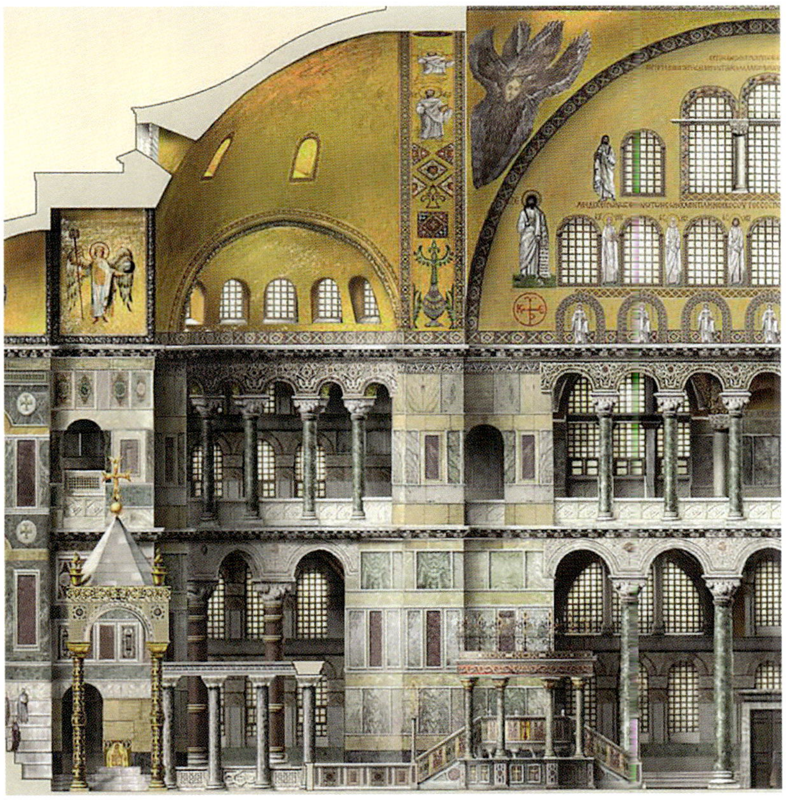

Cross-section of Hagia Sophia.
Reconstruction by Antoine Helbert, 1870.

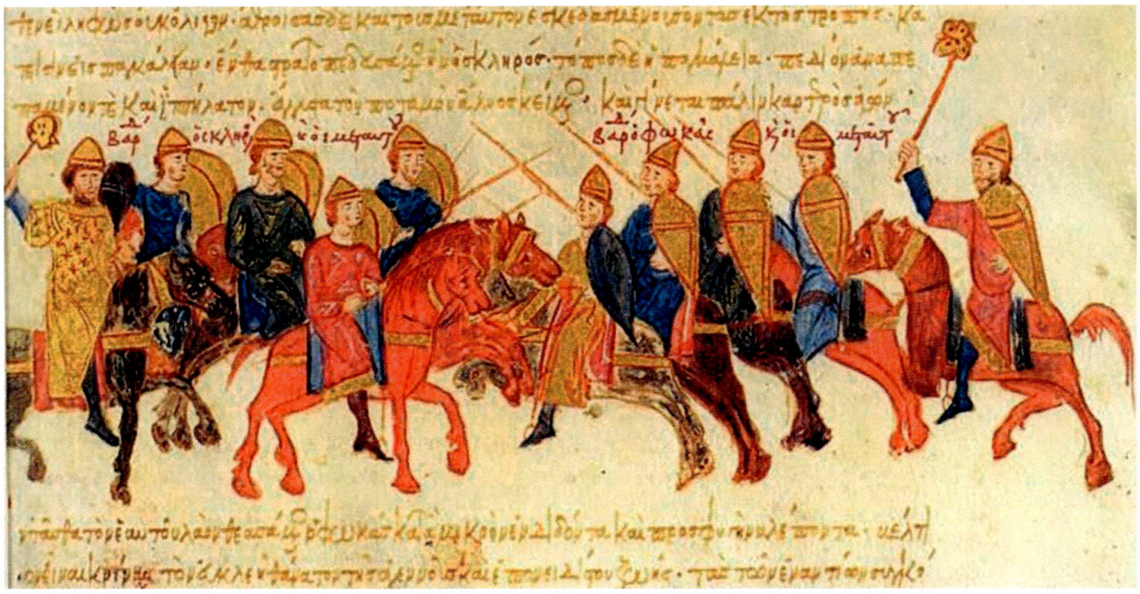

Clash between the aristocratic families of the "Dynatoi": the Skleroi and the Phokades.

Miniature from the Skylitzes Chronicle, 12th century, National Library of Spain, Madrid.

among themselves and remained vassals to their king. The common folk held the role of serfs, and those who were not "noble"—that is, people of humble origin—had no opportunity for social advancement. Everyone was born into their fate. Over the past hundred years, however, even in our own society, the so-called *Dynatoi* (the strong) had appeared, and certain landowning families had gained an almost exclusive claim to the imperial throne. Families such as the Phokas, the Skleroi, the Komnenoi, the Kantakouzenoi, the Laskaris, the Doukai… Yet this was something that prevailed as a custom, not as an institutional principle.

Antigone, Manuel's sister, was a gentle and kind young woman who quickly formed a friendship with my sister, Iphigenia. I was struck by her gracious upbringing, her breadth of knowledge—despite having received only a basic education—and, above all, by her keen interest in learning and in contributing to society. She admired and respected my decision to become a physician and confided in me that she, too, deeply wished to become a doctor. Yet, this was nearly unthinkable for her family. Her father was pleased to see his sons—especially Manuel—take an interest in letters and the sciences. Yet his social and financial standing was not high enough to afford higher education for his daughter as well. Antigone understood this and held no resentment toward her father. The only way for her to pursue serious studies would have been to enter a convent known for its support of learning and the arts. But she felt no such calling. Together with my sister, they never missed the chance to read whatever books came into their hands—whether mine or Manuel's—and they also offered their volunteer services at the nearby Xenon of the Pantocrator, considered the model hospital of the Empire, where I later had the joy and honor of serving myself.

The commercial partnership of Vlemmides–Messenes was doing fairly well, thanks to my father's connections with the markets of Italy and Vlemmides' ties with those of the northern Balkans and the Rus' of Kiev. However, the silk and purple dye trade was in crisis due to the extensive customs privileges granted to the Italian maritime cities, which resulted in unfair competition. These economic pressures, coupled with the Crusades, eventually stirred up deep resentment between the Romans and the Latins and led to very unpleasant events—ones I would come to experience firsthand later on.

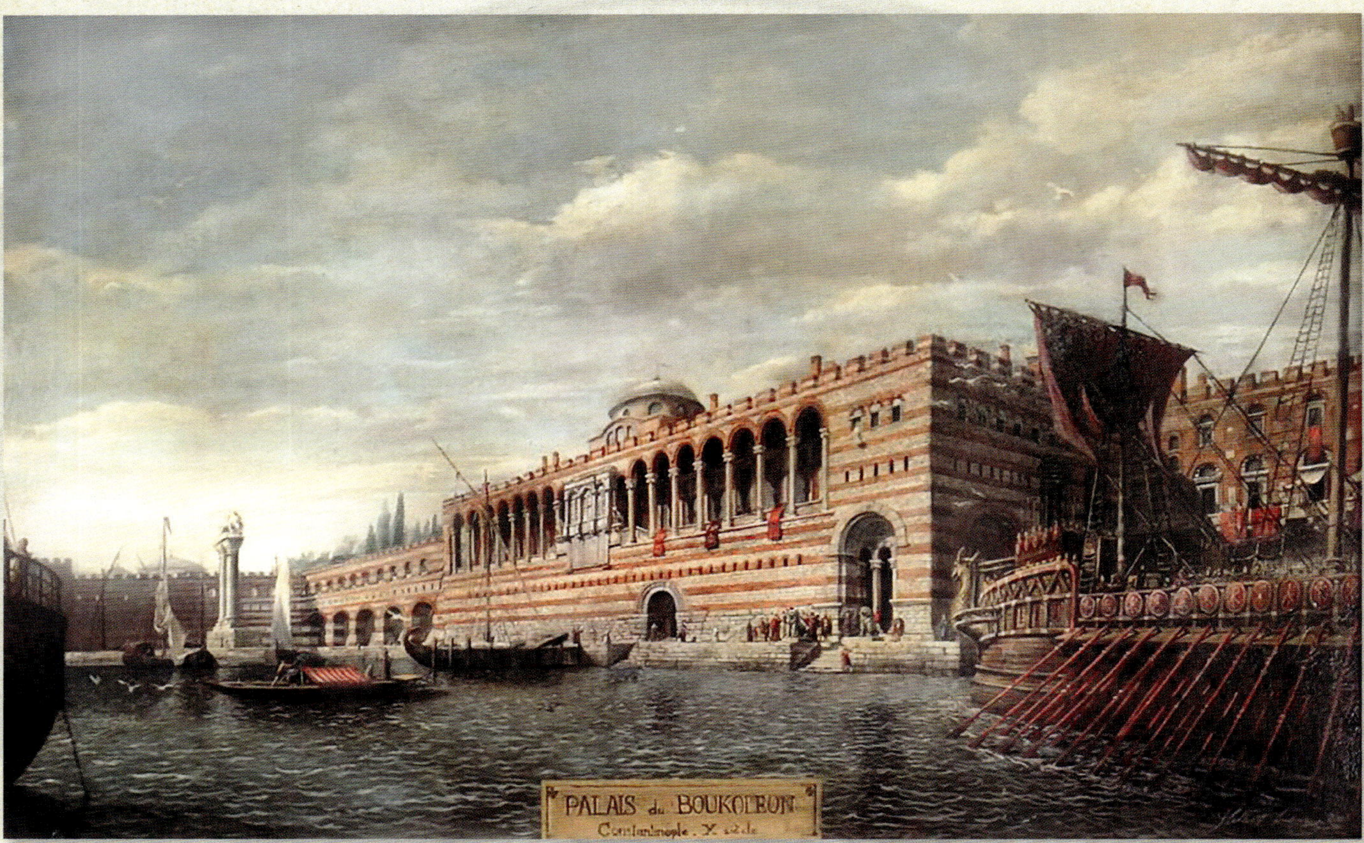

The Palace of Boukoleon.

Reconstruction by Antoine Helbert, 1870.

Medical Studies and Hospitals

After the first dazzling impressions of Constantinople, I began to explore the educational system and the operations of the various Schools. At the School of Magnaura, courses were offered in Philosophy, Rhetoric, Mathematics, Geometry, Music, Astronomy, and Law. In the teaching of Medicine, the writings of great physicians—from antiquity up to our own time—were used. After completing their basic studies at Magnaura, future physicians underwent practical training in the Xenones, that is, the hospitals, of which there were quite a few in Constantinople. There, students would observe the physicians at work, care for the sick themselves, receive instruction from specialized teachers, and study in the rich medical library that each xenon possessed.

In our time, the most prominent and renowned *Xenones* (Hospitals) were the Imperial Xenon of the Mangana, the Xenon of the Pantocrator, that of Myrelaion, the Xenon of Sampson—which was also the oldest—that of Narses, of Euboulos, and of Saint Irene. There were also many others, less well-known. The first three were the most sought after by students, as they offered the highest quality education. The Xenon of the Mangana was founded in 1050 by Constantine IX Monomachos, who, although he was a clumsy—even poor—ruler in political and military affairs, proved to be a great patron of letters and the arts. He upgraded and strengthened the School of the Magnaura and established, in the nearby palace of the Mangana—where the Monastery of Saint George was located—the Imperial *Xenon* (Hospital). The chief physician who directed the *Xenon* held the title of *Aktouarios* (Actuarius) and was also the

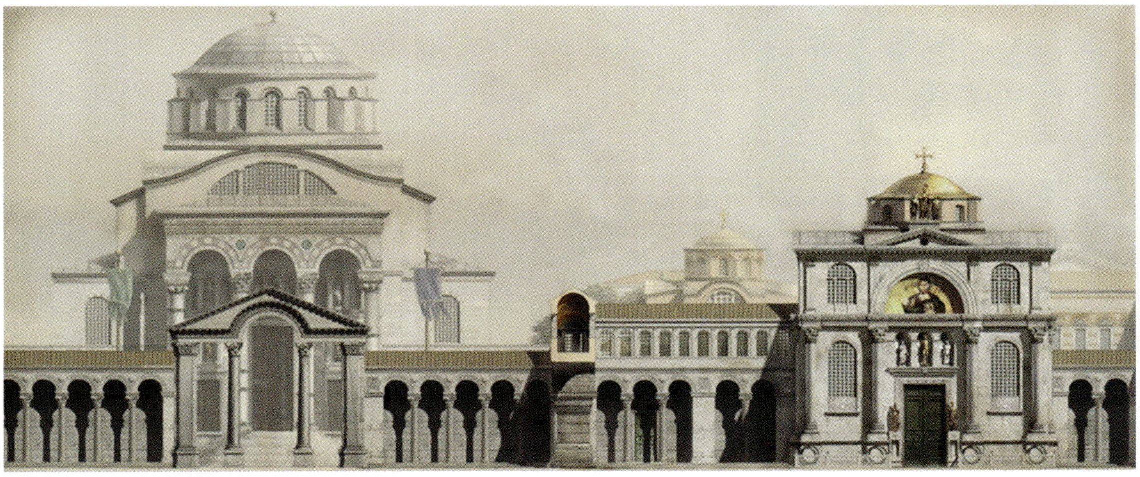

The Palace of Magnaura and the Chalke Gate.

Reconstruction by Antoine Helbert, 1870.

personal doctor of the Emperor. The quality of care was such that Emperor Constantine himself was hospitalized there at the end of his life. Moreover, seventy years later, when Alexios Komnenos fell gravely ill, the *Aktouarios* Ioannes transferred him to the *Xenon* for more complete and improved treatment. This was unthinkable for the corresponding medical institutions in Western Europe, which were merely shelters for the poor and in no way would aristocrats condescend—or risk—to be hospitalized there. The second *Xenon*, that of Myrelaion, had been founded earlier, in the 10th century by Romanos I, within the complex of a palace located above the Port of Theodosius—precisely where we had disembarked upon arriving in Constantinople. This too was an Imperial *Xenon*, and the chief physician who administered it held the title of *Megas Kourator* (Grand Curator).

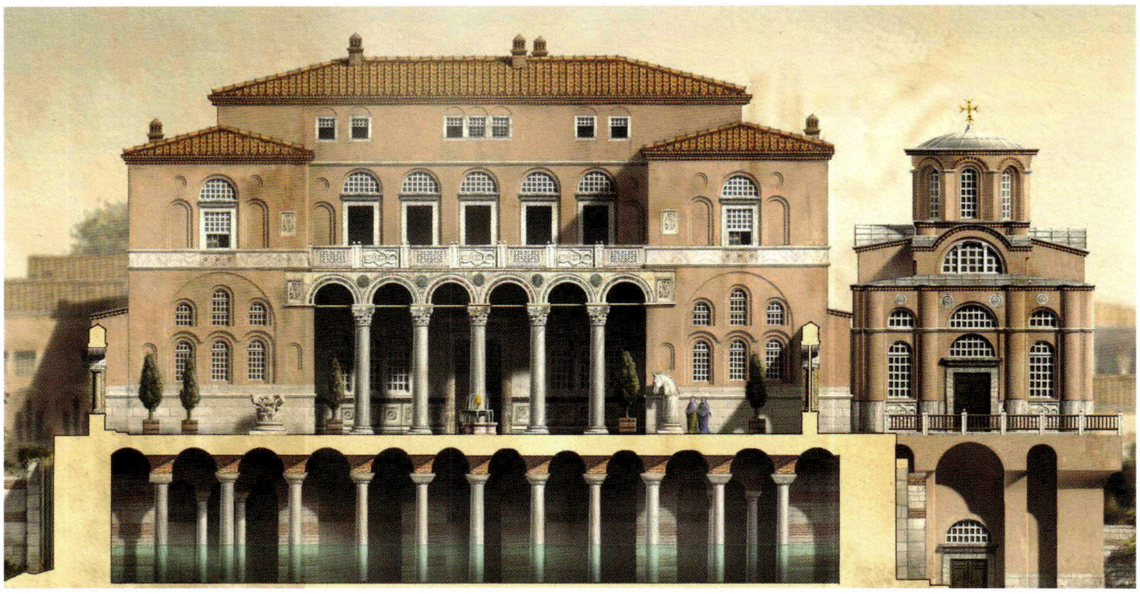

The Monastery and the Xenon of Myrelaion.
Reconstruction by Antoine Helbert, 1870.

Finally, the *Xenon* of the Pantocrator, the most renowned of all, was the creation of John II Komnenos just thirty years ago, in the northern part of the City, near the Golden Horn and the district of Vlachernae. Each Xenon had its own *typikon*, that is, its own organizational charter, though many of these *typika* were quite similar. The most detailed and comprehensive among them was that of the Pantocrator. This is only natural, since its compiler had at his disposal all the earlier *typika* to consult and build upon. I completed the practical part of my studies at the Xenon of the Mangana, but afterward I had the great fortune to work as a physician at the Xenon of the Pantocrator as well. I came to know its operations intimately, and I will have the opportunity to describe them. To preempt any misunderstanding, let me say that although the *xenones* were, for the most part, Imperial institutions and occasionally treated people of high rank, they were primarily intended for and served the common people. Medical care was provided free of charge, and all who were in need were admitted.

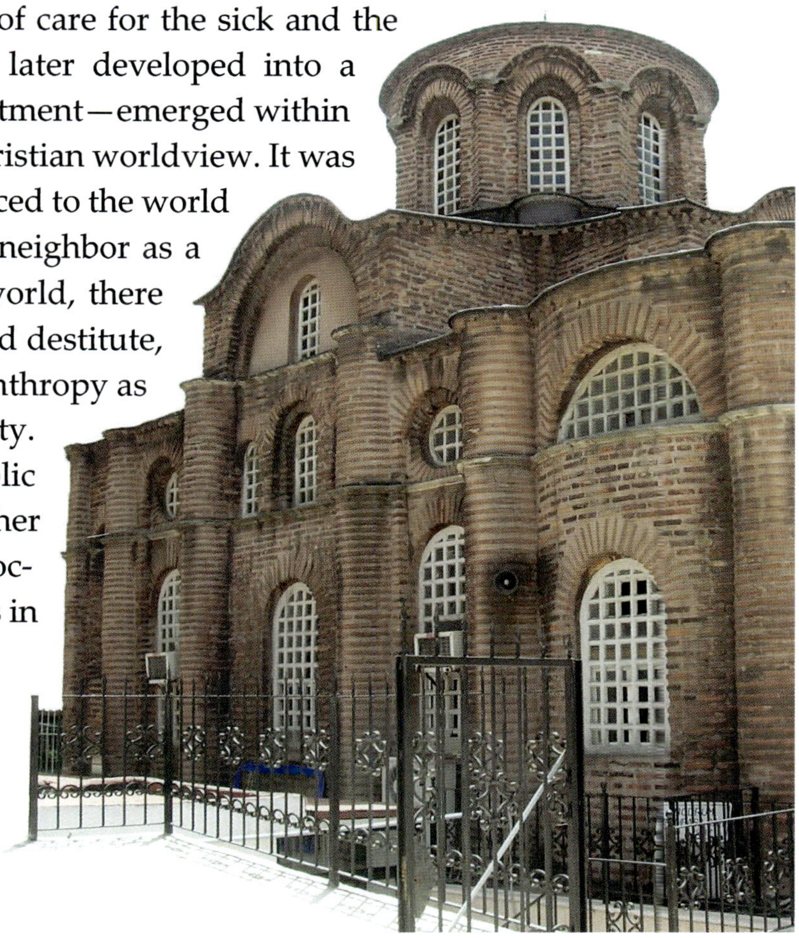

The concept of the *xenon* as a place of care for the sick and the homeless—initially rudimentary but later developed into a system of comprehensive medical treatment—emerged within our Roman Empire as a fruit of the Christian worldview. It was the Christian Church that first introduced to the world the notion of love and care for one's neighbor as a duty and obligation. In the ancient world, there was no social provision for the sick and destitute, nor was there any conception of philanthropy as a personal or communal responsibility. In Ancient Greece, there were no public hospitals. Medicine was practiced either by private physicians or by public doctors who would visit and treat patients in their homes. Of course, there were the Asclepieia, but these were primarily religious healing sanctuaries intended mainly for well-off citizens. In the Hellenistic period, they even evolved into true resorts for the wealthy, featuring baths, libraries, and entertainment halls.

In ancient Rome, the only healthcare institutions that existed were a type of infirmary for wounded individuals, primarily soldiers or slaves, known as *Valetudinaria*. However, neither the Asclepieia of Greece nor the Valetudinaria of Rome were true hospitals in the modern sense. They lacked the organized and comprehensive medical care that later developed in the *Xenones* (Hospitals) of the Byzantine Empire.

Monastery of Myrelaion.

Photo: Darwinek, 2009.

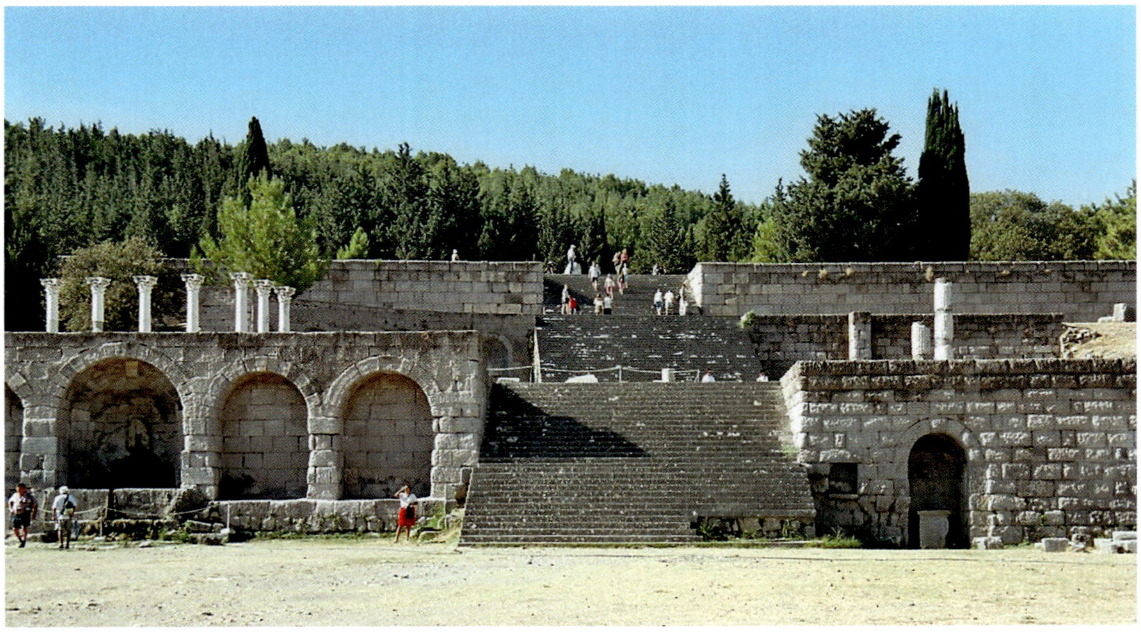

The Asclepieion of Kos.

Later, while I was studying at the *Pandidakterion*, our teachers described to us how social welfare developed in the Roman Empire and how various philanthropic institutions gradually evolved into well-equipped hospitals, known as *xenones*. This history was deeply fascinating, and I would recount it with great enthusiasm to the two young women of our extended family—my sister Iphigenia and Antigone. In the afternoons, when I returned home, they would await me with eager anticipation. The unfulfilled desire of both young wom-

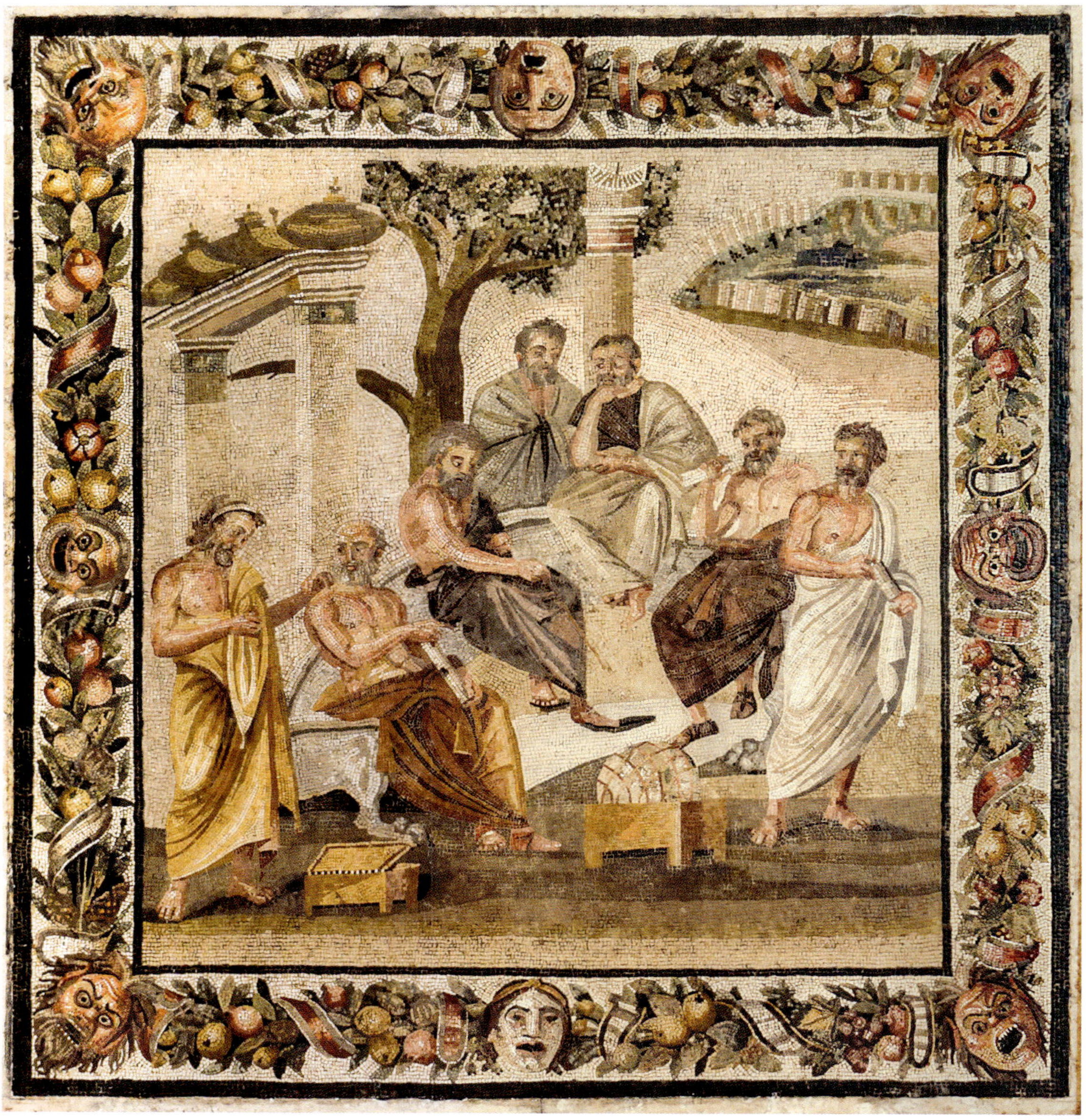

The Academy of Plato.

Mosaic from Pompeii, 1st century B.C. Archaeological Museum, Naples.

en to pursue studies found a partial expression in the "interrogations" they conducted when I returned home, asking about everything I had learned. I recounted it all with pleasure—and, I must admit, with a touch of pride—as best I could. Deep down, I was flattered by their admiration, especially that of Antigone, which stirred within me the first flutterings of love. And so, I would tell them:

When, in the 3rd century, Emperor Caracalla's decree granted Roman citizenship to all inhabitants of the Roman *oikoumene*, a striking social phenomenon occurred: the large-scale internal migration of rural populations. In the great cities, which until then had enjoyed a system of partial self-governance and prosperity, the distinction between native citizens and foreign settlers ceased to exist. The poor rural populations thus began migrating freely to the large cities in search of a better life. This phenomenon was observed primarily in the eastern part of the empire, where great cities such as Alexandria, Antioch, Edessa, Pergamon, and of course Constantinople, were located. In the western part, there was no major city other than Rome. Thus, in the Greek-speaking East, there was a notable increase in population, a mass migration into the cities, and consequently a large rise in the number of unemployed and impoverished people—something that did not occur in the Latin-speaking West. This gave rise to urgent social needs in the East. While Christianity was still persecuted, bishops practiced charity in secret, usually in their own homes or in the homes of well-to-do believers.

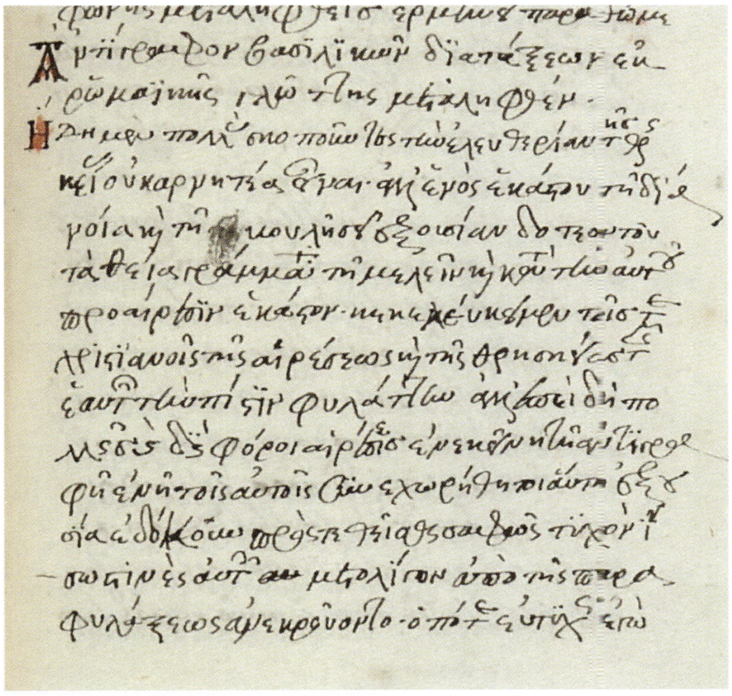

The Edict of Milan.

Manuscript, 16th century. Ecclesiastical History by Eusebius of Caesarea. British Library, London.

When, through the Edict of Emperor Constantine the Great in 313, Christianity was recognized as a free and equal religion, the Church took care to establish institutions where the poor, the elderly, the sick, and others in need could be cared for. This initiative began very early, with corresponding decisions of the First Ecumenical Council, and initially concerned only Christian communities, since it was an initiative of the Church, which at that time still operated independently from the state. It is characteristic that just a few years later, Julian the Apostate—the tragic and unrealistic visionary Emperor who attempted to revive the ancient religion and its former glory—wrote to his friend Oribasius, the most renowned physician of the time: "We must organize ourselves and care for the weak just as the Christians do"... Sadly, he did not live long enough to implement it.

When Christianity was established as the official state religion in 380 by Emperor Theodosius I, the Church's earlier philanthropic initiative was embraced and supported both by the Emperors and by many wealthy individuals. The political attitude toward vulnerable groups changed radically. A wealthy person who, for various reasons, wished to make a donation to a city no longer built fountains or monuments, as was customary in antiquity, but instead

> *The personal physician and friend of Emperor Julian, Oribasius, was sent to the Oracle of Delphi to inquire about the emperor's reforming mission. The oracle's response was as follows*
>
> Tell the king, the splendid hall fell to the ground.
> Phoebus no longer has his house, nor the prophesying laurel,
> nor the speaking well. The speaking water has dried out.
> — *Passio Artemii* 96.1284.45–7, *Cedrenus* 1.532.8–10)

constructed or supported charitable institutions. Social care came to include not only the sick and the poor, but also widows, orphans, people with special needs, and others in vulnerable situations. The first such charitable institutions appeared in Antioch and were called *katagogia* or *xenodocheia* (hostels or shelters). They did not offer medical care but served primarily as asylums providing basic shelter and food to those in need. Depending on the groups of people they served, they were named accordingly: *gerokomeia* (homes for the elderly), *orphanotropheia* (orphanages), *ptochokomeia* (poorhouses), *vrefokomeia* (infant care homes), *leprokomeia* (leprosaria), etc.—words that appeared for the first time in the Greek language. The great innovation, however, was that now these institutions offered care to everyone, without any distinction of gender, race, or ethnicity—unlike antiquity, where only specific groups were cared for. Another remarkable innovation was that women actively and equally participated in the operation of these charitable institutions. Alongside the social foundations, the monasteries also contributed significantly to philanthropic work. Every monastery could offer shelter to the sick and to travelers, at least for a period of time.

Iphigenia and Antigone, who—as I have already written—had a deep desire to study medicine and serve their fellow human beings, naturally knew nothing of the history of medicine and nursing in the Empire. They listened to me with wonder as I recounted the precious knowledge I had received from Tornikes in Patras, as well as what I was now learning at the Magnaura.

Oribasius, "Prologue to Julian".

Moscow, 1808.

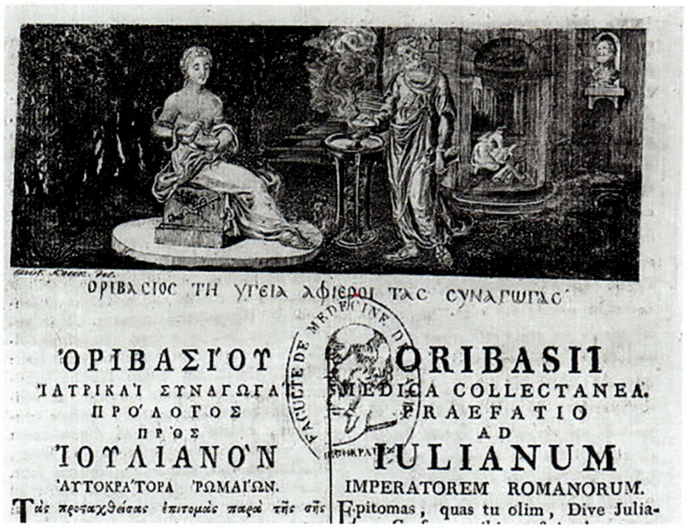

"And when did the first real hospitals appear?" Antigone would ask me, hanging on my every word. Her interest gave me a deep sense of satisfaction. Trying not to show my excitement and to appear composed, I would say to them:

"The first healthcare institution that had professional physicians and official medical care," I would begin, "was founded by St. Basil the Great in 370 AD. He himself called it *Katagogion*, a place of shelter. But after his death, in his honor, it became known as the *Basileias*—and by that name it passed into history. Basil himself was a physician, educated at the School of Athens, yet in his institution, he also employed other doctors, nurses, and support staff." The *Katagogion*, in addition to its wards for the sick, also included facilities for the care of the elderly, the disabled, travelers, lepers, and others in need. It was a veritable city in itself, where one could even learn a manual trade—thus *serving also as a center for social rehabilitation*. The *Basileiad* was a titanic, groundbreaking endeavor, truly worthy of a man called Great. A few years later, John Chrysostom founded the first medical care institutions in the Queen of Cities (Constantinople), which he called *Nosokomeia* (Hospitals). These were the earliest to resemble modern-day *xenones* (hospices or hospitals), staffed with physicians, paramedics, administrators, cooks, nurses, servants, and more. Their directors were clergy. In the centuries that followed, the *xenones* (or hospitals) became independent from the Church and came under the jurisdiction of the state. Nevertheless, the monastic *xenones* continued to operate, and the state hospitals were usually built within the grounds of a monastery, which significantly supported their functioning through the charitable and voluntary work of the monks."

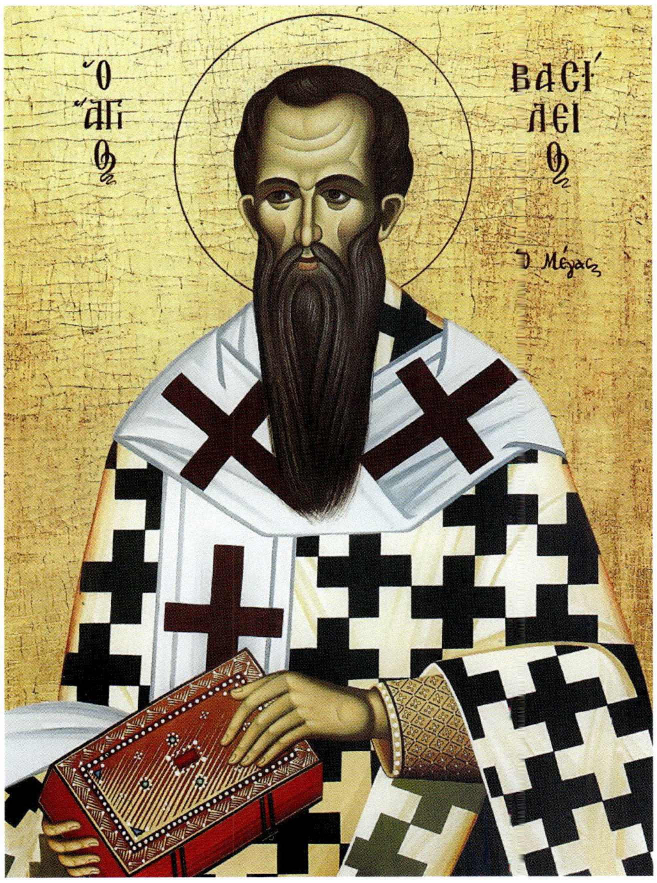

Saint Basil the Great.

Modern icon.

The story had sparked the girls' interest, and they were full of questions.

"When did doctors begin working exclusively in hospitals?" asked Iphigenia, equally enthusiastic about the account.

"Emperor Justinian, with his great political insight," I answered her, "made a historic shift in the 6th century. Until then, the best doctors, following the ancient model, were either private practitioners or public physicians employed by the cities, where they practiced medicine for high salaries paid by the city councils, known as the *Curiae*. Justinian, however, issued a mandate that transferred all public doctors to hospitals, where they were now required to provide their services exclusively. The funds that the state had previously allocated to the Curiae for doctors were now redirected straight to the hospitals, which were further protected by new laws and supported through tax exemptions. The results of this reform were striking. Both the medical capabilities and the prestige of the *xenones* (hospitals) grew significantly. Until then, hospitals primarily served the poor and destitute, with services offered free of charge, while wealthier individuals sought out renowned private physicians. Now, however, even members of the well-off middle classes began turning to the hospitals. From that time onward began a golden age for the *xenones,* which evolved to such a degree that in our own era, even members of the imperial court's aristocracy—as well as the Emperors themselves—when seriously ill, are admitted to these hospitals for treatment.

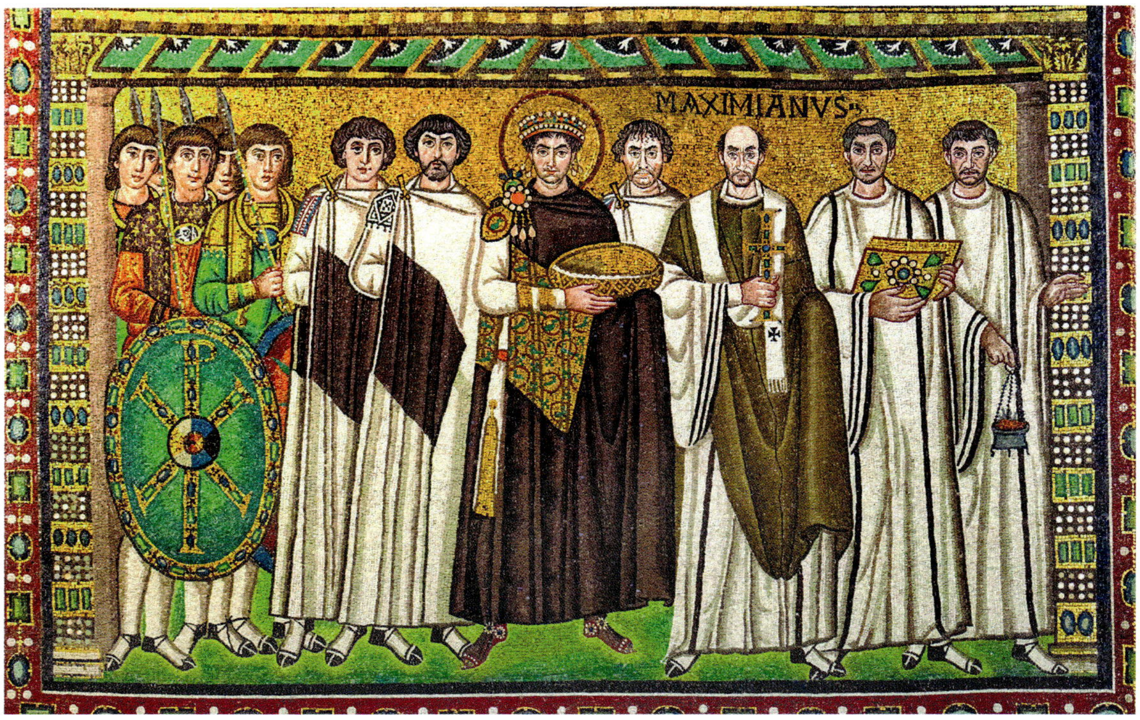

Justinian with his physician Aetios of Amida at his right.

Mosaic, 6th century, San Vitale, Ravenna.

My listeners showed no signs of fatigue. Enthusiastic and carried away by their eager eyes and attentive silence, I continued:

From the 5th century onward, more and more *xenones* (hospitals) were established in Constantinople as well as in many provincial cities. The oldest among them was the *Xenon of Sampson,* which was even burned down during the Nika Revolt. Its founder, the physician Sampson, had healed Emperor Justinian himself from a serious illness. As a result, the Emperor ordered the complete reconstruction of the hospice from the ground up. In the same century, the *xenones* of *Euboulos* and of *Marcian* were also built in Perama. The construction of *xenones* continued into the 6th century, with the establishment of those of *Kosmidion, Christodotus,* and the *general Narses*. In the 7th century, with the emergence of the Arabs, the Empire was shaken to its core following the destruction of our army at Hieromyax. Some *xenones* were forced to close, but in the 8th century, two more were added. Then, during the 9th and 10th centuries, under the Macedonian emperors, the second flourishing of the Empire began. All the older *xenones* were repaired and renovated, and new ones were founded: the *Xenon of Myrelaion* and the *Xenon of the Mangana,* within the complex of the *Pandidakterion*. Finally, in our own century, our Emperor Kyr John Komnenos, together with his wife Irene, built in the year 1136 the pride of Byzantine medicine—the most complete hospital that has functioned to this day—the *Xenon of the Monastery of the Pantocrator...*"

In the eyes of the two girls I could see admiration and excitement. I promised them that I would tell them more about the xenones and about the physicians—both ancient and contemporary.

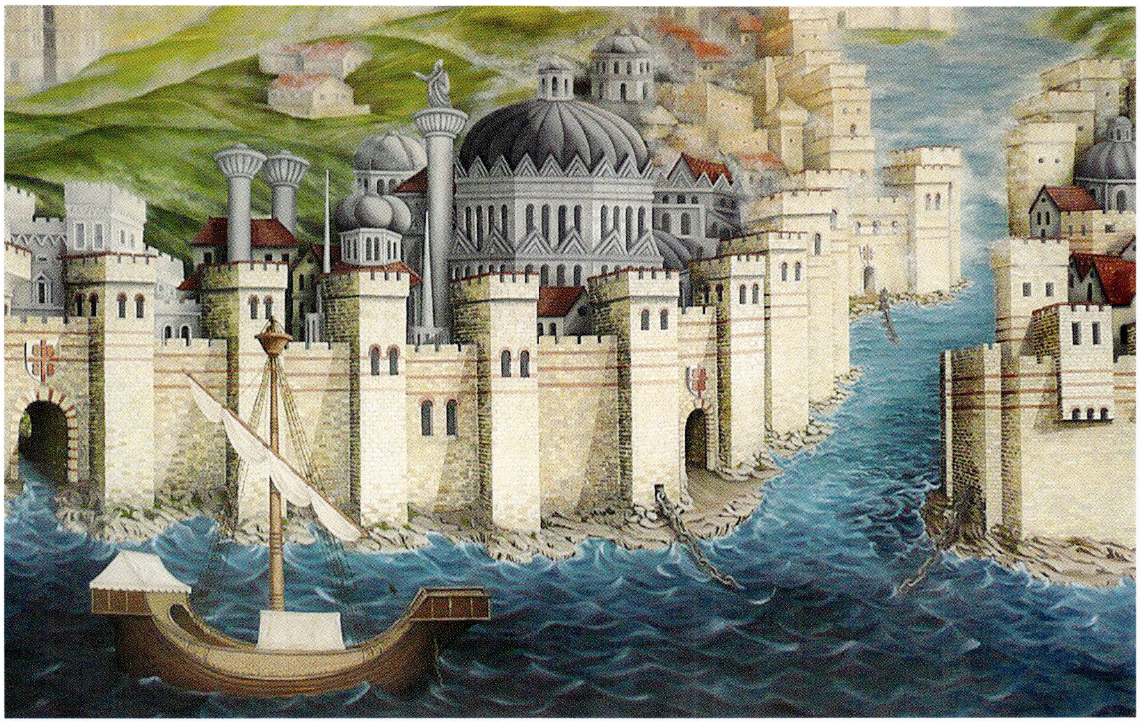

The sea walls of the City, 14th century.

Fresco, Archaeological Museum, Constantinople.

I was fortunate to meet Manuel Vlemmydes, for not only did he initiate me into the secrets of the capital, but he also opened new horizons through the world of art—and especially painting—which had flourished greatly, particularly in Constantinople, but also throughout the regions of Greece, especially Macedonia, the northern Balkans, Byzantine Italy and Sicily, and Asia Minor. My own education and interests, of course, leaned more toward the sciences—Medicine, Mathematics, Geometry, and Astronomy. I had already read nearly all the writings of the great Hippocrates. Manuel, on the other hand, was inclined toward the theoretical sciences and the arts. He was interested in Philosophy, Law, Theology, and Rhetoric. He had a talent for painting and practiced it as an amateur. Yet due to his deep interest, he possessed profound knowledge in the history of art—especially architecture, mosaic work, and painting. Thus, our conversations were endless and never lost their charm, as each of us enriched the other with insights born from the paths our interests had taken us.

I did not have significant experience with our Byzantine art, which had not particularly flourished in the Peloponnese. However, my father, who traveled

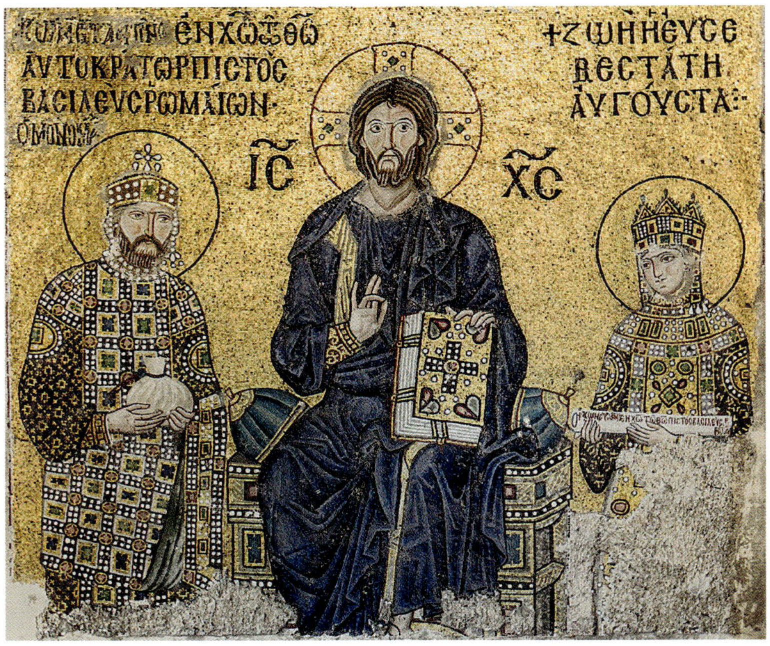

Empress Zoe.
Mosaic, 10th–11th century, Hagia Sophia.

to Italy and Sicily, had spoken to me and described the astonishing mosaics found there—in Ravenna and Palermo. Ravenna had been recaptured from the Ostrogoths by the forces of General Belisarius in 540 and remained the seat of Byzantine rule in Italy for two centuries, until it was conquered by the Lombards. There, the famous church of Saint Vitale was built—adorned with magnificent mosaics depicting Emperor Justinian, Empress Theodora, and their entourages. Other churches and baptisteries were also built, either by the Orthodox Romans or by the Arian Ostrogoths, all decorated with equally beautiful mosaics crafted by our own artisans.

In Palermo, more recently, when the Normans conquered Sicily, Roger built his palace and the "royal chapel" (Cappella Palatina), which was adorned by Greek artisans with mosaics of astonishing artistry. Likewise, the Church of Martorana in the city was built by Roger's Greek admiral, George of Antioch, around the same time, in 1142. The mosaics bear Greek inscriptions, and Roger himself is depicted being crowned king by Christ, with the Greek inscription «ΡΟΓΕΡΙΟC ΡΗΞ». Manuel knew all this from friends of his father and spoke to me with great enthusiasm about the art of mosaic as it had developed in the Empire.

"The mosaics," he told me, "first appeared very long ago, as early as the 8th century before the birth of the Savior, in Asia Minor and more broadly in the Eastern Mediterranean. They are made using a particular technique in which surfaces are covered with small tesserae—usually square—crafted from natural stones or colored glass. These tesserae are affixed onto a prepared substrate coated with a special mortar, forming intricate decorations or figurative compositions. Mosaics became beloved in Ancient Greece, especially during the Hellenistic period, and later, from the first century onward, in Ancient Rome, where they adorned the walls and floors of palaces and villas, even courtyards and sidewalks. After the fall of the Western Roman Empire to the barbarians, the mosaic art flourished greatly in our Eastern Empire, which preserved the civilization of antiquity. Mosaics nowadays are made chiefly in churches, and the scenes they depict are religious in nature. The Byzantine craftsmen are renowned across the world and adorn not only the churches of Constantinople and the wider Romanía, but also temples commissioned by other Christian rulers. They have worked in *Akyïsgranon*—that is, Aachen, as

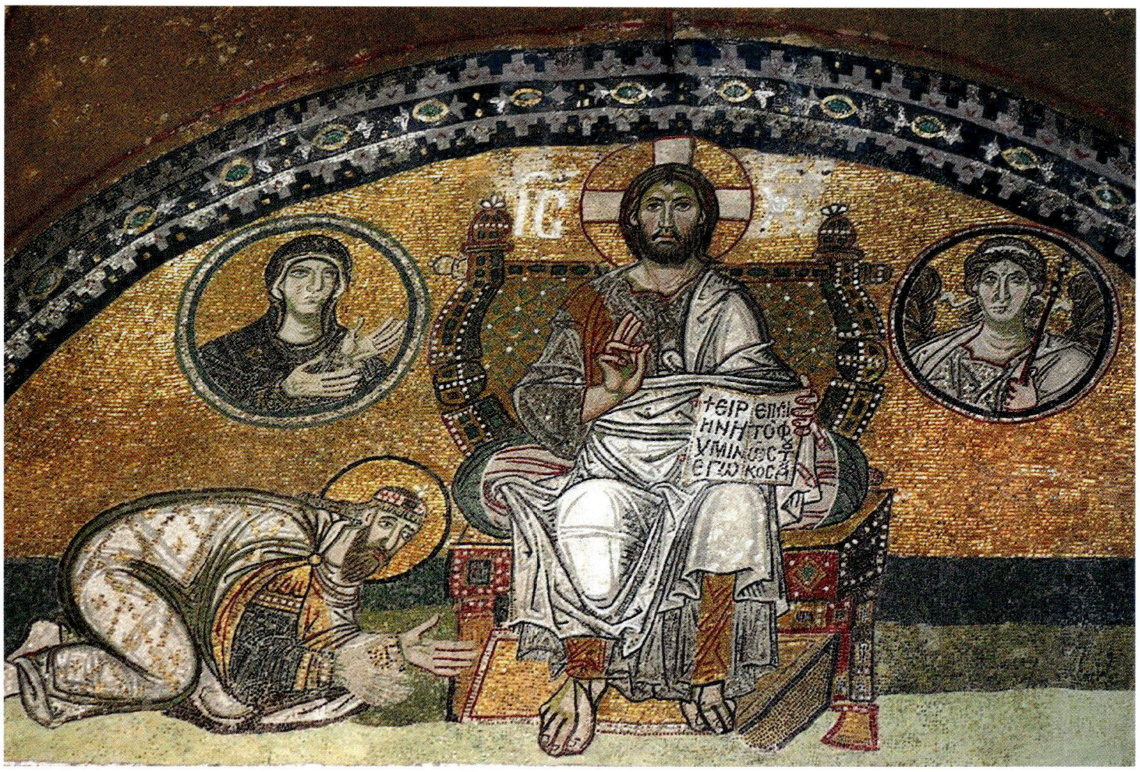

Leo V (886–912) venerating Christ.

Mosaic, 10th–11th century, Hagia Sophia.

the Franks call it—the capital of their ruler Charlemagne, who usurped the title "Emperor of the Romans." They've also contributed to churches throughout Germany and, more recently, in Sicily, in the kingdom of Roger, where our artisans have produced nothing short of masterpieces. Their skill and artistry proclaim not only beauty but also the faith of our Empire.

The Byzantine craftsmen adorned churches as far as Venice, Georgia, Kiev, and Bethlehem. Of course, the true flourishing of mosaic art occurred chiefly within our own dominion, centered around the Hagia Sophia and other churches of Constantinople. One finds them also in Thessaloniki, in Ravenna, in Boeotia, in Attica, and on the island of Chios. What is especially fascinating is that mosaicists from Constantinople were commissioned to decorate even Muslim monuments: the Great Mosque of Damascus, the Dome of the Rock in Jerusalem, and the Mosque of Córdoba—all of which bear traces of our tradition. In some cases, the mosaic tesserae themselves were transported from the Queen of Cities."

I was astonished by all this information—much like the young girls who had listened with wide-eyed wonder when I recounted to them the history of medicine. My young friend, seeing the depth of my interest, spoke with fervor about the art of mosaic-making:

"In preparing the mosaic, three different layers of mortar are made, and the tesserae are selected and fixed onto a rough preliminary drawing. For the faces and the bare parts of the body, small tesserae are used to depict the details. For the clothing and the objects in the background, larger ones are chosen. Bright colors are selected—blue, green, red, purple—which give liveliness

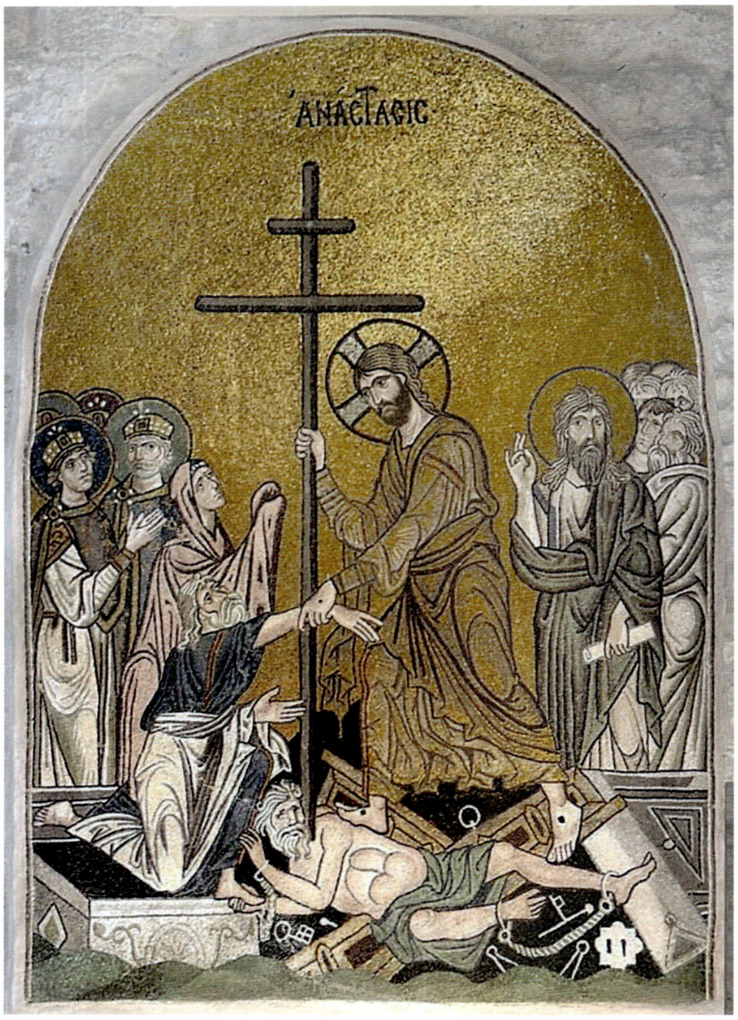

The Descent into Hades.

Mosaic, 11th century, Daphni Monastery.

and grandeur to the images. The background is always rendered in gold so that the glory of the Heavenly King and His saints may be visible. Byzantine mosaic art produced masterpieces that inspire awe—especially the depiction of Christ Pantocrator, whose gaze from the church's dome seems to hold you fast. In fact, the tesserae are affixed in such a way that each one's surface tilts ever so slightly from its neighbors, maximizing the reflection and interplay of light."

That last detail thrilled me—never had I imagined that the shimmering brilliance of the figures, especially the golden backgrounds of the mosaics, was due to the careful angling of each tessera. My friend's narratives left a deep impression on me, and naturally, at the first opportunity, I would visit Hagia Sophia and other churches to savor the beauty of the mosaics, as well as the painted icons—another inheritance of Greek antiquity, which Manuel later explained to me in rich detail.

Alongside these pursuits that so captivated me, I had to begin preparing for my studies in medicine. Here, I had the opportunity to engage with the writings of the great physicians—both those of antiquity and their Byzantine successors—who not only preserved the knowledge of the classical masters but enriched and refined it by adding their own insights and experiences. The history of medicine in the Roman oikoumene is, in truth, an almost exclusively Greek affair. Following the conquests of Alexander the Great, Greek culture and language had spread throughout the Eastern Mediterranean. In the great cities that flourished—Alexandria, Antioch, Pergamon, and others—many eminent physicians emerged as heirs to the Hippocratic legacy. Following his vision of a scientific medicine, one unburdened by metaphysical interpretations, they advanced the field significantly and left behind valuable treatises. In the Hellenistic kingdoms, science and the arts thrived. The Ptolemies, the Seleucids, and the Attalids competed in their patronage of learning, resulting in a remarkable blossoming of mathematics, astronomy, medicine, and the fine arts.

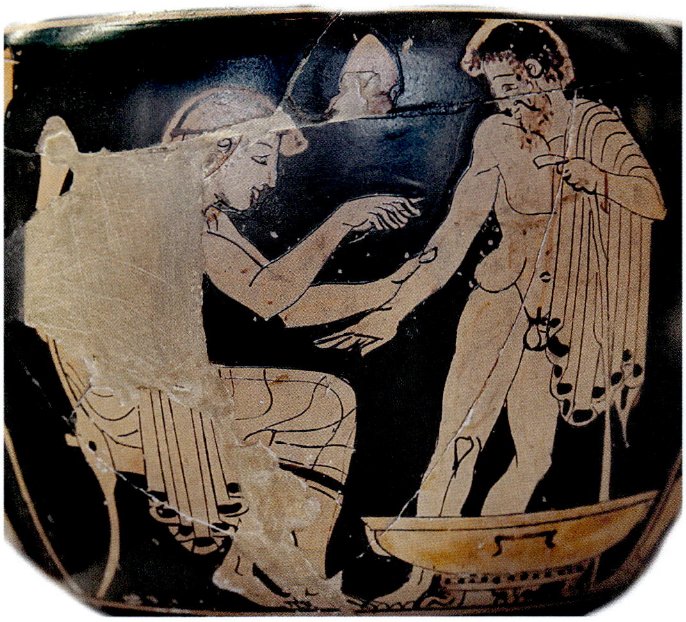

Doctor treating a patient.

Attic aryballos, 5th century B.C.
Louvre Museum, Paris.

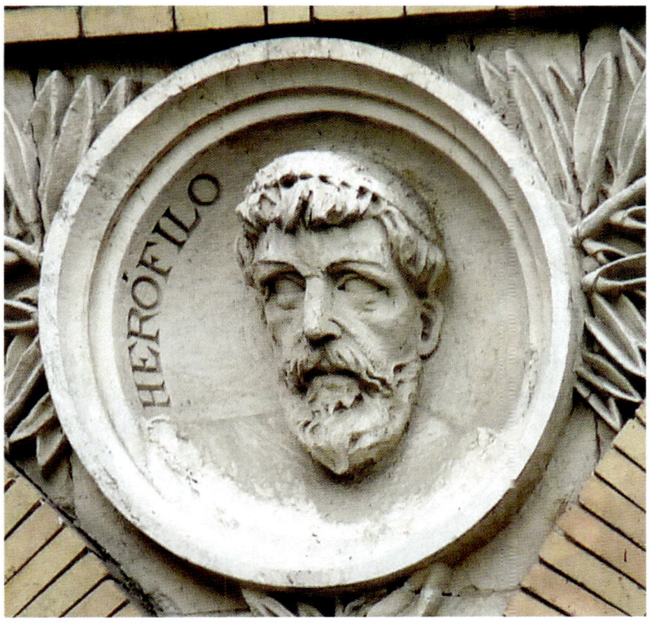

Herophilos of Chalcedon.

Relief at the Old Medical School
of Zaragoza, Spain.

As I had promised, I recounted the story of the ancient and more recent physicians to the two girls, who awaited it with eager anticipation. Naturally, it was impossible to mention them all—for they are far too many. So I chose, selectively, those I considered the most significant. Before speaking to them, I made sure to refresh my memory by leafing through my books and notes, for I did not want to disappoint Antigone. And so, one afternoon, after our time at the Pandidakterion, the three of us sat together at home, and I began my narration.

"One of the most eminent physicians of the Hellenistic era was Herophilos of Chalcedon, who lived during the 4th to 3rd century before the coming of the Savior.

He conducted dissections on human bodies—typically those of condemned criminals—with special imperial permission. Let me remind you that dissection of human corpses was forbidden both in antiquity and in our own time, and most of our anatomical knowledge derives from animals. Herophilos greatly advanced anatomical understanding, particularly of the brain, which he regarded as the seat of thought. He also studied and described in detail the eye and its structures, including the optic nerve. Moreover, he examined and documented the reproductive organs, the intestines, and the internal viscera with remarkable precision. We owe to him the terms *duodenum*, *prostate*, and *choroid plexus*. In fact, a formation within the brain still bears his name: the "torcular Herophili" (Herophilos' winepress).

A contemporary of Herophilos and equally significant was Erasistratos of Ioulis, who also engaged in anatomical studies and was the first to distinguish

Agnodice, student of Herophilos.

Lithograph by F. Villain after a work by A. Foucaud, 1833.

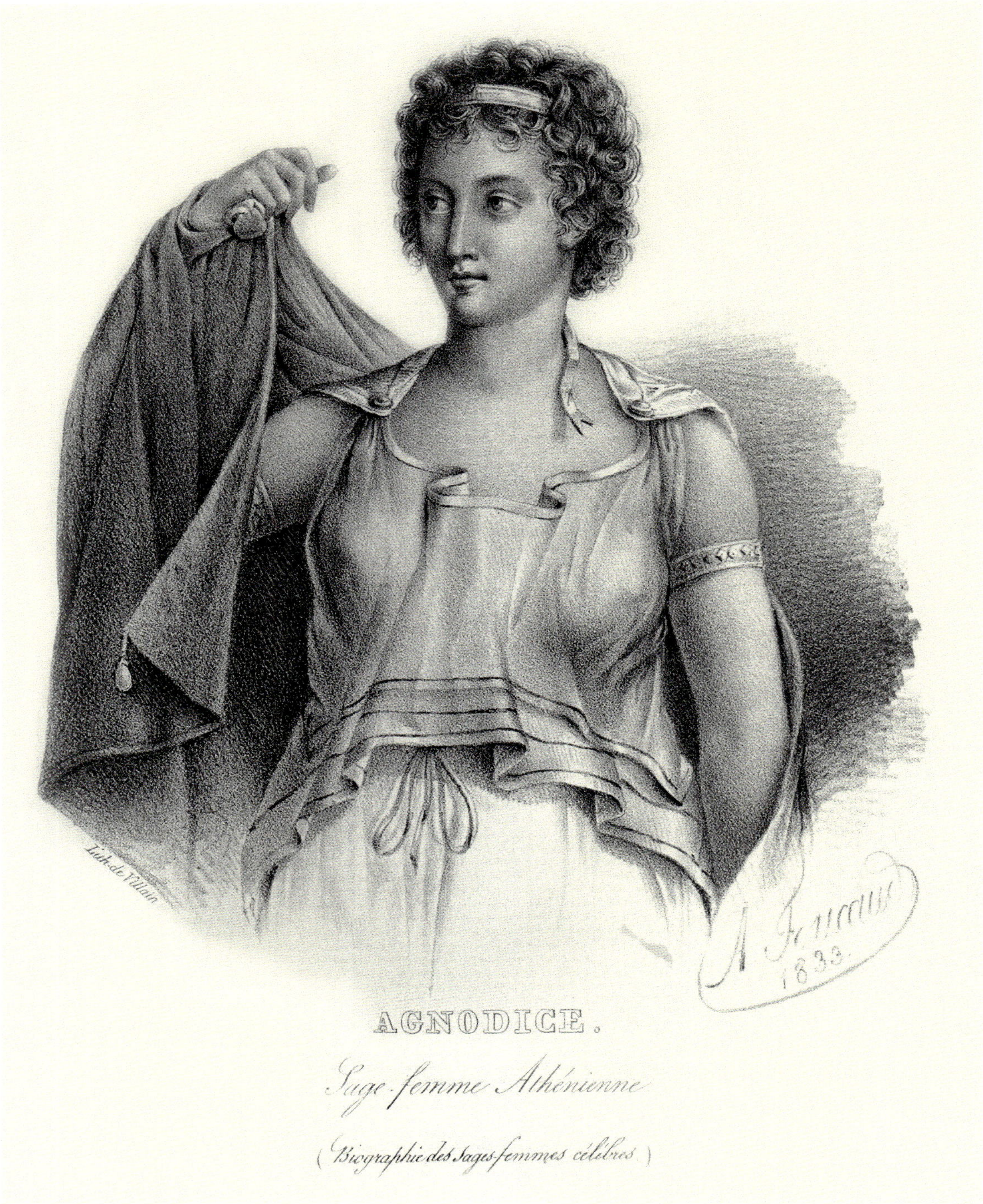

between motor and sensory nerves. He served at the court of the Seleucids in Antioch and later at the Ptolemaic court in Alexandria. A slightly younger figure, Eudemos, also gained fame for his medical achievements. In the 1st century before Christ, Asclepiades of Bithynia lived and practiced. He moved to Rome, where he established a prominent medical career and became well known. To him we owe the introduction of the medical terms *tetanus* and *opisthotonos*. He was also among the first to perform *tracheotomy* in order to relieve airway obstruction and restore breathing.

There was also a remarkable woman, Agnodice. She lived in Athens at the end of the 4th century BCE and, disguised in men's clothing, studied medicine as a pupil of the great Herophilos. She practiced medicine in Athens, treating only women—and with great success. When her true sex was discovered, she was brought to trial, as it was forbidden at the time for women to practice medicine. However, many men came to her defense, including prominent officials whose wives she had treated or delivered in childbirth. Thanks to their testimonies, she was acquitted in a triumphant verdict. As a result of her acquittal, the law was revised, and from that point on, women were permitted to study medicine. Thus, Agnodice was able to continue her medical practice freely.

"What an extraordinary woman!" said Antigone. "I admire her courage and skill. How I would love to be like her..."

"Anything is possible—you never know," I replied [with a smile].

"May it be so," she answered softly. "But go on with your story—it's absolutely fascinating."

"All those physicians I've just mentioned wrote medical treatises, though unfortunately only a few have survived. Still, we know of them through the writings of later doctors, who often refer to them—either praising their accomplishments or critiquing their errors."

"But what about the ancient Romans?" Antigone asked with a puzzled look. "Didn't they contribute to medicine too?"

"The ancient Romans," I replied, "were primarily preoccupied with military affairs and legal matters; medicine did not particularly interest them. By the time Rome had conquered the known world and the entire oikoumene was gathered under the unified imperial rule, the fame and legacy of the Greek physicians were already so firmly established that medicine was practiced almost exclusively by Greeks. The finest physicians migrated to the new heart of the world—Rome—and thus, Greek doctors came to dominate the empire. During the centuries of late antiquity that followed, the language of the intellectuals, philosophers, artists, scientists, and even merchants was Greek. In Rome, all educated individuals spoke Greek, and even among the lower classes, many were Greek-speaking—especially among merchants and sailors. It is no coincidence that the Apostle Paul addressed his *Epistle to the Romans*—that is, to the Christians living in Rome—writing it in Greek, the language they best understood. At that time, many distin-

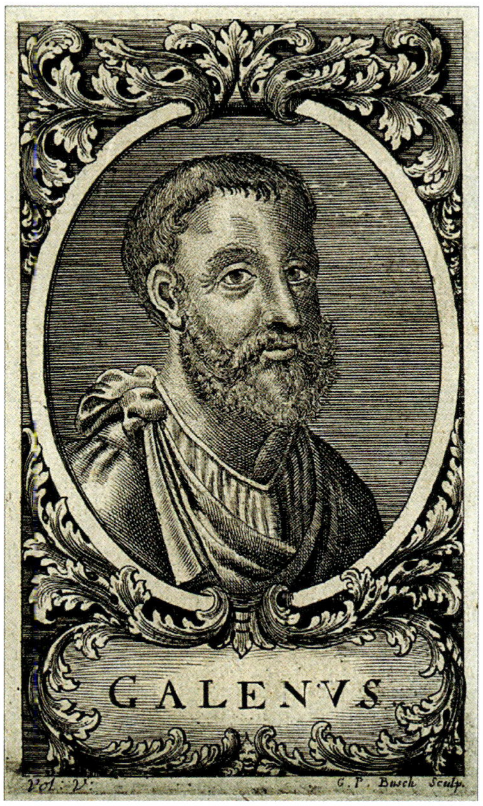

Claudius Galenus

Engraving, 18th century by Georg P. Busch.

guished physicians emerged, practicing either in Rome or in the great cities of the Eastern Empire. They were so numerous that listing them all would only cause confusion. Some of the most notable names you may have heard include Archigenes, Rufus, Aretaeus, Leonides, and Heliodorus. These were all significant physicians who left behind substantial contributions to the field. Yet all of them were eventually overshadowed by the greatest figure after Hippocrates—the brilliant Galen.

"It's not easy to remember so many names," said Antigone. "But tell us about Galen."

"Claudius Galen was born in Pergamon in A.D. 129 into a prosperous family. He first studied Platonic and Stoic philosophy, and later medicine—initially in his hometown and subsequently in Alexandria, the renowned center of culture and science. He traveled extensively and taught in many cities of the Roman Empire, successfully practicing medicine and surgery. At the age of thirty-three, he settled in Rome, where he became physician to four emperors: Marcus Aurelius, Commodus, Septimius Severus, and Caracalla. Galen shared the views of Hippocrates, holding that the human body is governed by four humors [body fluids], and that health depends on their proper balance—what he called *eukrasia*. These humors are: *blood*, *phlegm*, *yellow bile*, and *black bile* (melaina chole). The predominance of one humor over the others, he taught, gave rise to four types of temperament: the *sanguine*, the *phlegmatic*, the *choleric*, and the *melancholic*.

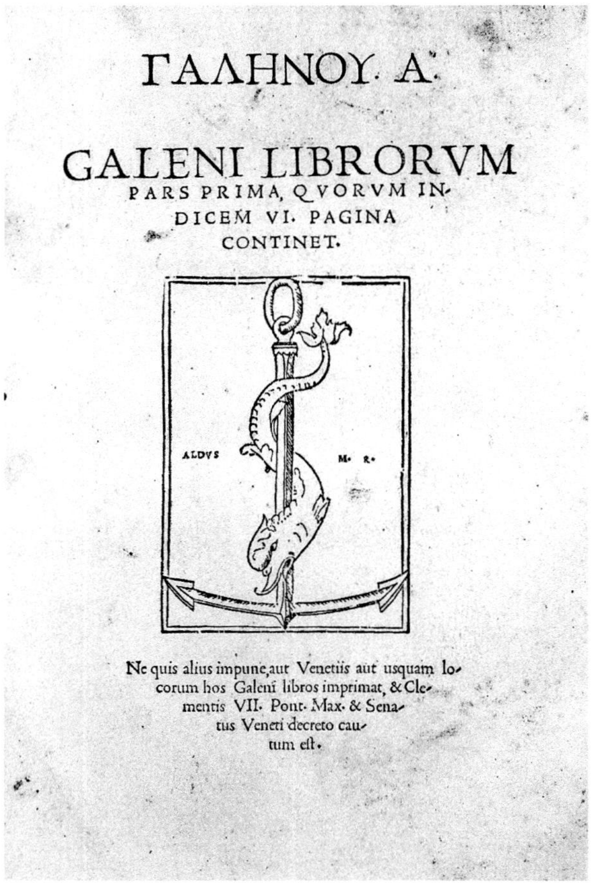
ΓΑΛΗΝΟΥ Α.

GALENI LIBRORVM PARS PRIMA, QVORVM INDICEM VI. PAGINA CONTINET.

ALDVS M. R.

Ne quis alius impune, aut Venetiis aut usquam locorum hos Galeni libros imprimat, & Clementis VII. Pont. Max. & Senatus Veneti decreto cautum est.

Books of Galen.
Published by Aldine Press, Venice, 1525.

He performed animal dissections, primarily on monkeys and pigs, since human dissection was prohibited in his time. Through these, he greatly advanced anatomical knowledge. In fact, his anatomical work remains unsurpassed, and even a thousand years later, we still rely on much of his understanding. Galen discovered that veins and arteries contain different types of blood. He described muscles and nerves, internal organs, and various bodily systems, including the mechanism of speech originating from the larynx. He documented numerous diseases and their treatments, and he conducted successful surgical procedures, particularly for treating wounds, which were common in the war-torn empire. With remarkable dexterity and boldness, he treated cataracts by removing the clouded lens of the eye—a daring and impressive operation for his time. He wrote an extraordinary number of treatises in which he gathered all the accumulated medical knowledge of the previous seven centuries, while also introducing his own innovations. Yet Galen was not only a physician—his philosophical knowledge ran deep. He had studied the various schools of philosophy—Platonists, Peripatetics, Stoics, and Epicureans—and sought to integrate philosophical thought with medical practice. He firmly believed, and frequently emphasized, that *a good physician must also be a philosopher*. For Galen, medicine was a multifaceted field of inquiry, where *theory*, *observation*, and *experimentation* must be brought into harmony. But, as he insisted, experimentation leads nowhere unless it is guided by sound theoretical understanding."

I began to worry that I had spoken too much and that my young listeners might have grown tired. So I suggested that we pause for the day and continue tomorrow.

"We're not tired at all!" they both exclaimed. "We want to hear the rest—don't leave us in suspense!" And so, encouraged by their eagerness, I took heart and continued my story.

"Galen is regarded as equal to the great Hippocrates and, to this day, remains unsurpassed throughout the world. His works were translated into Latin and are used throughout the Western lands, but also into Arabic, where they are studied by the Arabs—who, after their violent and barbaric expansion into the civilized lands of Asia (Persia, India) and Africa (Egypt, Cyrenaica), came to adopt the culture of the Persians, Indians, and Greco-Romans and went on to develop it with notable merit

They translated all the ancient Greek authors—physicians, astronomers, mathematicians, philosophers (with the exception of poets and tragedians, as

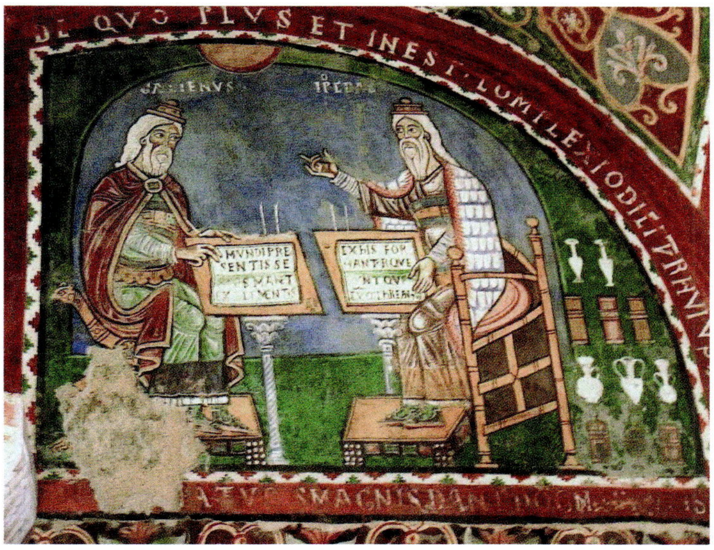

Hippocrates and Galen.

Fresco, 12th century, Anagni, Italy.

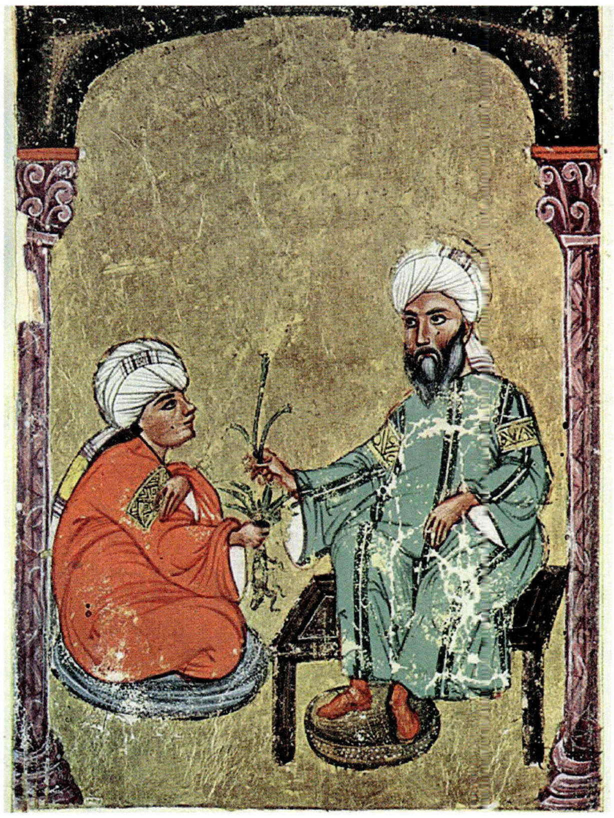

Arab physicians.

Miniature from De Materia Medica *by Dioscorides, Arabic translation, 13th century. Topkapi Museum, Constantinople.*

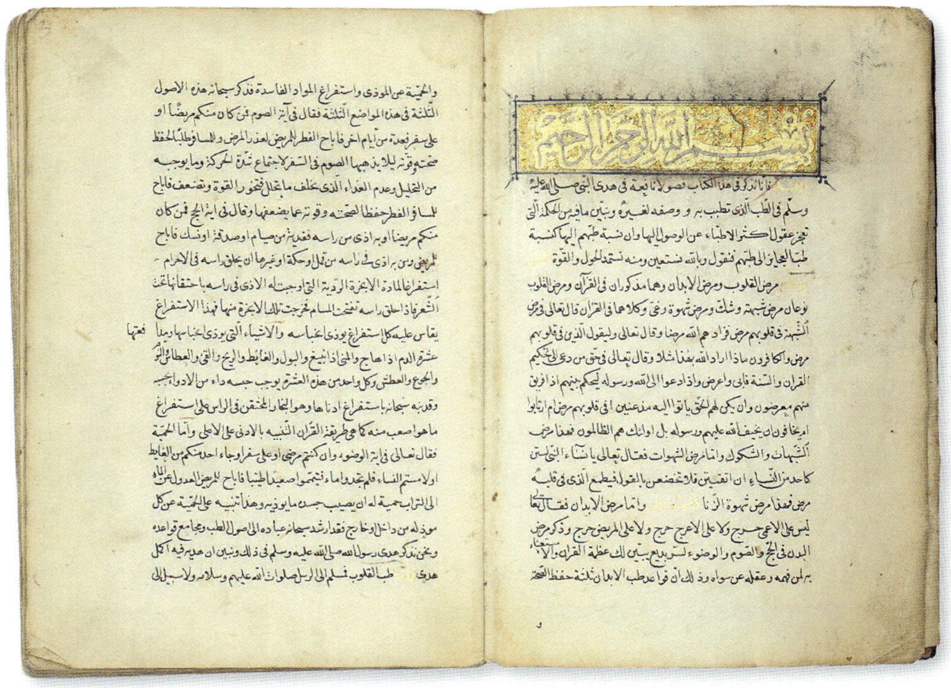

Treatise on the Medicine of the Prophet.
16th-century manuscript, N. Khallili Collection of Islamic Art, London.

their interest lay solely in the practical sciences)—and upon this foundation they continued and advanced knowledge to an impressive degree. In medicine, they drew much from us, but we also benefited from them. Even today, Arab physicians occasionally come to the City, just as Romans—whether physicians or philosophers—travel to and establish their careers in the lands of the caliphates.

I did not wish to tire my young listeners with further details, even though they followed my narrative with great interest. So, we began to discuss and reflect upon what I had just shared. They asked me many questions, eager to better understand certain medical details. I answered gladly, with a quiet sense of pride. Later, I noticed them discussing it among themselves, repeating the names of the great scientists of Greek antiquity.

Here, I would like to offer a clarification regarding the complex fate of the name "Greek" (*Hellēn*) and the adjective "Greek" (*Hellēnikos*) within the Roman Empire. Before the time of Alexander the Great, the Greeks lived in dense populations primarily in the Greek peninsula, along the western coast of Asia Minor, and in Southern Italy and Sicily. Scattered in colonies, they also inhabited many coastal regions of the Mediterranean and the Black Sea. The ancient Greeks cultivated their language to a marvelous degree, using it to express the highest concepts of philosophy, science, art, and politics. They referred to those who spoke other languages as *barbaroi*, a term which originally bore no pejorative meaning—it simply denoted someone who spoke in an unintelligible tongue. However, once the Greeks became conscious of the superiority of their own civilization in comparison to most of their neighbors, the word gradually took on its modern sense: that of the uncivilized, the coarse, or the rude.

With the conquests of Alexander, the Greeks—their civilization and language—spread throughout Syria, Egypt, Mesopotamia, all the way to India and Bactria. Ethnic barriers were dismantled, and people everywhere strove to learn Greek, which had become the language of administration and culture. From that time forward, the name "Greek" was no longer limited to ethnicity; it applied to all who partook of Greek culture, education, and way of life. Thus, Hellenism became synonymous with Greek customs and traditions, as well as with their religion, which by then had evolved into a syncretic blend of elements—from the ancient Olympian pantheon to Egyptian, Eastern Iranian, and Indian deities.

When Rome conquered Greece and, eventually, the entire known world, the Romans recognized the value of Greek civilization and fully embraced it, while contributing their own significant cultural achievements. Thus was born our marvelous Greco-Roman civilization. Latin became the language of administration and the military, but Greek remained the language of philosophy, art, and science. Later on, all the subjects of the Empire were granted Roman citizenship, and from that point onward we were all called Romans—regardless of our ethnic origin or native tongue—throughout the vast Roman State.

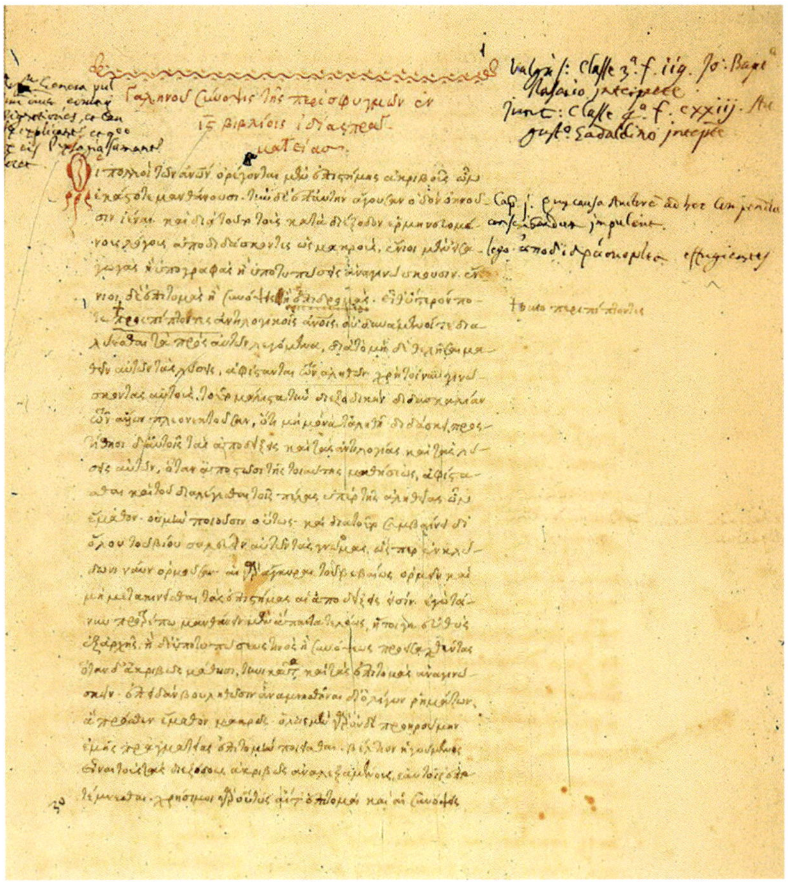

Manuscript of Galen in Greek and Latin, Venice, ca. 1550.

National Library of Medicine, Maryland, USA.

Thus, within the Roman *Oikoumene,* the name "Greek" (*Hellēn*) lost its ethnic significance and became synonymous with cultural achievements, philosophy, and the religious beliefs of the ancient Greeks. When Christianity spread throughout the Roman Empire and reached all its peoples, it came into sharp conflict with the pagan state, which still upheld the religion of the Greeks. As a result, once the State embraced Christianity, the remnants of paganism were closely associated with the adherents of Greek ideas. The term "Greek" became synonymous with "pagan." The Fathers of the Church—except for a few, though significant, exceptions such as the Great Cappadocians—often spoke vehemently against the "Greeks" and their doctrines. And they did so in impeccable Greek, for that was the language most people understood and the one capable of articulating complex philosophical and dogmatic concepts.

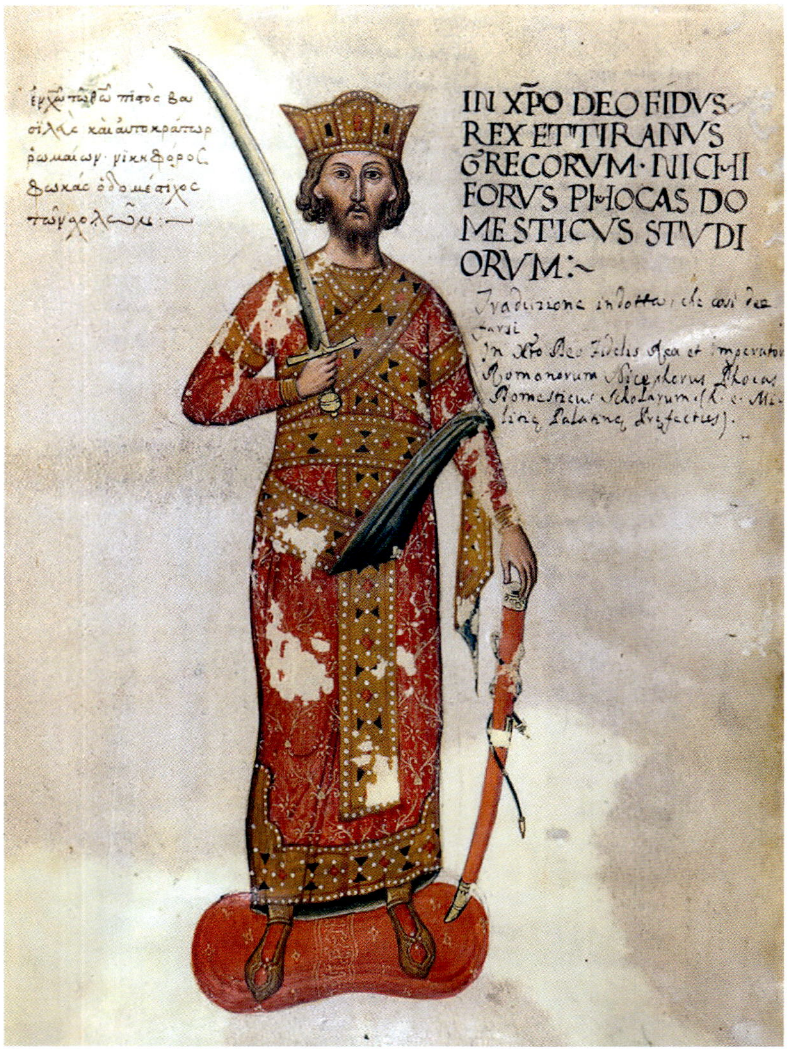

Nikephoros Phokas is called "Basileus of the Romans" in the Greek inscription and "Tyranus Grecorum" in the Latin.

Miniature, 15th century, Marciana Library, Venice.

The first Christian emperors—especially Theodosius I and Justinian—persecuted pagans with great severity, as well as Christian heretics of every kind, because they believed that a unified religion guaranteed the unity and therefore the strength of the state. Unfortunately, along with the ancient religion, the magnificent works of art from antiquity were also identified and thus destroyed: temples and statues of unsurpassed beauty were demolished by zealots. The ancient philosophical schools were also shut down, though until the sixth century, both pagan and Christian intellectuals had studied there—including the great Fathers of the Church in the fourth century. Fortunately, the enlightened Emperor Theodosius II, in the fifth century, founded a Higher School in Constantinople to which he gave unique prestige. There, ancient Greek philosophy and Roman law were taught—this institution was originally known as the *Auditorium* and later as the *Pandidakterion*.

But things changed over the centuries. After the division of the Empire into East and West, a significant divergence occurred between the Latin-speaking

West and the Greek-speaking East. In the East, we spoke the Greek language, and Latin was gradually forgotten, while in the West the opposite occurred. Westerners began to call us *Graeci*—Greeks—as the ancient Romans had referred to the *Hellenes*, assigning the term an ethnic rather than a ethnic connotation. Already by the sixth century, when the armies of Belisarius reconquered Rome and the rest of Italy from the Ostrogoths and North Africa from the Vandals—thus restoring these regions to the unified Roman Empire governed from Constantinople—the local populations, having developed their own distinct identity, claimed that those who had conquered them were not Romans but *Greeks*. Even though we spoke Greek and took pride in our Greek cultural heritage, we rejected the official designation Graeci, for it called into question the universality of our Roman Empire, whose rightful heir and uninterrupted successor was the Emperor in Constantinople. We insisted—and we continue to insist—on the name Romans [Ρωμαίοι], for we are the true heirs of the Ecumenical Empire, which we inherited and have always rightfully claimed. The Russians and, more broadly, the Slavic peoples—whom we civilized, for whom we created an alphabet based on the Greek, to whom we gave Greek names, and whose language we enriched with a multitude of Greek words—call us *Greki* (Greeks). Meanwhile, the Arabs and the peoples of the East call us Rum, that is, Romans.*

Now, in the era of the Komnenoi, when the territory of the Empire has been reduced to exclusively Greek-speaking regions and the danger of paganism no longer looms, Greek studies have flourished greatly, and the name Hellene has become an honorary title. We feel ourselves politically and officially to be Romans, while at the same time the true heirs of the great Hellenic civilization.

* The name Byzantium and the adjective Byzantine were never used by the inhabitants of the Eastern Roman State themselves, who identified as Eastern Romans (*Eōoi Rhōmaioi*) or simply Romans. The term is a clever invention of the German historian Hieronymus Wolf, who coined it in 1557, drawing inspiration from the name of the ancient Greek colony Byzantion, on whose site Constantinople was built. The narrator of this text, Messenes, would not have known the term Byzantine, but it is employed here to assist the modern reader. (*Editor's note*)

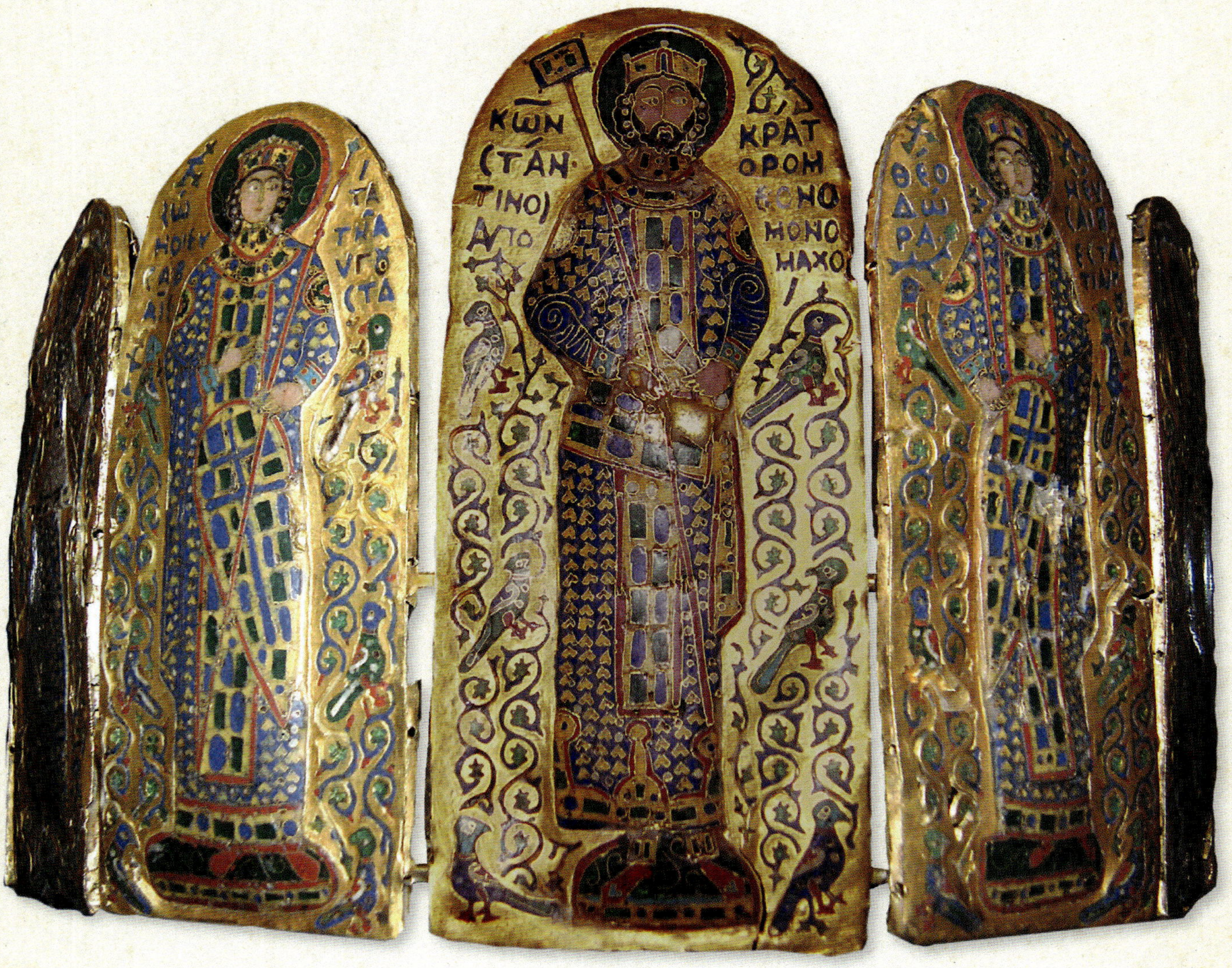

Crown of Monomachos. Emperor Constantine IX Monomachos, Empress Zoe, and her sister Theodora.

Enamel, 11th century, National Museum, Budapest

Medicine and Physicians in the Eastern Empire

October of 1168 had arrived, and at last, I began my studies at the Magnaura School. Thankfully, Theodore Vlemmydes had arranged for my enrollment, as well as for his son Manuel, who would be studying in the School of Philosophy. Tuition was free, but strong recommendations were necessary. With a mix of emotion and fear, I passed through the great doors of the former Imperial Palace, now the "Ecumenical School of Learning."

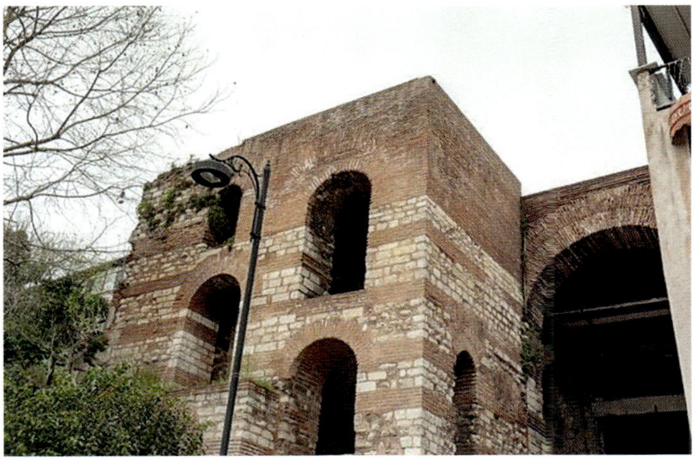

The Magnaura Palace as it stands today.
Photo: Afurkcnakin, 2022.

The Pandidakterion was founded in 425 by Emperor Theodosius II. Ironically, history dubbed him "the Younger," in contrast to his grandfather, Theodosius I, who is remembered as "the Great." Theodosius the Great left a dual legacy: on one hand, the establishment of Christianity as the sole and obligatory religion of the empire and the suppression of heresies through the convocation of the Second Ecumenical Council, which aimed to secure the unity of the vast state; on the other hand, his legacy is also shadowed by the ruthless massacre of the population of Thessaloniki, the harsh persecutions of pagans, the destruction of their temples, and the abolition of the Olympic Games. "Theodosius the Younger" also left behind a significant legacy: the construction of the famous Theodosian Wall of Constantinople—a unique feat of its time—which protected and still symbolically guards the city as an impregnable stronghold; the compilation of the Codex Theodosianus, the first systematic collection and recording of Roman laws, which preceded the definitive compilation under Justinian; and, most notably, the founding of the Pandidakterion of Constantinople—the first institution of higher learning in Europe. It was initially named *Auditorium*, since Latin was still the official language of the Empire. Though Theodosius II was known for his weak character, he was fortunate to be surrounded by two remarkable women: his older sister Pulcheria, who

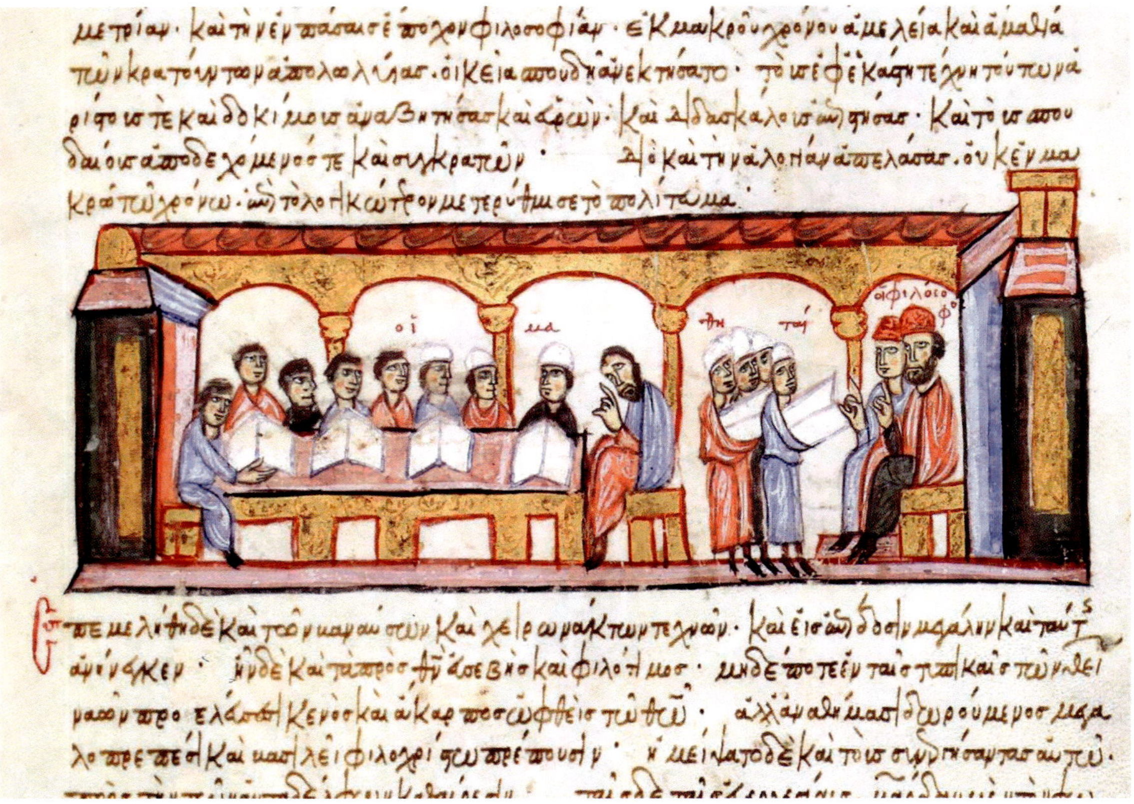

Students and Philosophers. Teaching of Law at the Pandidakterion.

From the Skylitzes Chronicle, 12th century, National Library of Spain, Madrid.

served as his regent during his youth, and his wife, Aelia Eudocia. Eudocia—originally named Athenais—was selected by Pulcheria as a suitable bride for her brother. She was a pagan by birth, the daughter of Leontius, a distinguished professor of rhetoric at the School of Philosophy in Athens. Upon her baptism into the Christian faith, she took the name Eudocia. Like her sister-in-law Pulcheria, she was exceptionally intelligent and possessed a profound philosophical education. These two women played a pivotal role not only in the establishment of the *Auditorium*—known in Greek as the *Oikoumenikon Didaskaleion* (Ecumenical School)—but also in shaping the broader legacy of Emperor Theodosius II. The main coordinator of this monumental endeavor was the Greek poet and philosopher Cyrus of Panopolis, who also held the office of Praetorian Prefect.

The *Didaskaleion* (School) initially had thirty professors in total: fifteen taught in Latin—covering Roman literature, philosophy, and law—while the other fifteen taught in Greek, focusing on grammar, philosophy, and philology.

Its operation was interrupted several times, especially in the early 7th century during the Arab invasions. However, it was revived by the late Emperor Heraclius in 610, who summoned the philosopher Stephen of Alexandria to Constantinople for this very purpose. From the reign of Heraclius onward, Latin studies began to decline until they eventually disappeared altogether. The institution endured great trials during the dark years of Iconoclasm, yet its function was never entirely suspended. In the 9th century, in the year 863 during the reign of Michael III, through the efforts of Caesar Vardas, the Ecumenical School was relocated to the Magnaura Palace and thereafter took on that name. Its revival and expansion were undertaken by Leo the Mathematician from Thessaly, who taught the "external education" and the *Quadrivium*—that is, Arithmetic, Geometry, Astronomy, and Music. A few years later, the enlightened Emperors Leo the Wise and his son Constantine Porphyrogenitus established free education at the Pandidakterion, provided respectable salaries to the professors, and granted scholarships to students in need.

In the 11th century, under Constantine Monomachos, the Ecumenical School was divided into two faculties: the School of Law (*Didaskaleion of the Laws*) and the School of Philosophy (*Gymnasion*). The term Pandidakterion was given much later. The head of the School of Philosophy was the *hypatos ton philosophon* ("consul of the philosophers") Michael Psellos, followed later by John Italos. The director of the School of Law was John Xiphilinos, the *nomophylax* (guardian of the laws) of the state. Other distinguished professors who adorned the institution included Patriarch Photius the Great, George Choiroboskos, the enlighteners of the Slavs Cyril and Methodius—who invented the Slavic alphabet based on Greek—and my fellow countryman, Arethas of Patras. The School was purely secular; theology was not taught there but was reserved exclusively for the Patriarchal School.

The atmosphere within the Pandidakterion was akin to that of a sacred temple. The professors were venerable figures, dressed in a distinctive garb—not ostentatious or luxurious, but dignified—which, combined with their beards, rendered them deeply respectable. We, too, were required to be dressed "modestly and decently." We addressed them with the utmost reverence, using titles such as *logiotate* ("most

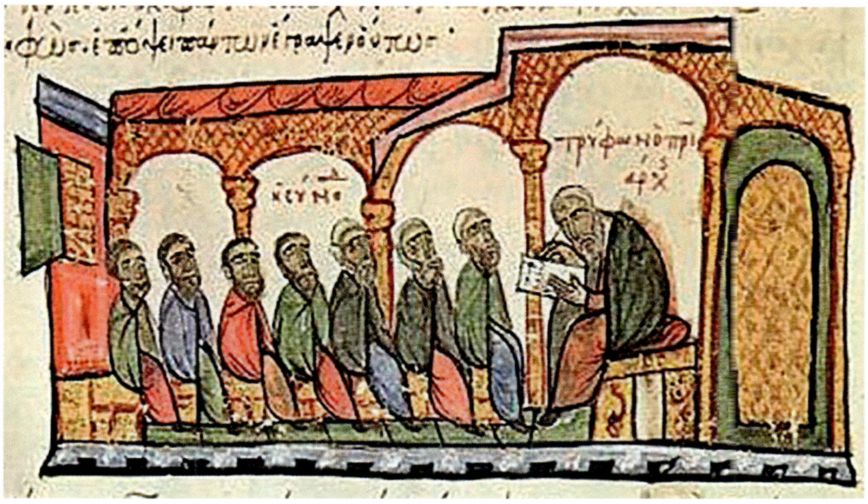

Teaching. Miniature, 11th century,
Museum of Byzantine Culture, Thessaloniki

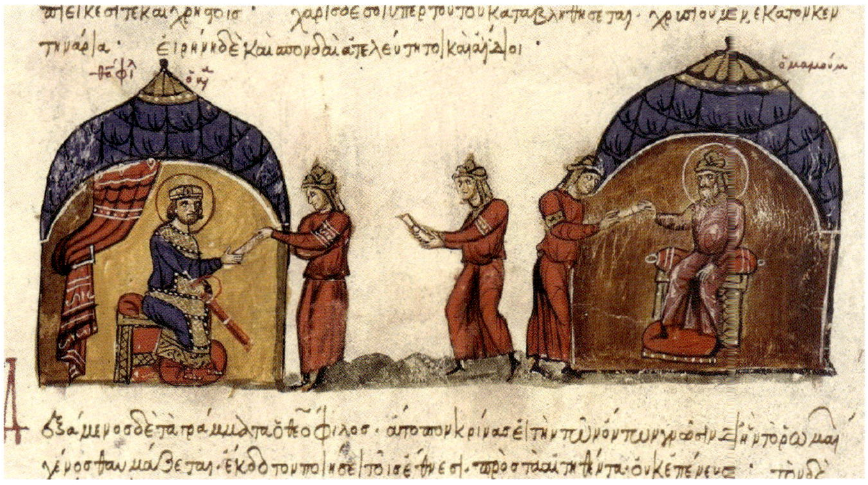

Leo the Mathematician, envoy between Emperor Theophilos and Caliph Al-Ma'mun.

Miniature, Skylitzes Chronicle, 12th century, National Library of Spain, Madrid.

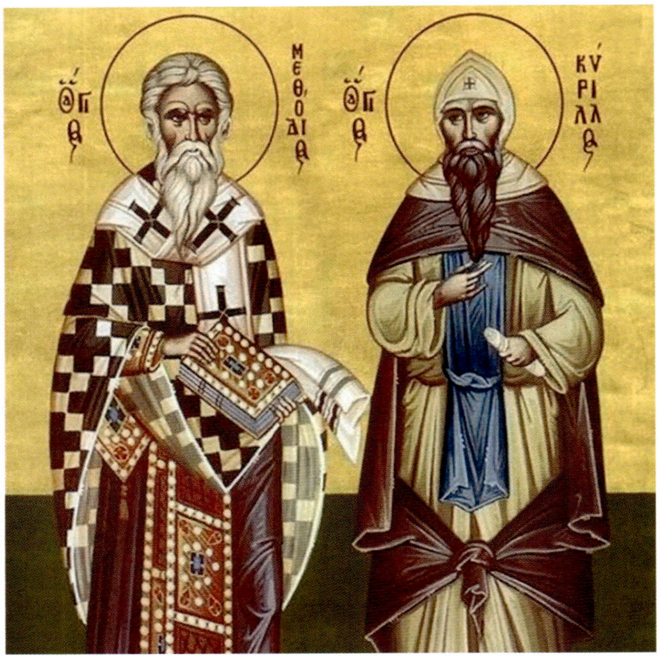

Saints Cyril and Methodius.

Modern icon.

learned"), *eklamprotate* ("most illustrious"), or *epiphanestate* ("most eminent"). To become a professor, one had to demonstrate eloquence, vast learning, and teaching experience. The title of professor or *didaskalos* was held in high esteem. There were also secondary-level instructors, called *hypogrammateis* ("undersecretaries"), who provided supplementary lessons. In order to complete their studies, students were required to submit a scholarly treatise with legal or rhetorical content, on a subject approved by their school's teacher. This was known as a *drakton*—their equivalent of a thesis or dissertation.

Medical studies had a particular structure: they began with fundamental courses in philosophy, mathematics, and astronomy, and continued with the study of the writings of ancient physicians—Hippocrates and especially Galen. Following that, students studied the works of the great physicians of our Roman Empire, from the founding of Constantinople to the present day, all of which were written in Greek. However, the primary training took place through practice—by observing experienced doctors in the *xenones* (hospitals), participating in the care and treatment of patients, and simultaneously engaging in study within the libraries housed in those same institutions. In addition to the doctors, the hospitals included special "medical teachers" (*iatrodidaskaloi*), who instructed us in both theory and practice and examined us in order to assess our knowledge.

The atmosphere of the Pandidakterion had truly captivated and deeply impressed me. I respected and admired my professors and held my fellow students in the highest regard. I considered myself greatly privileged to belong to this distinguished group of students at the most exalted intellectual institution in the world, and I was determined to prove myself worthy of this fortune. I immersed myself wholeheartedly in my studies, eagerly absorbing the knowledge imparted by our teachers—both theoretical and practical. I never

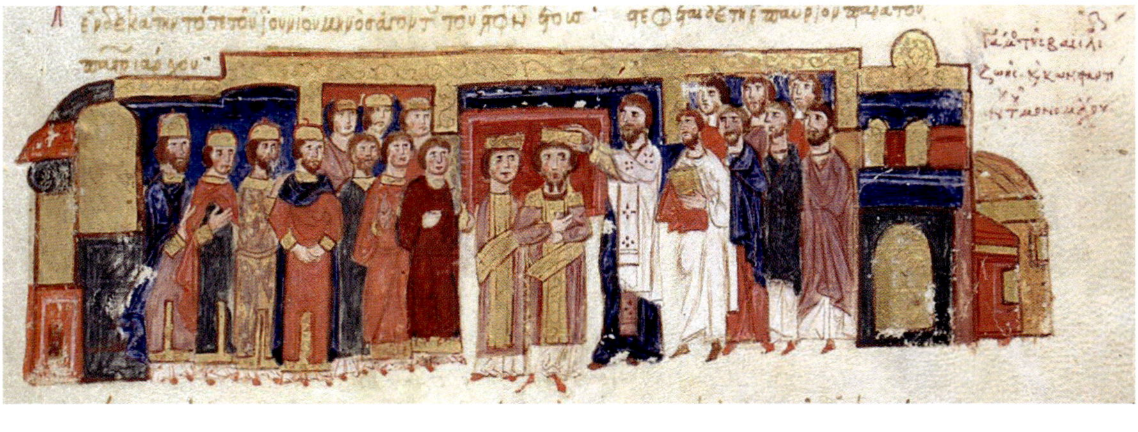

The Coronation of Constantine Monomachos.

Miniature, Skylitzes Chronicle, 12th century, National Library of Spain, Madrid.

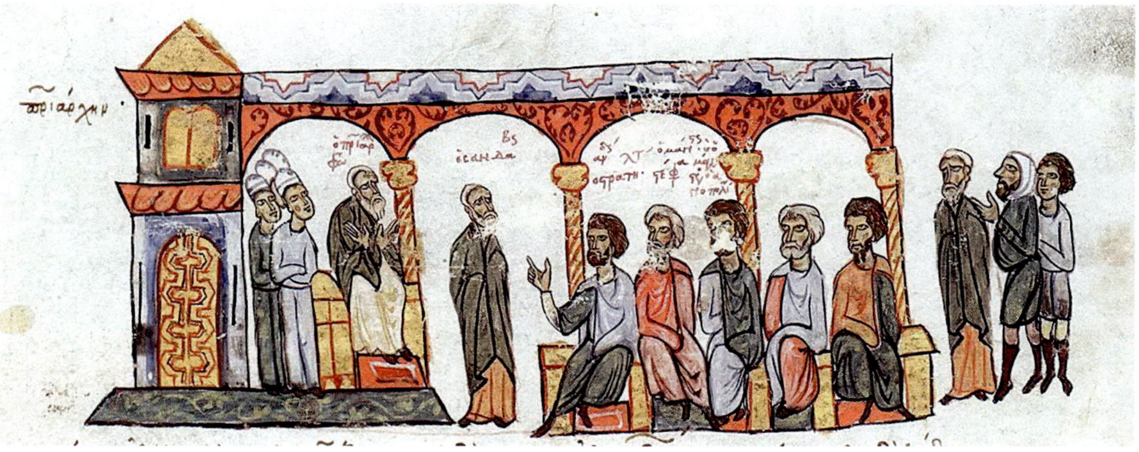

Patriarch Photius in Dialogue with His Students.

Miniature, Skylitzes Chronicle, 12th century. National Library of Spain, Madrid.

missed a lecture, and I could hardly wait each day to return to the Pandidakterion.

Something unique and unfamiliar to both of us had begun to blossom between Antigone and me for some time. What had started as friendship and mutual respect was slowly taking on a deeper character. I found myself thinking about her smiling face, her gaze, longing to be with her, to confide in her my thoughts, hopes, and dreams, and to hear her opinion—always expressed with seriousness and understanding. I wanted her to share in all my emotions, to hold in common with her all that was best within me. The thought of her love and esteem inspired me to become a better person. Many times during my studies, when I felt discouraged or weary, thinking of her gave me the strength to overcome those difficulties. It even happened that I changed my behavior to be a better version of myself for her sake. She confided in me that she felt the same way about me. Our siblings—and of course, first among them, Iphigenia—quickly understood what was still incomprehensible to me. And so, I found the companion of my life, with whom I would share all the years to come—both joyful and sorrowful—along the challenging path of a physician's life, a life that daily confronts pain and death.

Every morning, as I prepared to go to the Pandidaktērion, I would think about how I had to prove worthy of the love and admiration that Antigone had for me—as well as my sister and my parents. I considered my studies a

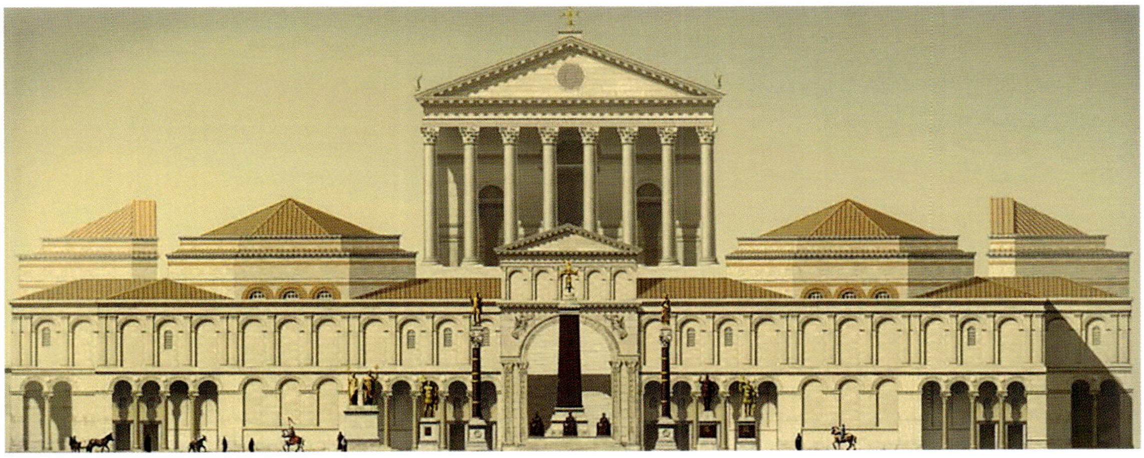

Capitolion and Philadelpheion.

Reconstruction by Antoine Helbert, 1870.

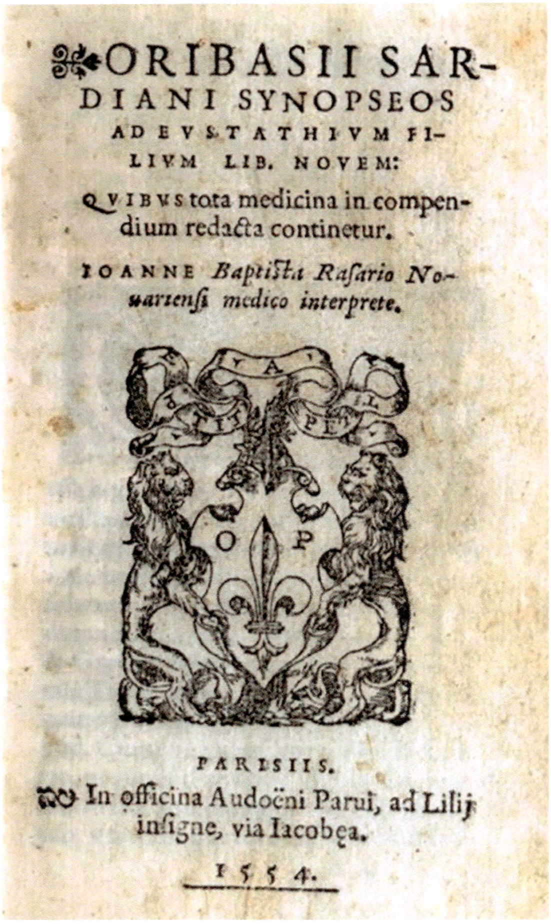
ORIBASII SARDIANI SYNOPSEOS AD EVSTATHIVM FILIVM LIB. NOVEM:

QVIBVS tota medicina in compendium redacta continetur.

IOANNE *Baptista Rasario Novarensi medico interprete.*

PARISIIS.

In officina Audoëni Parui, ad Lilij insigne, via Iacobea.

1554.

Left: Works of Oribasius. *Paris, 1554.*

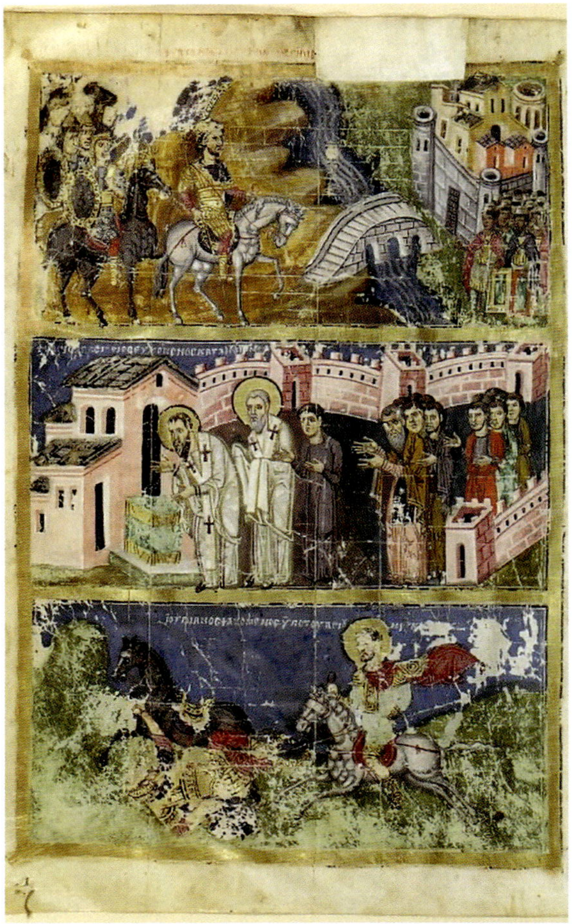
Right: Julian before Ctesiphon in Persia. *Miniature from the Homilies of Gregory the Theologian, 9th century, National Library of France, Paris.*

sacred calling entrusted to me by God and by fortune, and I felt compelled to live up to it. What I was learning was astounding—the miracle of the human body was gradually being revealed before my eyes. Yet so too was the calamity of illness and decay, which destroys the harmony and beauty of creation. In the afternoons, many of the things I had learned I continued to share with my two "pupils," who eagerly awaited the moment they could hear about them. They too longed to learn how to serve those who suffer, and they listened to me with great attentiveness.

I spoke to them about the greatest of our more recent physicians—those who not only preserved the knowledge of Hippocrates, Galen, and the other ancient doctors, but also advanced it and enriched it, adding their own insight and experience. Science never ceased to evolve in our Eastern Empire; the treasures of Greek thought were safeguarded, expanded, and then passed on to the Arabs, who put them to excellent use and developed them further. Only recently have the arrogant Franks and the Italians begun to recognize the value of our learning. So I would say to my devoted "students":

"The first significant physician of the Empire after the transfer of the capital to Constantinople was Oribasius of Pergamon, who lived in the 4th century (325–403). He was a fellow countryman of the great Galen and a devoted follower of his thought. He studied in Alexandria and Athens during the same period when the future Emperor Julian the 'Apostate', Saint Basil the Great, and Gregory the Theologian were also studying there. He was a close friend of Julian and accompanied him as chief military physician on nearly all his campaigns. At the urging of the idealistic Emperor, he composed the *Seventieth Book Collection*, a vast medical encyclopedia that gathered all existing knowledge of Ancient Greek medicine, enriched with his own original observations. He also wrote many other treatises, which were later translated into Arabic and Latin. Oribasius devised many original methods for treating diseases. He developed special sutures for tying off arteries, treated wounds with antiseptic medicines, and cured varicose veins and phlebitis of the lower limbs through surgical removal of the great saphenous vein. He recommended treating vertigo with alkaloids derived from hellebore and nephritis with a water-based diet and milk. His work profoundly influenced our later physicians as well as the Arabs, especially the great doctor Abu Ibn Zakariya, known as Rhazes. I find it very significant for Oribasius' scientific rigor that he often revised his own writings, recording earlier methods he had used that were later shown to be mistaken. This reveals the boldness and honesty of a Great Man."

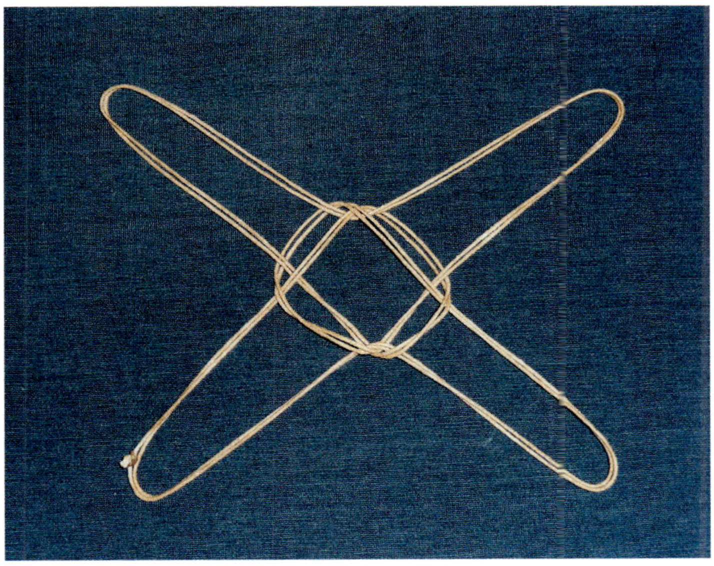
Reconstruction of Heraklas' Brick Loop (1st century A.D.) for the reduction of a jaw fracture, as described by Oreibasius.

"A contemporary of Oribasius was Saint Basil the Great, Bishop of Caesarea (330–379). This eminent Hierarch studied at the School of Philosophy in Athens, where he also received instruction in medicine. In fact, at that time, all philosophy students attended medical courses, in accordance with Aristotle's adage: 'A philosopher should begin with medicine, and a physician should complete his education with philosophy.' His remarkable and pioneering contribution was the renowned hospital in Cappadocia, the "Basileias"—the first healthcare institution in the Western world. Basil made medical observations with remarkable scientific precision. He offered significant insights into the rate of bodily growth, engaged in the study of the eye's function, and was among the first to explore the laws of heredity and biology. Above all, however, he stands out as the foremost representative of Humanitarian Medicine in those dark and troubled times.

"How remarkable," said Antigone, "that two such important figures could coexist on such opposite sides. On the one hand, the magnificent philanthropic and scientific work of Saint Basil the Great, and on the other, the great scientific contribution of Oribasius. What a pity that he remained a pagan..."

The great missionary Albert Schweitzer (1875–1965) on the work of St. Basil the Great

One evening at the hospital of Lambaréné in Equatorial Africa, a journalist praised the great doctor Albert Schweitzer for his work and remarked that Lambaréné is *"the first and oldest healing village in the world."*

Schweitzer replied to her: "You are mistaken by several centuries. Around 370 A.D., in Caesarea, in the heart of Asia Minor, there lived a man named Basil—a very educated man, a professor of Rhetoric, devoted to God, who became a monk and later a bishop. He envisioned an institution much like ours, to help the suffering people of his time. They called it the Basileias. It included a hospital for the sick, a hostel for traveling strangers, and a shelter for the disabled and homeless. There were many people working there—doctors, nurses, builders, craftsmen..." Basil wanted to bring together every human activity, every profession, so that the Basileias would be self-sufficient. Even the residents themselves took part, more or less, in the daily work of the institution—just like here, in our own community. The Basileias grew so vast and gained such renown that some jealous individuals slandered him to the Governor and dragged him to court. When he died, the entire populace wept and followed his funeral procession with sobs and lamentations. And Schweitzer added in a low voice, "Except for the Governor—and the other bishops, of course."

"We don't really know what he believed," I replied, "especially in that time, when everything was so fluid from a religious point of view. What is certain is that he was devoted to Julian, admiring both his military and intellectual virtues—while we know that Saint Basil the Great held no such admiration for Julian, despite the fact that they were classmates in Athens. But let us continue..."

"In the 6th century, when the empire reached the height of its power and territorial extent under Emperor Justinian, Alexander of Tralles (525–605) flourished. He was the brother of the great mathematician and architect Anthemios, who—together with his colleague Isidore of Miletus—designed and constructed that architectural wonder, the Hagia Sophia.

Alexander traveled throughout the Mediterranean, accompanying the army of the great General Belisarius, and practiced medicine in both Constantinople and Rome—truly a cosmopolitan figure. He authored many works, such as *Therapeutics*, *On Fevers*, *On Worms*, among others. His writings were translated into Latin, Hebrew, and Arabic. In them, he describes in detail 120 surgical procedures, including mastectomy and the removal of stones from the bladder. He possessed the boldness and scientific integrity to critique—even while admiring—the great Galen, considering some of his views to be mistaken. He is the first pioneering physician who dared to question the great teachers of antiquity."

"A truly remarkable family, the Trallians, to have produced two geniuses," commented Iphigenia.

"Indeed," I replied. "In fact, around the same period (5th–6th century), another great physician distinguished himself—Aëtius of Amida."

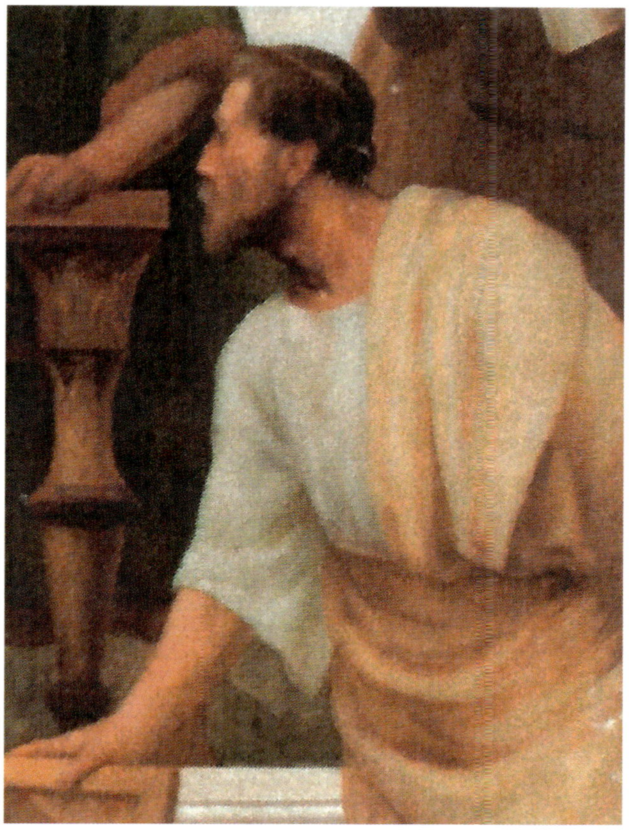

Alexander of Tralles.

Painting by Veloso Salgado, 1906, University of Lisbon.

He studied in Alexandria and practiced primarily in Constantinople, where he eventually became Chief Physician at the court of Emperor Justinian. He too composed a vast medical encyclopedia that encompassed all medical knowledge up to that time—especially the teachings of Galen—while also presenting his own theories. Aëtius is considered a pioneer in contraception, recommending intravaginal administration of astringent substances, as well as in the calculation of the fertile days of a woman's menstrual cycle. In his writings, he also mentions the midwife Aspasia, a valuable assistant in the fields of obstetrics and gynecology. In the mosaics of San Vitale in Ravenna, he is immortalized standing beside the great emperor. [see p. 66]

»During the time of Heraclius and his successors, the devastating Arab raids did not hinder the development of science and education. It was then that a

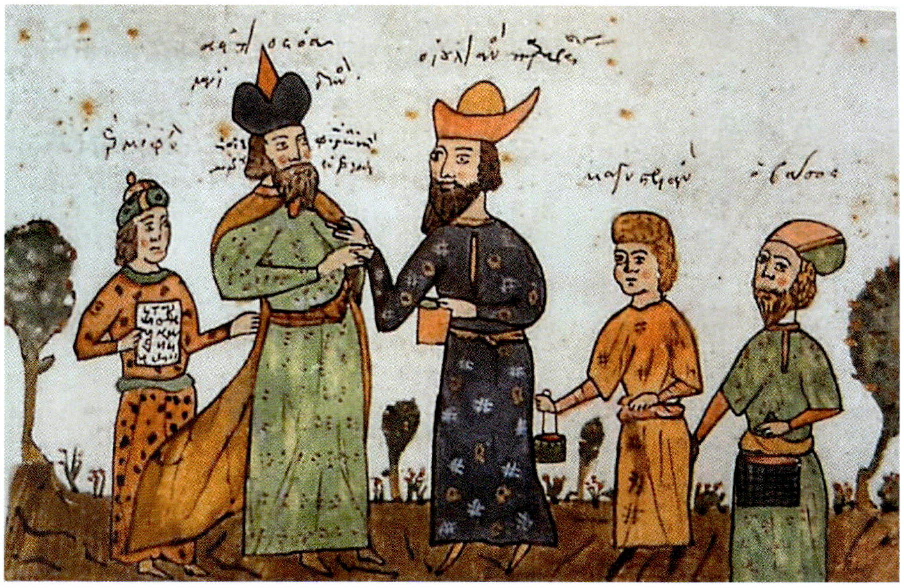

Aëtius of Amida Examines the Pulse of Emperor Justinian. Present are the physicians Hermophilus, Bassus, and Magistrianos.

Miniature, 15th century, University of Bologna.

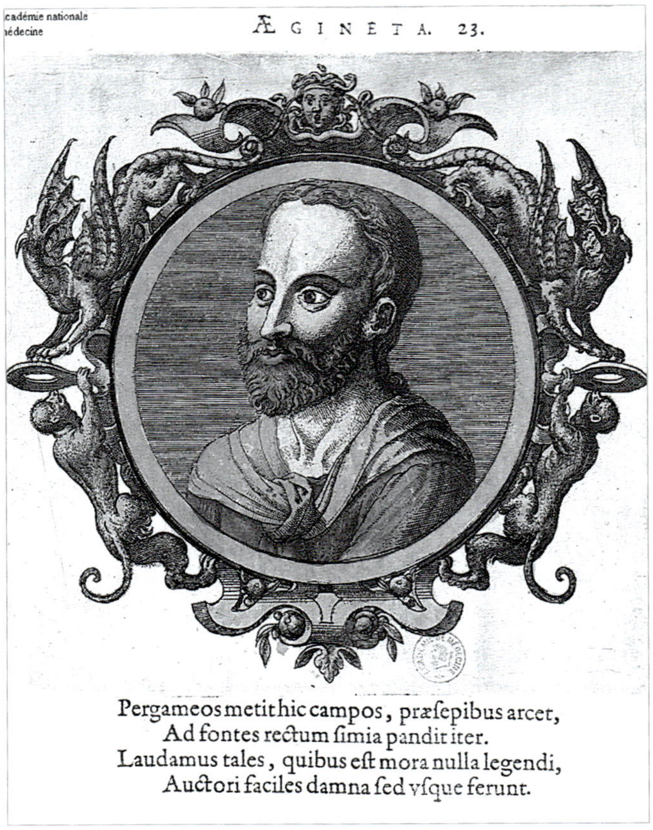

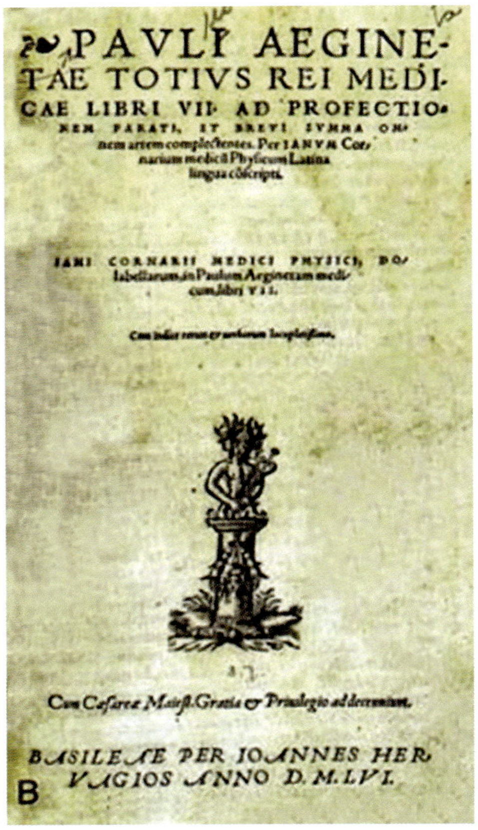

Paulus of Aegina.
Basel, 1556.

very important physician lived—Paul of Aegina (625–690). He was born on the island of Aegina and practiced medicine primarily in Alexandria, where he also died. He never went to Constantinople.

He is considered the last representative and continuator of the ancient Greek medical tradition. His written work, titled *Epitome of Medicine,* was highly esteemed by the Arabs, who translated it into Arabic in the 9th century. Through the Persian physician Rhazes (al-Rāzī) and the Arab Abu al-Qasim (Abulcasis), it made its way to the West in Latin translation. Paul of Aegina focused especially on surgery, developing his own operative techniques, including for the plastic repair of inguinal hernias. He describes various procedures such as lithotripsy, mastectomy, trepanation, tonsillectomy, and different types of punctures (e.g., for pleural effusions or other fluid collections). He performed tracheotomies and devised original surgical methods for treating vascular aneurysms, as well as for catarract surgery, where he used a special instrument known as the *parakeutērion* to remove the lens. The Arabs regarded him as the foremost obstetrician (calling him *Al-Qawābil*), because he had compiled and synthesized all existing knowledge on obstetrics.

Around the same time lived Theophilos Protospatharios, chief physician to Emperor Heraclius, who authored several medical treatises. One of his students was Stephanos the Athenian, a physician and mathematician born in Athens and active in Constantinople. Stephanos composed a work on the "*effect of medicines*" as well as a treatise on Hippocrates and Galen.

Paul of Aegina

In Chapter 45, "On Cancer", Paul of Aegina notes that the disease appears in many parts of the body, but most commonly in the womb and the breasts of women, and he explains the etymology of the term:

"It is called cancer (καρκίνος) because the veins around the tumor are stretched out in all directions, like the legs of the crab (*karkinos*), from which the disease also takes its name."

"The list continues throughout the long history of our Byzantine State. In the 9th century, a noteworthy physician was Leon the Iatrosophist, who performed tonsillectomies, provided a definition of asthma, and was the first to associate clubbing of the fingers with pulmonary diseases."

"What is pliktrodaktylia (clubbing of the fingers)?" Antigone asked.

"It is a condition where the tips of the fingers, around the nails, swell, and the fingers begin to resemble the rounded ends of drumsticks. Today we know it is caused by chronic lung disease, but it was Leo who first observed it, three hundred years ago. In the 10th century, Theophanes Nonnos appeared. He wrote an *Epitome of Medical Instructions and Treatment of Diseases*, in which he recognized that epilepsy was a brain disorder and not caused by metaphysical forces. However, the towering figure of the 10th century is the great Photius, who accomplished a vast philosophical, cultural, and philological mission. He also authored a critical assessment of the works of all prominent physicians from the 1st to the 6th century. Lastly, notable physicians of the 11th century include Nikitas Byzantios, Symeon Seth, and Michael Psellos. Byzantios authored the treatise *Surgical Compendium*, which contains many highly illustrative images. Symeon Seth, of Arab descent and born in Antioch, had a strong command of Arabic. He wrote a book describing the properties of new medicines coming from the East. He also published a noteworthy *Summary on Urine*, as well as treatises on smell, taste, and touch. He translated texts from Arabic and was instrumental in introducing numerous elements of Arab medical knowledge into Byzantium.

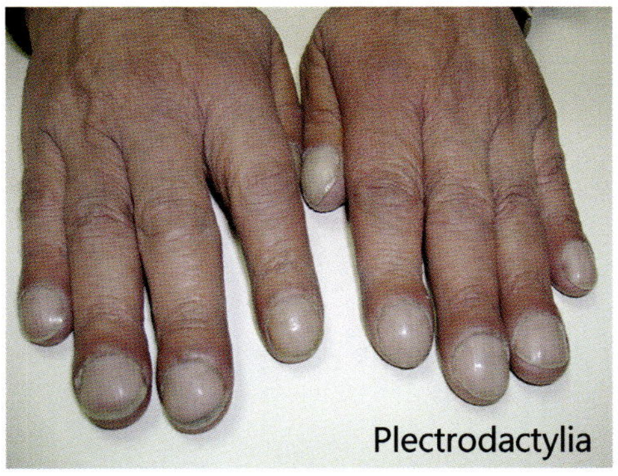

Plectrodactylia

I cannot overlook one of the most brilliant and multifaceted figures of our time, even though medicine was not his primary occupation—just as it wasn't for St. Basil the

Great. I speak of Michael Psellos (1018–1096), who was called the *Consul of the Philosophers*, and who, among many other roles, also served as Rector of our Pandidakterion. He produced a vast body of writings—on astronomy, philosophy, the natural sciences, and mathematics—and was also an outstanding chronicler. He held a deep admiration for classical antiquity and Platonic philosophy. His involvement in medicine was significant as well, and he authored works such as: *On the Power and Properties of Foods, On Lunar Disease (Epilepsy), An Anatomical Introduction* and *On the Interpretation of the Parts of the Body.*

My listeners, despite their interest, were probably growing a bit tired—and perhaps even dizzy—after hearing so many names and unfamiliar medical terms. Yet they followed my endless accounts without showing any sign of displeasure; on the contrary, they occasionally asked clarifying questions, eager to understand more.

"I won't tell you any more names because it might become too tiring," I told them. "These are the most prominent physicians up to today, whom I mentioned to you in brief. There were many others, less well known but no less worthy, whose works and accomplishments would take many pages to describe. All of them have brought medicine to the high level at which it now stands in Byzantium. What is particularly noteworthy about our physicians from the 6th century onward is that they no longer practice privately, but work in hospitals, in the xenones. There, they enjoy the privilege of collective labor and of applying their methods on a larger scale, which makes the evaluation of their results far more reliable. In the *xenones*, there is collaboration and ex-

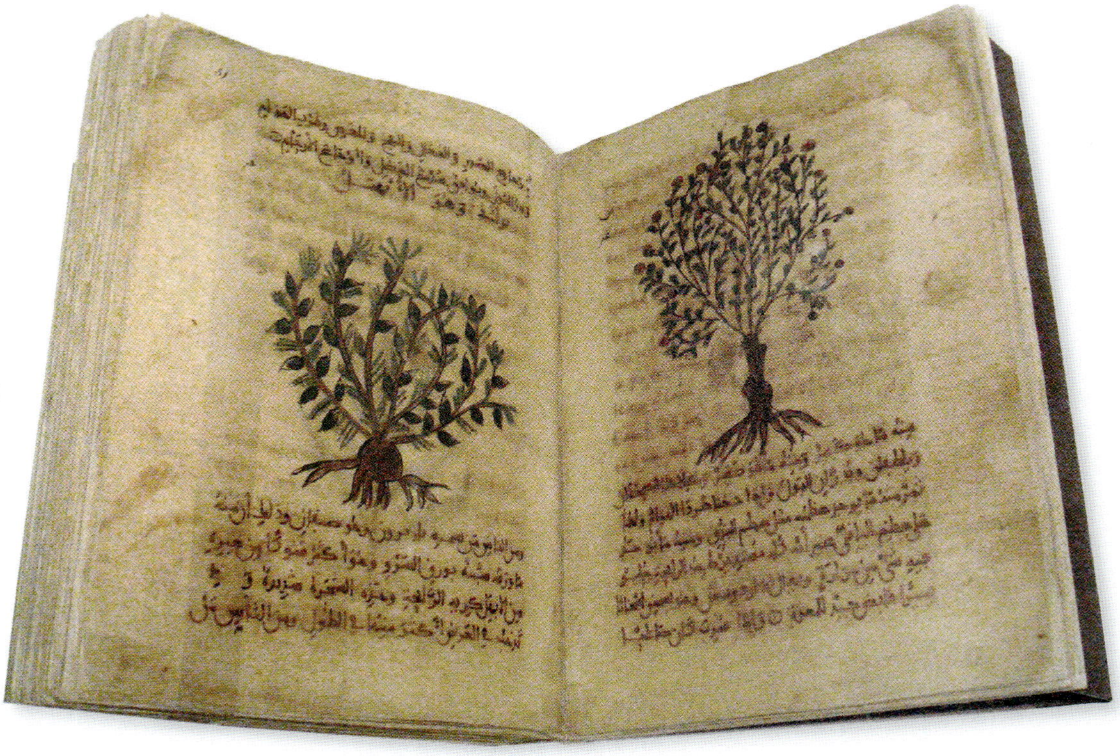

Dioscorides, On Medicine.

Arabic translation, 12th–13th century, Spain

change of knowledge and experience among physicians—something that has greatly propelled the advancement of medicine."

This truly was the defining distinction between our healthcare system and that of the West, where medicine remained largely a private affair. I felt deeply satisfied that my two listeners showed such interest in the stories I told them. And though they may have occasionally grown tired, they always followed with attention and admiration. What pleased me most of all was the look of wonder with which Antigone watched me—especially when, carried away by my own words, I would rise to my feet, almost moved, and describe with passion and detail the original treatments our renowned physicians applied to various illnesses.

Manuel Vlemmydes and I saw each other very often, especially in the early years at the Magnaura School, before I moved to the Xenon of the Mangana for my strictly medical studies. We were both filled with enthusiasm for our studies, our teachers, and the intellectual atmosphere that reigned at the Pandidakterion. Of course, there was great discipline, but these people loved their science, and you could see how devoted they were to the transmission of knowledge. Latin had long been abolished, and all the lessons were conducted in Greek. Our knowledge of Greek had become very deep through the continuous study of texts written in ancient or archaizing language. I had reached the point where I could comfortably understand the works of Plato, Euclid, and Hippocrates.

> "There are five branches of medicine: pharmacology, surgery, dietetics, diagnostics, and therapeutics. Pharmacology heals illnesses through the use of drugs; Surgery restores health by cutting and cauterizing; Dietetics relieves illness through regulated lifestyle and diet; Diagnostics through identifying the disease; And therapeutics provides immediate relief from pain by offering assistance."
>
> Aristotle, *On Divisions.*

Manuel and I used to exchange our knowledge and the plans we had for our lives. I would speak to him about the methods of medicine and the wondrous secrets of the human body, about the miracle of health and the proper functioning of the organism, as well as about the tragedy of decay and illness, which lead to death. Manuel was an artistic type. He was involved in painting and explained many things to me about that art during our long discussions as we walked back from Magnaura.

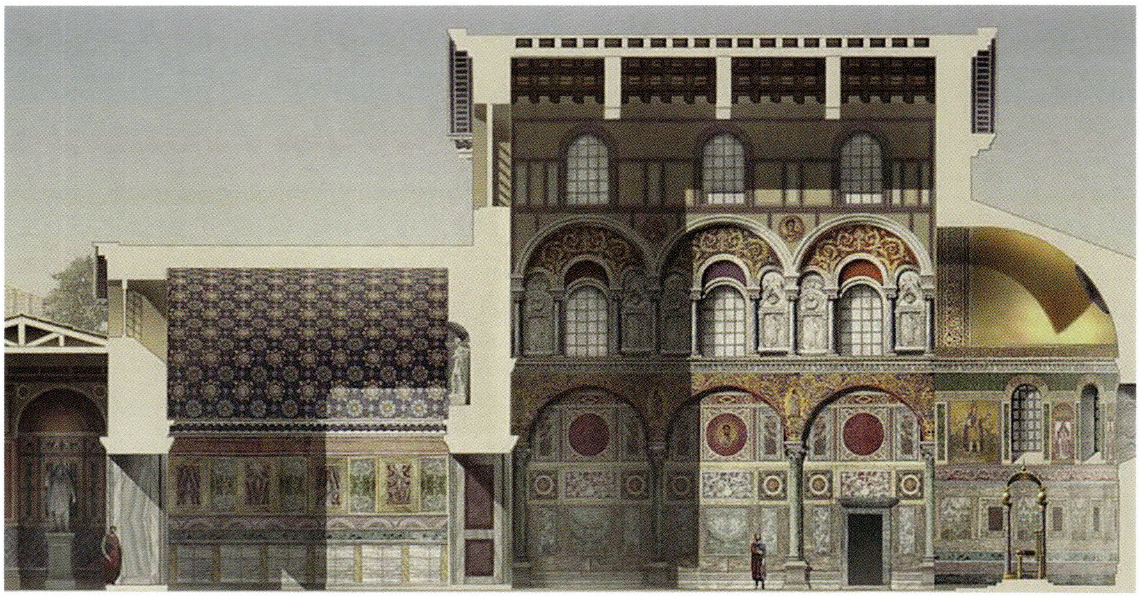

The Great Peristyle. *Reconstruction by Antoine Helbert, 1876.*

"I'm thinking, Nikiforos," he used to tell me, "of devoting myself to painting, which expresses me and gives me the means to 'speak' another language—the language of art, which does not simply depict, but transforms the world. The painter does not merely aim to reproduce the world as it is, but to offer his own perspective and emotional insight, to present the world as he sees it—or as he would like to see it. Painting in our time is primarily iconography, but I believe that through the depictions of scenes from the life of our Lord, or of the feats and martyrdoms of our saints, I will be given the opportunity to express my own artistic views—naturally within the bounds of our Byzantine style."

Speaking with genuine passion, he continued to reveal to me the secrets of his art:

"The artists of our Eastern Empire, influenced by ancient Greek painting and the Fayum portraits of Egypt—which are its natural continuation—strive to endow the depicted figures with an element of eternity, something that does not portray the marks of decay. The painting of our time, already from the 4th century, is almost exclusively ecclesiastical—that is, iconography."

Beyond the mosaics, which we have already discussed, icons are either wall paintings in churches using the fresco technique, or portable icons painted on wood. The depictions represent Christ, the Theotokos, or the Saints—either in full figure or just their faces—as well as complex scenes from the life of our Lord, such as the Crucifixion, the Resurrection, the Baptism, and so forth. Scenes are also depicted from the life of the Virgin Mary or of the Saints, whose martyrdom is often the subject portrayed. The wall paintings are created using the technique of fresco—what the Franks call *fresco,* meaning painted on fresh plaster.

This ancient technique is truly fascinating. The pigments exist in powdered form and are derived from processed stones, minerals, plants, and so on. They

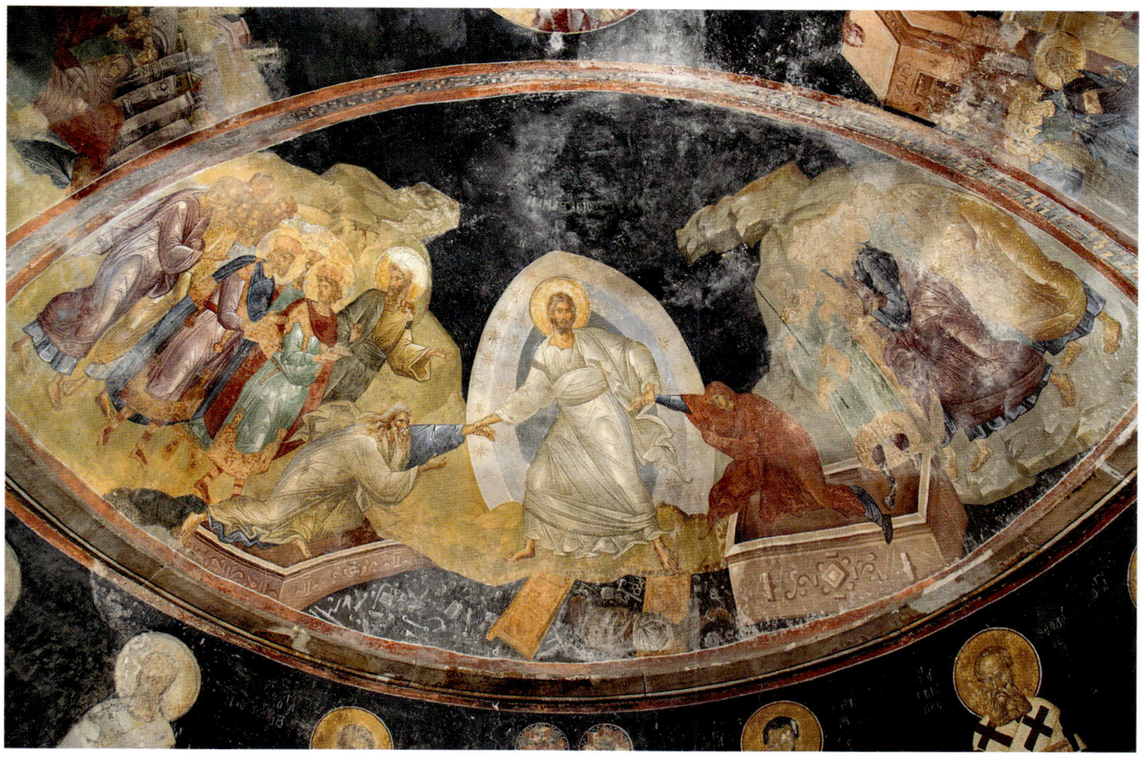

The Resurrection of Christ.

Fresco, 14th century, Chapel of the Chora Monastery.

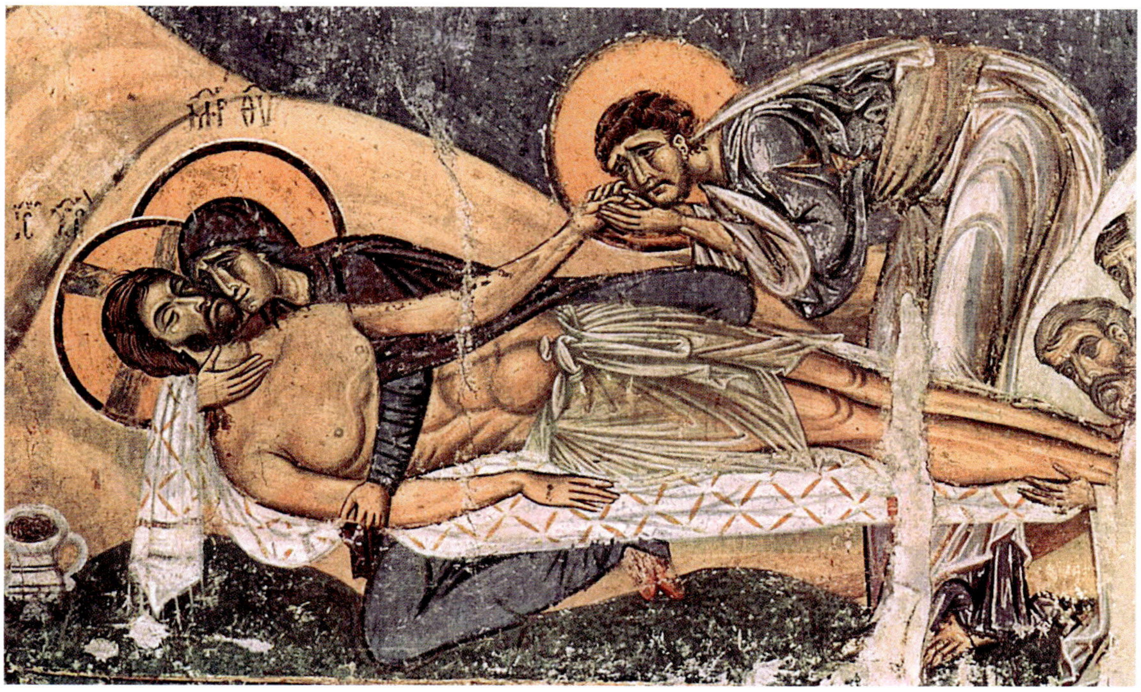

Lamentation over the Dead Christ.

Fresco, 12th century, Nerezi Monastery, Northern Macedonia.

bear curious names such as raw umber, burnt sienna, ochre, cinnabar, and others. These are dissolved in limewater and used to paint the wall. However, there is an essential detail: if paint is applied to a wall that has already dried, the color simply adheres like a crust, which, after some years and with moisture, will begin to peel off. Thus, the craftsmen follow this method: the painter estimates the surface he can cover in one day, and either he or the mason plasters just that portion with fine lime plaster (*psilo*). He then paints it while it is still fresh, so the color fuses with the plaster and is preserved for many

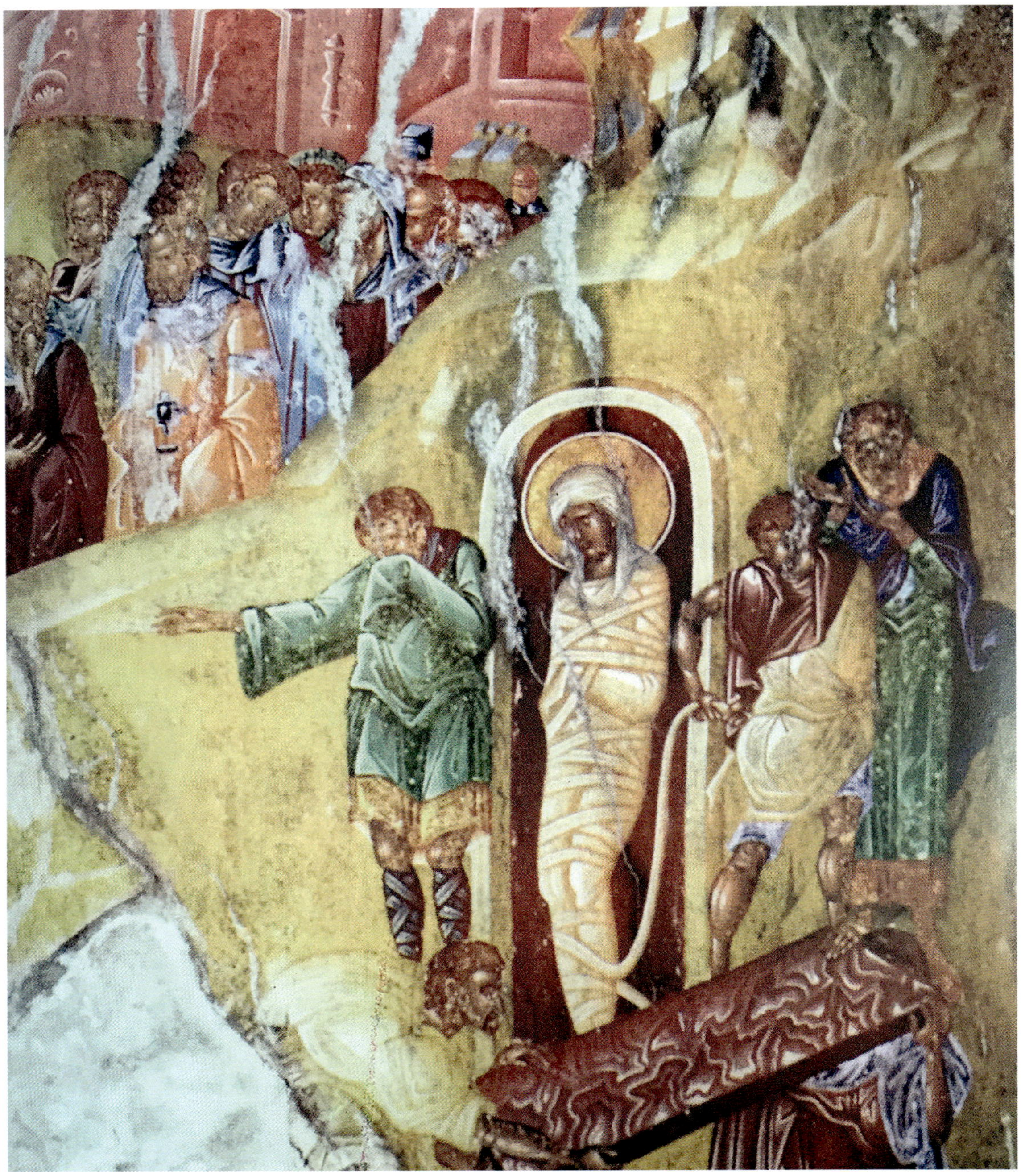

Raising of Lazarus.
Fresco, 15th century, Pantanassa Monastery, Mystras.

years. Fresco painting as a technique dates back to Minoan Crete. As for portable icons, the wood is first prepared by coating it with an animal-based glue, and the pigments are mixed with egg yolk and a bit of water. The earliest technique used in portable icons was encaustic painting, where the pigments were dissolved in melted wax and mastic, and the solution had to be used while still warm. This method was used to paint the *Fayum* portraits in Egypt and some early masterpieces of the 6th century, such as the Christ Pantocrator, the Enthroned Theotokos, and Saint Peter of the Monastery of Sinai. Today, this technique is no longer used, as it is technically quite difficult.

"Byzantine art is both a continuation and a development of classical Greek art. The choice of colors and themes is similar—there is a focus on the face—but now it is no longer a mere imitation of reality. Instead, it seeks to express an eschatological perspective of eternity. Anti-realist forms in painting began to prevail already in late antiquity, independent of Christian art, under the influence of Neoplatonic ideas espoused by Plotinus. Plotinus argued that true knowledge is attained by approaching the suprarational core of things, beyond the external attributes of matter. In art, this is achieved by eliminating space, perspective, the horizon line, targeted lighting, and the volume of forms. Christian art adopted these principles as well, aiming to transcend corporeality and sensory engagement with the natural world."

My friend spoke to me with passion about the uniqueness of Byzantine painting. His face lit up as he explained how the *proplasmos* is done—how they begin with the darker tones and then proceed with the *highlights* on the garments and the *flesh tones* on the faces, gradually illuminating the icon with increasingly lighter colors.

"The painter's journey moves from dark to light. At the end come the *psimmythia*—the delicate white touches of light added at the final stage of the work. The illumination is otherworldly; it comes from the front and falls perpendicularly onto the surface of the icon, with minimal shadows. The background is usually blue or azure in wall paintings, while in portable icons they favored orange, and later, gold. The expression of the face does not depict a fleeting emotion, but rather seeks to convey a sense of eternity. The faces of the saints are surrounded by a luminous golden halo, which is not a crown, but a circle of light, as if the face itself radiates divine brilliance."

"Iconography in our Eastern Empire expresses the Hellenic aesthetic perception of the human face. Its first flourishing spanned from the 4th to the 8th

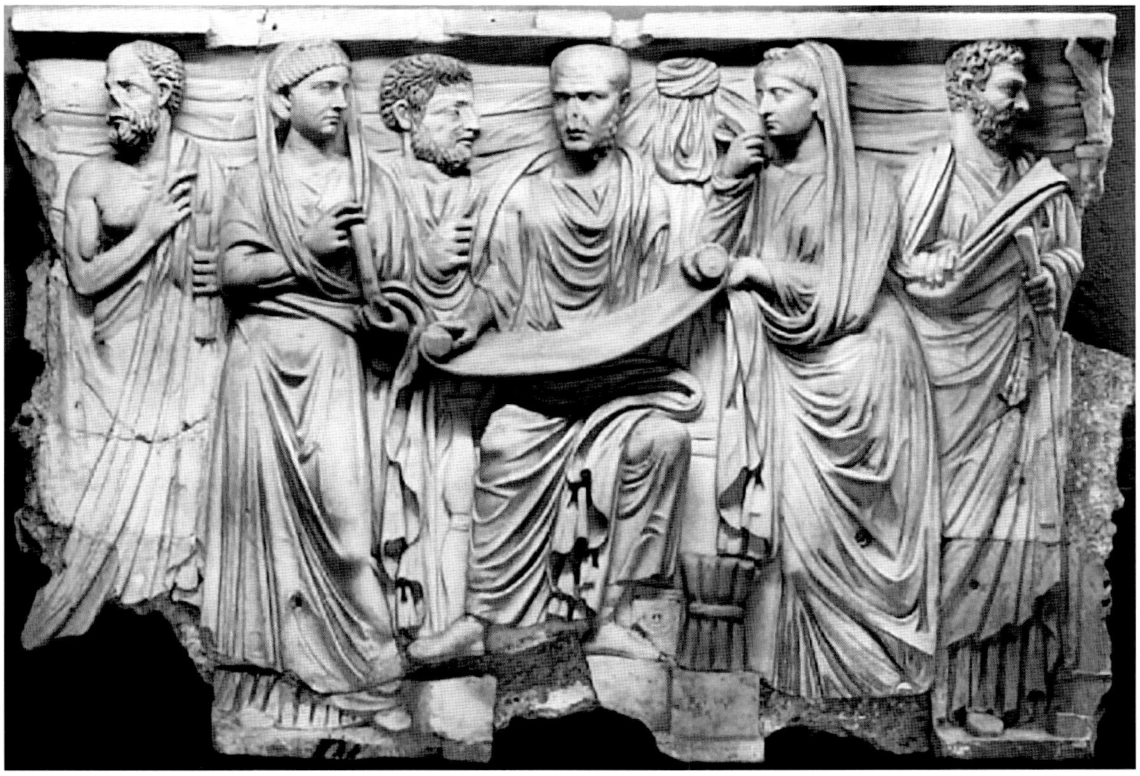

Roman Sarcophagus Depicting Plotinus and His Disciples.

Vatican Museums, Rome

century. The years from 730 to 843 are overshadowed by the dark period of Iconoclasm. Iconoclasm is a very significant and controversial phenomenon in the history of Christianity and Art. The aniconic notions of the eastern peoples, combined with the reaction against the excesses of popular superstition surrounding icons—which at times approached outright worship—led a series of politically and militarily capable emperors, along with a portion of the populace, first to the removal of icons from churches and later to their destruction. The veneration of icons and relics was regarded as idolatry. Invaluable works of art were destroyed in a resurgence of fanaticism. It is no coincidence that these emperors primarily came from the eastern regions of the Empire. This internal conflict—essentially a clash between the Eastern aniconic worldview and the Greco-Roman visual conception of expression—shook the Eastern Empire to its foundations. In the end, the iconophile view prevailed and was affirmed by an Ecumenical Council as the Orthodox position. Icons returned to the churches, and a great artistic renaissance took place during the blessed era of the Macedonian Emperors. Now, under the Komnenian dynasty, iconography is experiencing a second great flourishing, with masterpieces created in Constantinople, Venice, Thessaloniki, Nerezi, Kastoria, Patmos, Cyprus, Cappadocia, Sicily, and Kiev. Iconography has now reached marvelous aesthetic and spiritual heights. Especially in depictions of the Passion, the expression of suffering is rendered in astonishingly human tones—a new element that entered the art form. The movement, the drapery of the garments, the postures of the figures—these have all attained a level of refined elegance and profound inspiration. I believe, said Manuel, that in our day, our painting has reached an unmatched pinnacle."

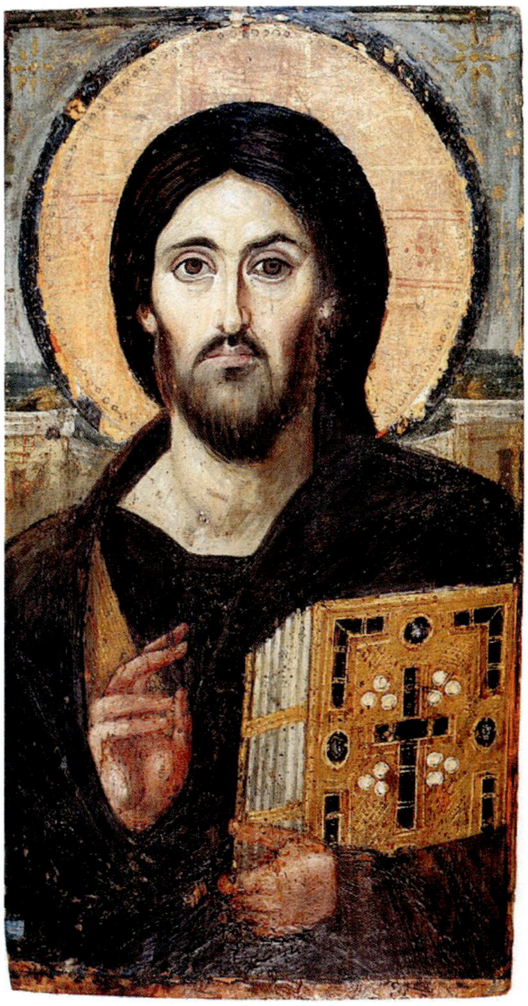

Christ of Saint Catherine's Monastery, Mount Sinai.

Encaustic Icon, 6th century.

The Komnenoi Emperors and Medicine in Byzantium

The years passed quickly, and I completed my studies in Medicine. My training took place at the Xenon of Mangana, where I finalized my theoretical knowledge, but more importantly, I gained substantial experience by observing treatments and taking part in the care of patients and in surgical operations. The Actuarios—the official in charge, who had direct access to the Emperor as his personal physician—oversaw our training alongside the medical instructors. By the time I graduated, I had learned all the diagnostic methods used today, the principles of dietary treatment, and the latest medications prescribed for various illnesses. I was capable of performing major surgical procedures, having acquired experience at the side of the esteemed doctors of the Xenon. I embarked on my medical career filled with dreams and hope. My profession had inspired me deeply. Although our science was powerless in the face of many diseases, there were not a few cases where proper and timely care truly saved the patient's life.

Floor plan of the Hospital of the Monastery of Varlaam at Meteora.

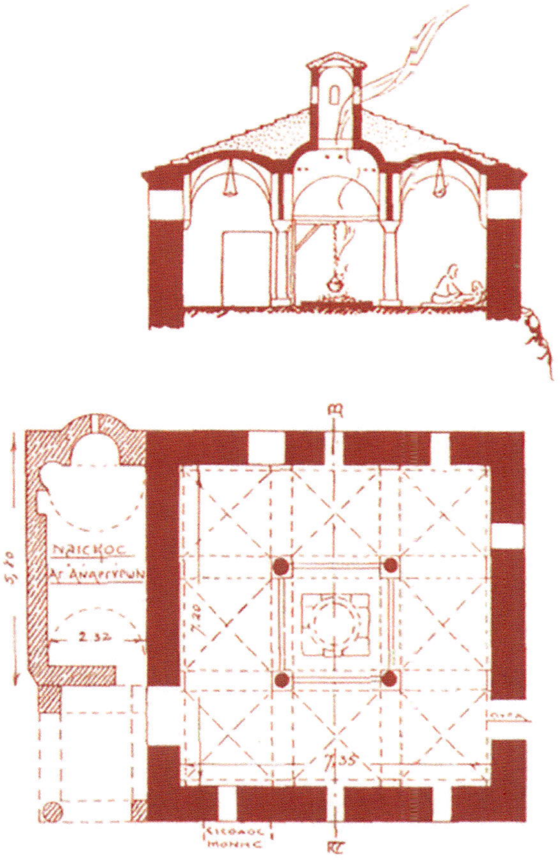

In all cases, however, as a physician I had the opportunity to offer support and comfort to those who were suffering—something that gave me strength and great satisfaction. A kind word, a piece of advice, a gesture of genuine care and concern, a presence beside someone in pain—these benefit the patient far more than we often imagine. Sometimes, even more than medicine itself. When a person becomes seriously ill, it is as if the ground beneath their feet vanishes. They are overwhelmed by the anxiety of pain and death, the fear of losing loved ones, of financial ruin. They lose the ability to govern themselves, become dependent on others, and are transferred into an unfamiliar environment that frightens them. In such a moment, it is vital that they hear a kind word, that they feel someone cares, that they are not just a number in a faceless crowd. I believe this is one of the

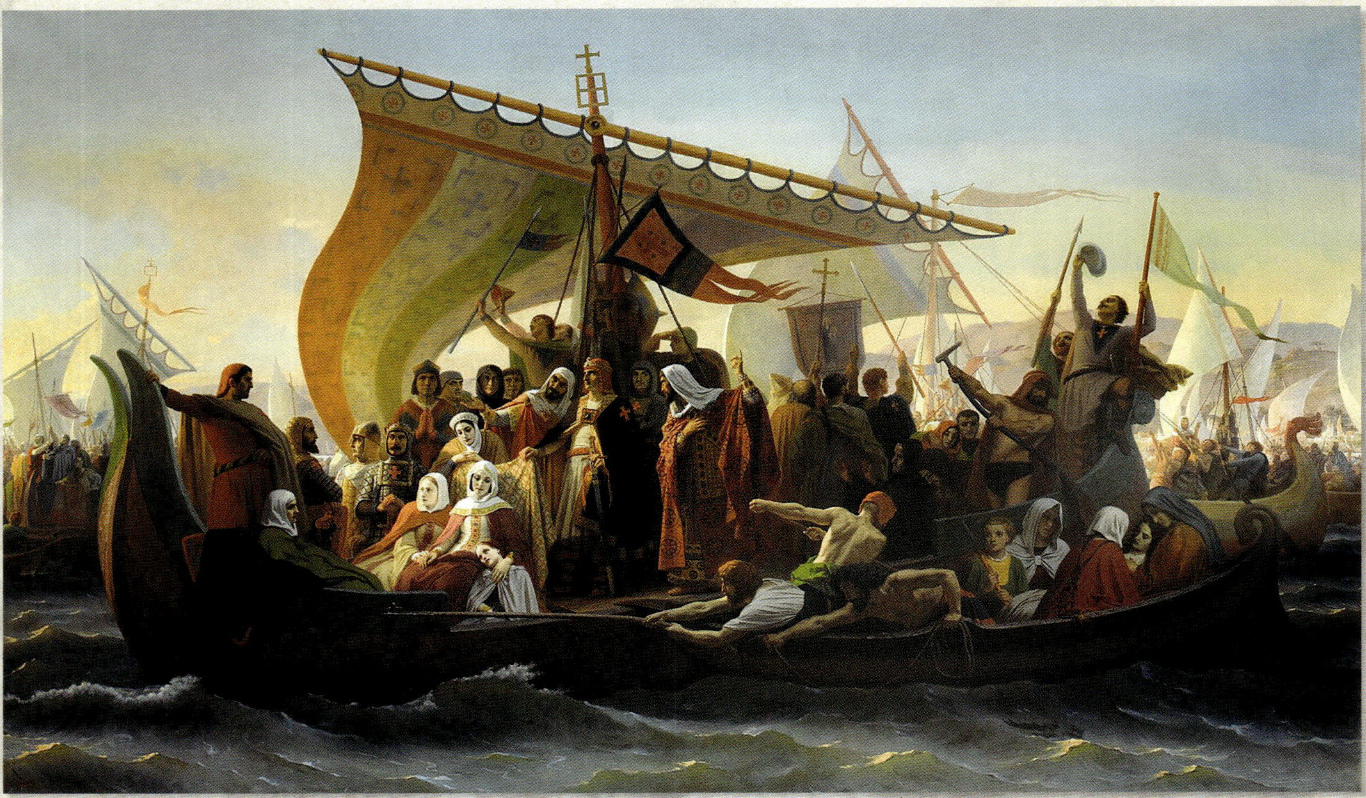

The leaders of the First Crusade cross the Bosphorus in Greek ships.

Painting by Emil Signol, 1854, Palace of Versailles, France

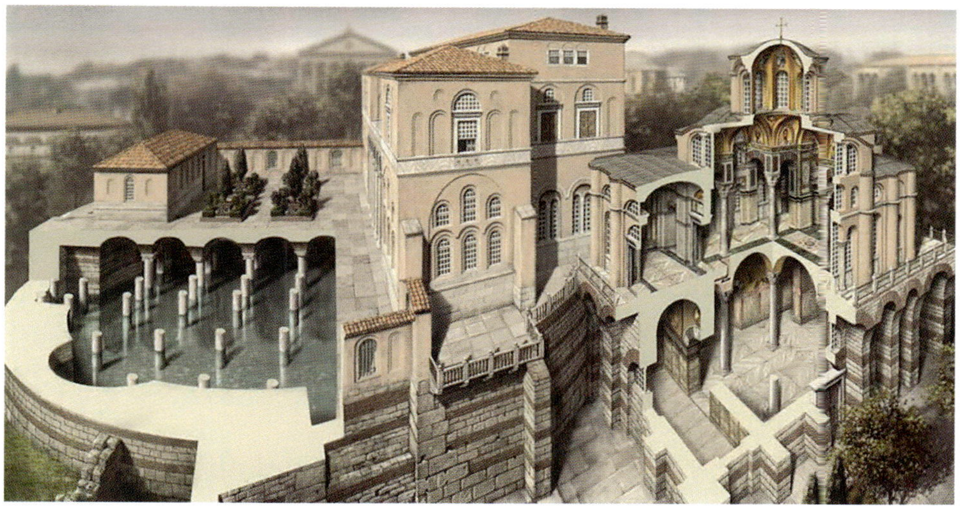

The palace of Romanos Lekapenos next to the Myrelaion, where the homonymous xenon (hospital) was located.

Reconstruction by Antoine Helbert, 1876.

most important roles of a physician.

Naturally, at the same time, the physician must be well-informed in his science so as to make an accurate diagnosis and prescribe the correct treatments. And if he cannot help, he should at the very least do no harm—a principle not always upheld, especially with the countless charlatans and quack doctors who roamed the City. It was first said by the great Hippocrates himself: "To benefit, or at least do no harm."

Of all the healing methods, surgery moved me most deeply. I watched my experienced teachers with awe as they prepared the patient and administered sedatives to ease the pain; then, with exceptional skill and swiftness, they would remove the cause of the illness—whether it was a purulent abscess, a diseased and damaged organ, or a tumor. The result was immediate and striking. The patient would feel relief at once. There were many specialized instruments used in the operations, which I will describe later. But they truly confirmed the second maxim of the great Master: "What medicines do not heal, iron heals." Indeed, Hippocrates in his work *On Fractures* writes that the art of surgery "is not for every man," meaning it is not something anyone can undertake.

At the head of the hospital is, as we have said, the *Aktouarios*, who in other xenones (hospices) is called *Primikērios*. Next come the assistant directors, known as *Protomēnitai*, followed by the specialized physicians, called *Koinoi* or *Embathmoi*, and finally we stu-

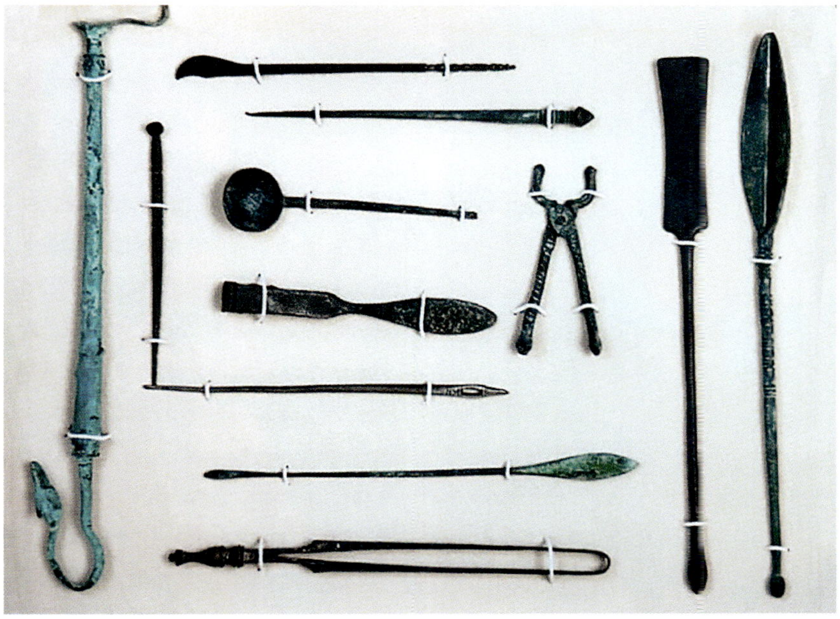

Imitation of Hippocratic surgical instruments.

National Archaeological Museum, Athens.

dents, referred to as *Perissoi* or *Hyperarithmoi* ("Supernumeraries"). We *perissoi*, along with the *koinoi*, would attend the xenon daily, and during the summer season—from the First of May until the Feast of the Cross (September 14)—we also attended in the evenings. In addition to the aforementioned physicians, there were also the *Teachers of Medicine*, whose exclusive role was our education. They primarily taught us theory, assessed our knowledge daily, and finally, once our training was complete, subjected us to a thorough examination, both theoretical and practical, and awarded us the diploma that certified our medical qualification and granted us the right to practice the profession.

When I completed my studies and received the much-coveted diploma, in the year 1173, I was twenty-three years old. I was proud to have succeeded in becoming a physician in the most civilized state of the oikoumene—the Eastern Roman Empire, our rightful heir to the Universal Roman Empire—within which existed the most advanced system of health care and the most esteemed physicians of the age. During my studies, I had shown great diligence and industriousness, and my teachers held me in high regard. As a result, I had excellent references that would help me find a position as an Embathmos, that is, a certified physician, in a good xenon. In Constantinople, there were many xenones of high-quality care, but the one that stood out above all was the Xenon of the Monastery of the Pantocrator, founded by our good Emperor, Lord John Komnenos, and his wife, the Augusta Irene. There was great competition among physicians for positions there, but I had very strong recommendations, and, with the connections of Theodoros Vlemmydes, I had every hope of being appointed.

I was eager to work as a head physician in a hospital. The idea of practicing privately never crossed my mind, even though in the City, those private phy-

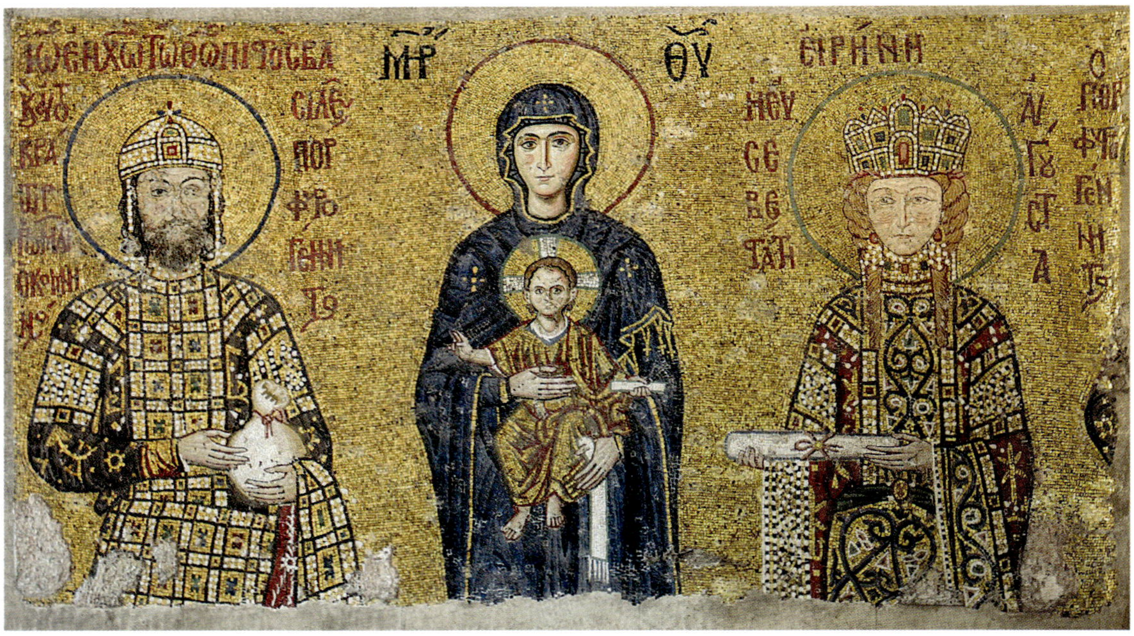

John Komnenos and Irene of Hungary.
Mosaic, 11th century, Hagia Sophia.

sicians who built up a clientele earned far more than hospital doctors, who—as full-time employees—were not permitted to work privately or to accept gifts (the so-called "blessings" or "tokens of love") from patients. I believed that medicine was a mission and a sacred calling, not a means of getting rich. Besides, the physicians of the xenones were held in great esteem and respect by the people, unlike private doctors, who were seen as greedy and exploitative, and were generally disliked. With youthful zeal, I believed then that I could change the world. That I could put into practice the principles my teachers had instilled in me—from Father Porphyrios and Tornikes in Patras, to the great instructors at the School of Magnaura and the Xenon of the Mangana. Foremost among these principles was the virtue of love for the one who suffers—for the *neighbor,* as it flows from Christian teaching. Secondly, there was the principle of healing the sick, rooted in the Hellenic perspective that man is not an isolated individual, but a member of a harmonious whole. Healing aims to restore not only the body's dysfunctions but also the disturbances of the soul. Man is called to restore his relationship with nature and with God, to bring his existence into harmony with the cosmic order. The physician's role is to guide him toward that restoration—not merely to correct a physical ailment.

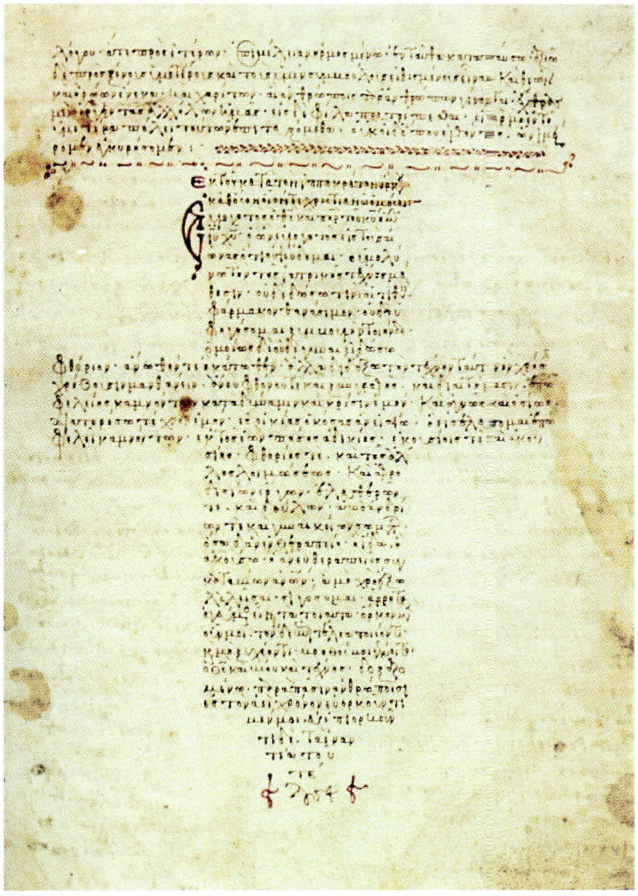

The Hippocratic Oath in the Shape of a Cross.

Manuscript, 12th century, Vatican Library, Rome.

During my years of study, my relationship with Antigone blossomed into a strong bond of love, mutual admiration, and respect. Gradually, we began seeing each other more often—and eventually, without the presence of my sister. Sensing what was unfolding and loving us both, she would kindly find a reason to step away and leave us alone. Our parents viewed our relationship very favorably, and so, once I had completed my studies, we were married in the beautiful church of the Monastery of Chora. The atmosphere was deeply spiritual and celebratory. Our parents, siblings, family friends, and many of my fellow students were present—friends who had come to know her well, especially during the last year when our relationship had become official and she would often accompany me to the Xenon of the Mangana, where she came as something of a nursing apprentice.

My relationship with Antigone ultimately had a deeply beneficial effect on my life. There was a positive atmosphere surrounding us that greatly strengthened me in my struggle to practice medicine faithfully. Her support sustained me during the difficult moments—when a patient's case had a poor outcome, or in the face of rivalry from certain colleagues. Through her steady demeanor, she helped me avoid slipping into pride or arrogance, or chasing after wealth and power. She remained the pure idealist who believed in me—and this belief of hers, in a certain way, "obliged" me to live up to her expectations.

In 1173, when I was beginning my career, our state was in one of its finest periods. In the 850 years that had passed since the founding of Constantinople, it had witnessed eras of flourishing greatness as well as times of humiliation and decline. In the 10th century, under the Macedonian dynasty, there was a remarkable period of military and cultural flourishing. Byzantine art had reached its peak, and our state stood as the most powerful and cultured in all of Europe. Then came the disaster at Manzikert in 1071, followed by a string of defeats by the Turks and the Normans, which led to a contraction of the Empire. Fortunately, in 1082, the blessed Komnenos dynasty rose to power, beginning with the great Emperor Alexios I, who reigned for nearly 40 years until 1118. He halted the decline that had gripped the state under the previous inept emperors, reorganized the army and the economy, halted the Norman advance, and with the aid of the Crusaders managed to reclaim vast regions of Asia Minor that had been seized by the Turks. He also restored the prestige of the Empire, though still diminished compared to earlier times. He was followed by the brilliant reign of John II, known as Kalojannis, from 1118 until 1143, and since then, the throne has been held by Kyr Manuel, who through his prudent governance and military victories over the Turks has brought the state to a radiant flourishing.

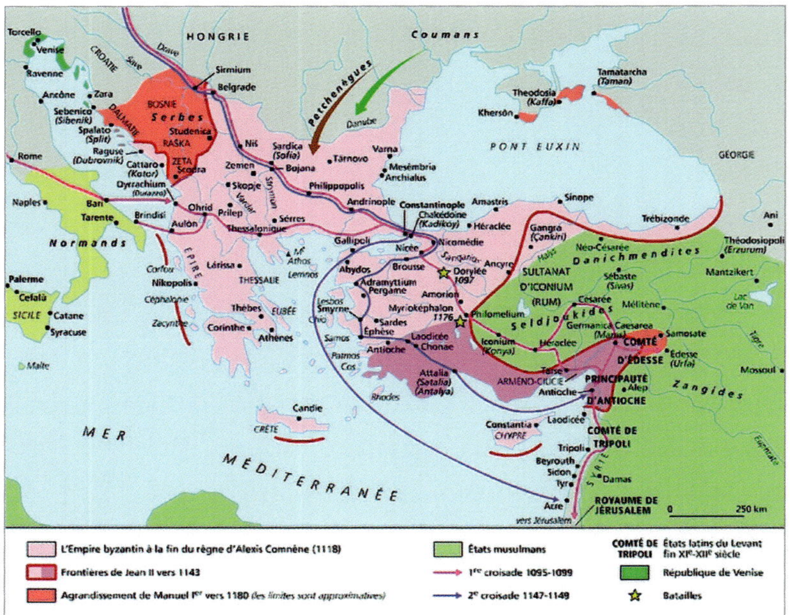

The Empire under the Komnenoi, 12th Century.

Map, Larousse Archive.

When Alexios I ascended the throne in 1081, the Seljuk Turks, during the decade following the defeat at Manzikert, had taken over nearly the whole of Asia Minor, sparing only a narrow strip around the Sea of Marmara. The Normans had seized Sicily and Southern Italy and had landed in Epirus, laying siege to Dyrrhachium. The army was in disarray, and the currency—the *solidus*—was plummeting in value. Alexios reorganized the army, brought the provincial lords—who had begun to show separatist tendencies—under control, and restructured the economy by strengthening trade.

Peter the Hermit Leading the First Crusade (of the Poor).

Miniature, 14th century, Avignon, France.

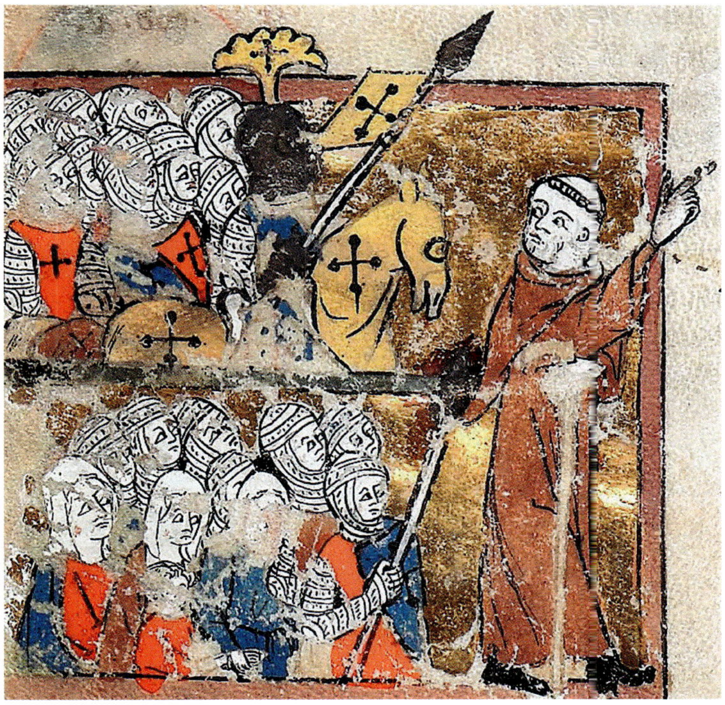

He also minted a new gold coin, the hyperpyron. In order to bolster commerce, he was, unfortunately, compelled to grant many privileges to the Italian trading cities—Venice, Genoa, and Pisa—and as a result, many Italian merchants settled in Constantinople. This proved to be a poor decision in the long term, bringing great misfortunes upon the Empire, though at the time it seemed necessary. Particularly masterful was the way in which he dealt with the arrogant and aggressive Crusaders of the First Crusade.

The first unruly waves of Crusaders, led by Peter the Hermit, arrived in Constantinople in the summer of 1096. The Emperor swiftly arranged for their passage across the Bosphorus into Asia Minor. There, they were scattered and decimated by the Turks, with only a handful of survivors returning to the City—humbled and broken. A few months later, in November, the real army of the Crusade began to arrive—well-organized and led by prominent nobles: Godfrey of Bouillon, Raymond of Toulouse, and Bohemond of Taranto. Their presence signaled a new, more formidable phase of the First Crusade, and the Emperor had to navigate with both tact and firmness the challenges they brought to the Empire's doorstep.

The Crusaders were proud and aggressive, but Alexios, with a masterful use of both "carrot and stick," managed to bring them under control and use them to his advantage. He transported them across to Asia Minor, providing them

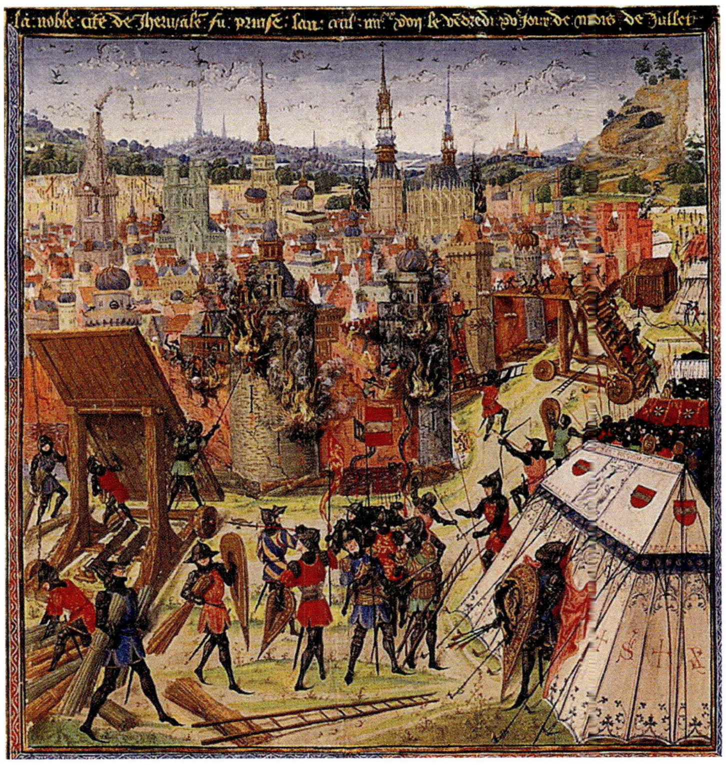

The First Crusade in 1099.

Miniature by Sébastien Mamerot, 15th century, National Library of France, Paris.

with guides, troops, and provisions, and in return secured their oath to hand over to him all the lands they would conquer, up to and including Antioch. With the support of our imperial forces, the Crusaders defeated the Turks, seized Antioch, and eventually went on to capture Jerusalem. They refused to hand over the possessions they had promised and organized the so-called overseas (*outre mer*) Latin principalities, such as the Kingdom of Jerusalem, the Principalities of Antioch and Cilicia, and the Counties of Tripoli and Edessa. As was to be expected, many misunderstandings and hostilities arose on both sides, which fostered distrust and animosity between the Westerners and the Byzantines. In the end, however, Alexios succeeded in reattaching a large part of Asia Minor to Byzantium.

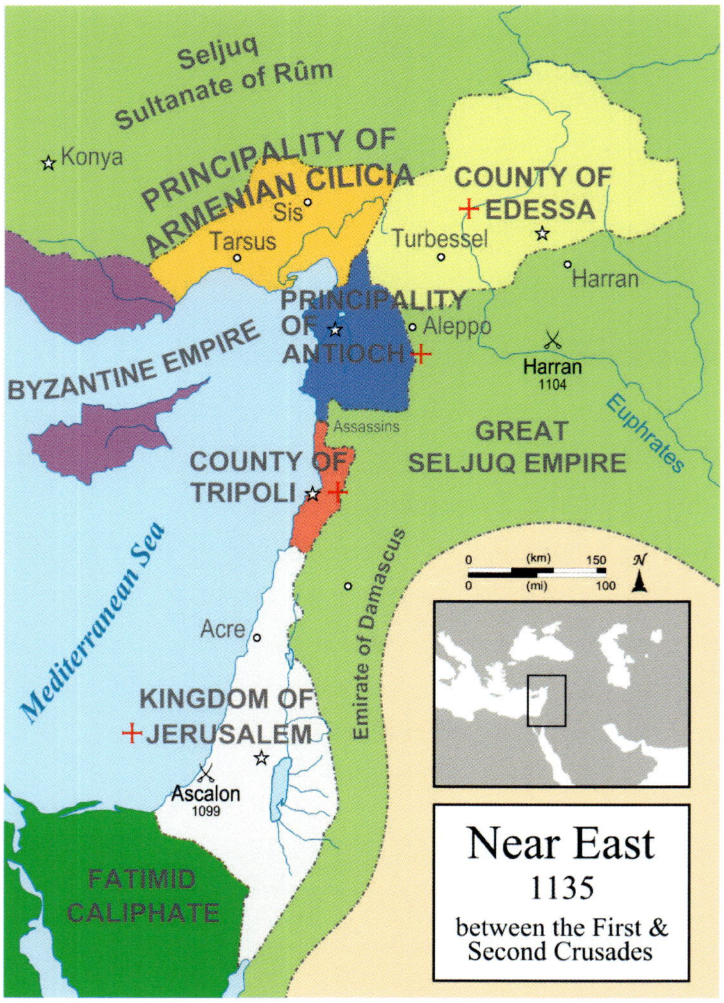

The Overseas Latin States in the East (Outremer), after the First Crusade, 1197.

Map by MapMaster.

There was no shortage of unpleasant aspects within the Imperial family, proving once again the well-known truth: that social and intellectual cultivation does not correct weaknesses and passions—especially ambition and pride. Alexios, together with his wife Irene Doukaina, had eight children: three sons and five daughters. The firstborn was Anna, a gifted and remarkably intelligent young woman, but highly ambitious. She received an exceptional education within the palace, married an aristocrat from her mother's lineage—Nikephoros Bryennios—and harbored the ambition to become co-emperor alongside her husband in place of her brother John, who was the eldest son and the natural heir. At the age of 68, Alexios fell ill, and when his condition worsened, he was transferred to the Xenon of the Mangana for better care. Anna, with the support of her mother, attempted to seize the throne by coup and to have her brother killed—but John acted swiftly. He went to his dying father, who gave him his blessing and the imperial ring. Taking the conspirators by surprise, John immediately assumed power, taking possession of the palace and being crowned Emperor of the Romans. It was then that he revealed the noble character for which he earned the epithet *Kalogiannis* ("John the Good"). Although his mother and sister once again tried to overthrow him, he forgave them. Vryennios, who had conducted himself honorably and did not share his wife's ambitions, was allowed to retain his position. Anna retired to a monastery, where she composed a large historical work in imitation of the Iliad, the *Alexiad*, recounting the deeds of her father. The reign of John the Good was a blessed time for Byzantium. He was deeply pious, lived a life of austerity and modesty in private, yet carried himself with imperial dignity in public. His justice became proverbial. During his reign, no one was condemned to death or mutilated for political reasons. He was a highly capable general and warrior—the very model of the emperor-soldier.

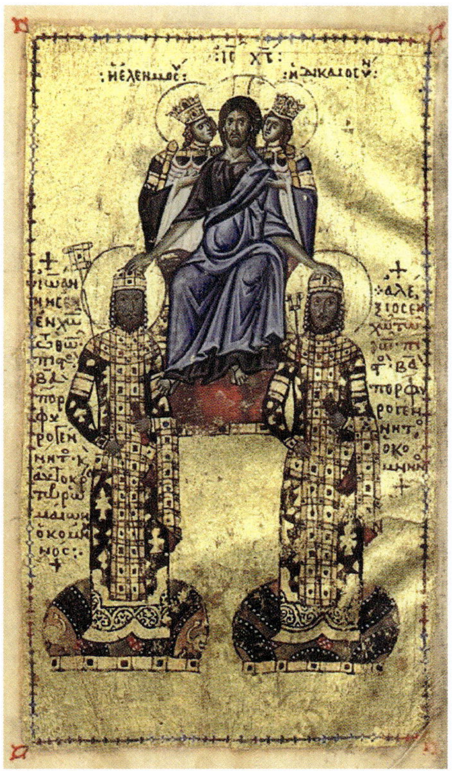

John II Komnenos and his son Alexios, "Co-Emperor."

Miniature, 12th century, Vatican Library, Rome.

He allied himself with the Germans of the so-called Holy Roman Empire and, with their help, halted the advance of the Normans. He defeated the Pechenegs, the Hungarians, and the Serbs in the Balkans, as well as the Seljuk Turks in Asia Minor, reclaiming most of the peninsula. The Crusader states of Antioch, Tripoli, and Edessa declared vassalage to the Roman Emperor. The economy grew stronger, and the population of the Empire increased. Together with his wife, Irene of Hungary, he undertook many public works, the most important of which was the founding of the Monastery of the Pantocrator. This grand complex included a hospital, a home for the elderly, and a leper asylum.

All this was recounted to me by Manuel's father, Theodore Vlemmydes, who, as I mentioned, though a merchant by trade, had many interests—especially in history. He would often speak to Manuel and me about the history of our Empire, describing events and interpreting their meaning and consequences. He used to tell us that history is the great teacher, helping one to interpret current events and foresee what might yet come to pass. The evenings spent discussing history with Kyr Theodore were truly a delight, and of course, the two young women would also listen in when they didn't have pressing duties around the house. Master Theodore would say to us:

"Kaloyannis, always fighting on the front lines alongside his sons, after 25 years of reign, had the misfortune during a wild boar hunt to be wounded in the arm by a poisoned arrow and died of sepsis in April of 1143.

John II Komnenos on the fatal boar hunt.

Miniature by the Maître de Fauvel, 13th century, National Library of France, Paris.

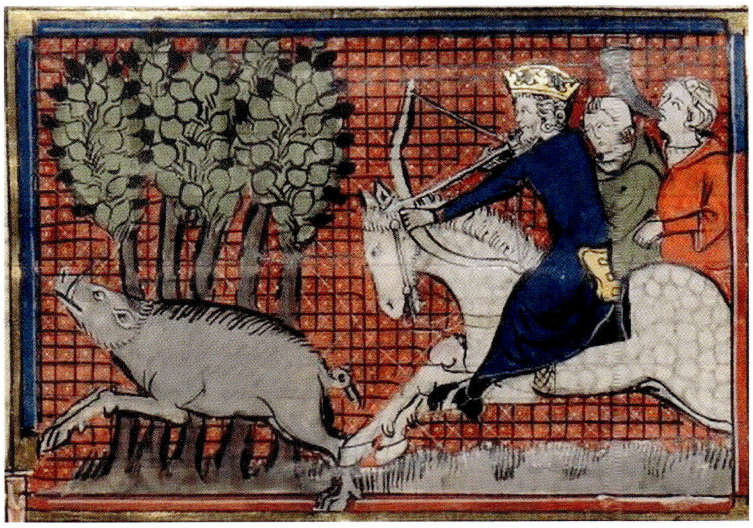

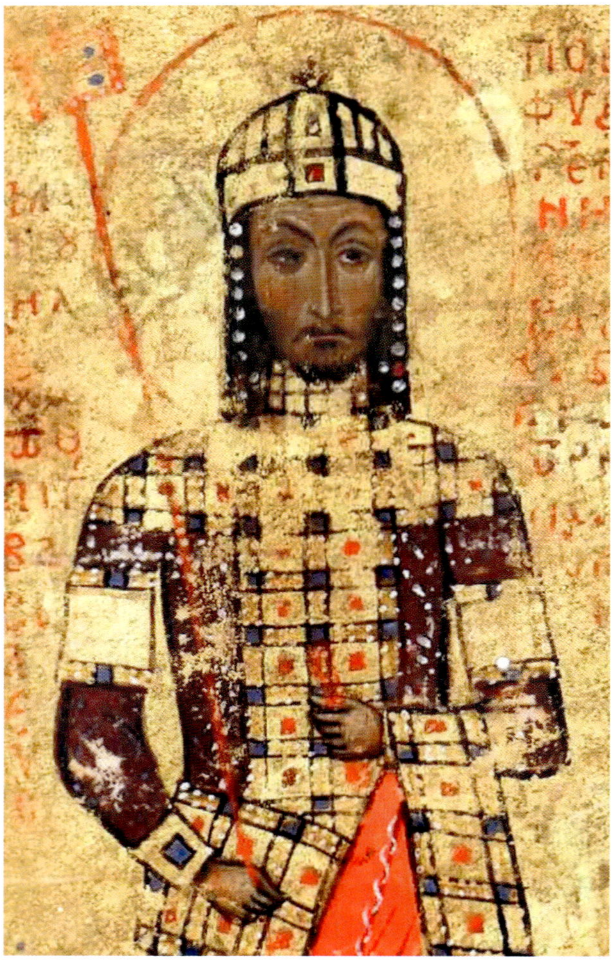

Manuel Komnenos.

Miniature, 12th century, Vatican Library, Rome.

The people mourned him like a father. Fortunately, he was worthily succeeded by his second son, Manuel, whom his father had chosen as heir due to his capability and bravery—and everyone accepted that choice. The reign of Lord Manuel was the most illustrious of the Komnenoi. Manuel was an irresistible warrior; the tales of his exploits in battle are countless. The Westerners respected and honored him. He himself organized jousting tournaments in the Hippodrome, where he had defeated many Frankish and Italian knights. You see, the old chariot races that once thrilled the people have now been forgotten. When he ascended the throne, the Normans had taken over all of southern Italy and Sicily, the Seljuks had conquered nearly all of central Asia Minor, and in the Middle East, a new power had arisen—the "overseas" Crusader states in Syria and Palestine, the legacy of the First Crusade. His empire was in danger from every side. Nevertheless, his stance toward the rulers of the West was that of a suzerain Emperor—the only legitimate heir to the crown of the Roman Augusti. In 1144, he secured the formal submission of Raymond of Antioch, who was under threat from the Muslim Emirs, and in 1146 he repeatedly defeated the Turks, driving them almost entirely out of Asia Minor."

"A few years after his ascent to the throne in 1147, the Second Crusade began, led by Conrad III of Germany and Louis VII of France. Louis, as an honor, invited Manuel to participate—an offer made to no other Byzantine emperor. Conrad of Germany requested permission to lead his troops through the lands of Byzantium, and Manuel granted it. However, the Germans behaved as if they were sovereigns over the people, and when they reached the City, they practically laid siege to it. Manuel marched out with his army beyond the walls and taught them a firm lesson. The Crusaders scattered, and Conrad hastened to be ferried across to the Asian side of the Bosporus with his army. The Second Crusade, unfortunately, ended in failure, and its only lasting result was to deepen the hostility between Byzantines and Westerners and to widen the rift between the two peoples.

The armies of the Crusaders, lacking organization and discipline, were crushed by the Turks without achieving anything of real significance. Nevertheless, Manuel—who had a great fondness for the Latins and their customs—formed an alliance with Conrad due to their shared enmity toward the Nor-

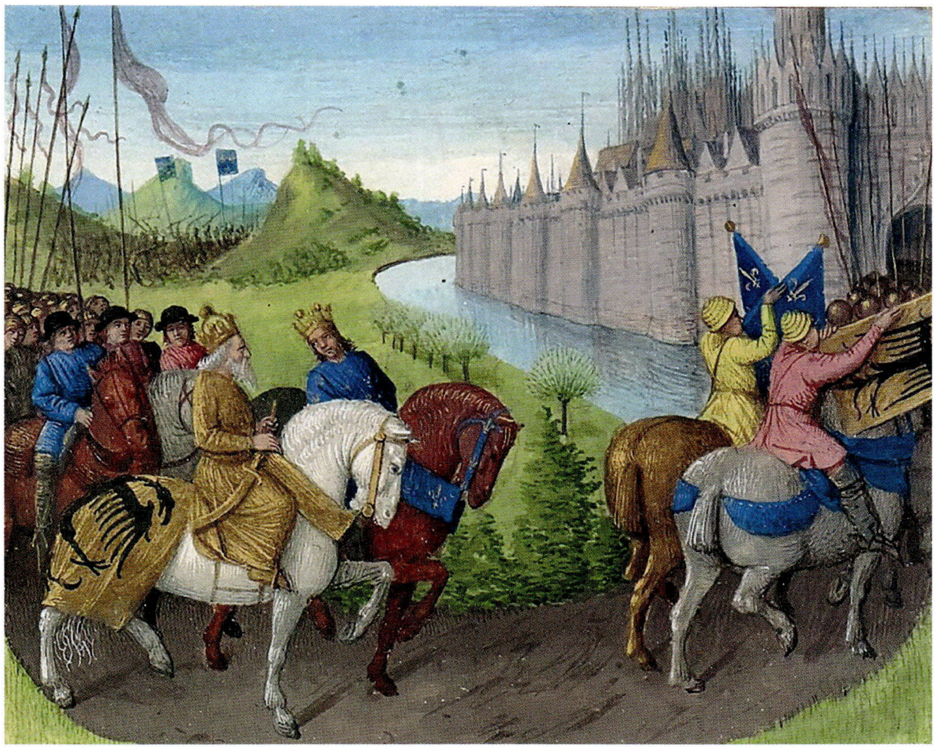

The knights of the Second Crusade arrive in Constantinople.

Painting by Jean Fouquet, 1455–1460, National Library of France, Paris.

mans. In fact, he married Conrad's niece, Bertha of Sulzbach, who was renamed Irene upon her arrival in Constantinople. The purpose of this alliance was to curb the power of the Italian Normans, a goal that he successfully achieved. Queen Irene was virtuous, modest, and humble. She carried out many charitable works alongside her husband, but she neglected her appearance. The pleasure-loving Emperor respected and loved her, yet he was not entirely faithful to her. When she died in 1159, he mourned her sincerely, but he did not delay in replacing her with the beautiful Maria of Antioch, from the House of Poitiers, who was only sixteen at the time—while the Emperor was forty-three. By 1173, the same year you, Nikephoros, completed your medical studies, Manuel had scored repeated victories against the Turks and had reclaimed much of Asia Minor. He had also defeated the Serbs in the Balkans and reconquered part of southern Italy from the Normans. The Byzantine Roman Empire had become a superpower in the Eastern Mediterranean, respected and acknowledged by all."

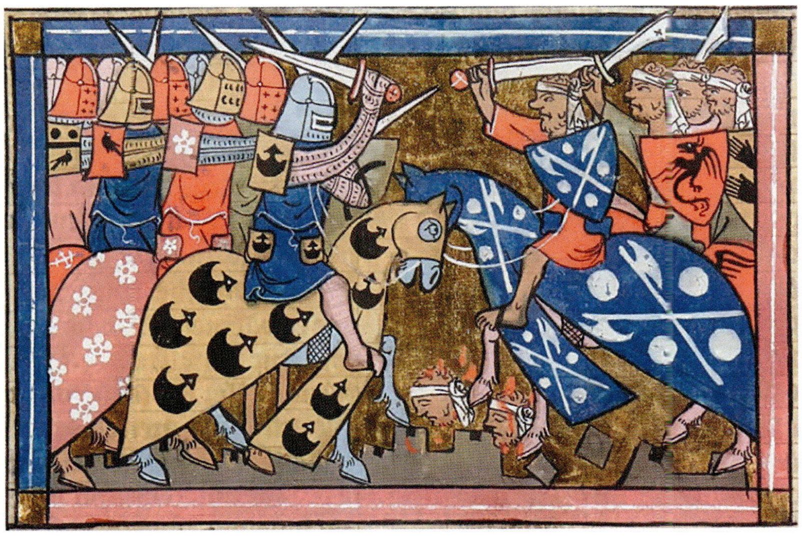

Battle of the Knights of the Second Crusade.

Miniature, 14th century. National Library of France, Paris.

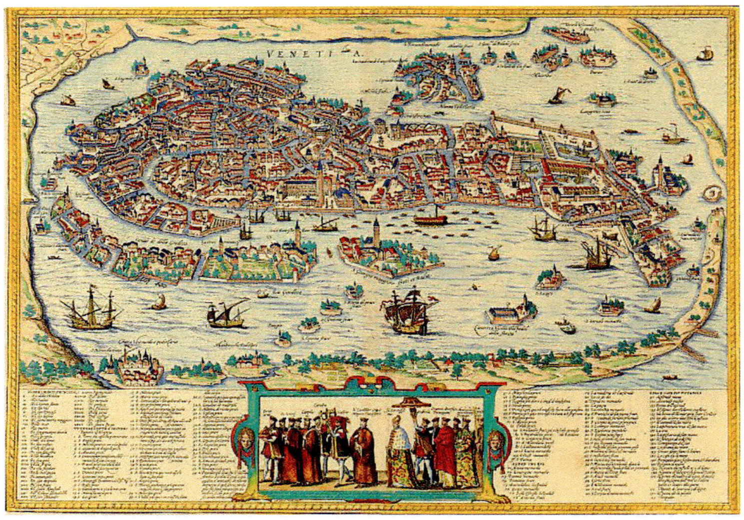

Venice.
Engraving by Bolognino Zaltieri, 16th century, National Library of Israel.

We all listened to the stories of Theodoros Vlemmydes with great attention. Amid this general atmosphere of prosperity within the Empire, I too experienced a great success. As soon as I completed my studies and received my Certificate from my medical teachers, I submitted it to the Xenon of the Monastery of Pantocrator, the hospital of my dreams ever since I had come to know the educational institutions and hospitals of the Queen of Cities. I awaited the response with anxious hope, and Antigone—who shared in my dreams—encouraged me and prayed for my success. After a month of anxiety and hopeful anticipation, the response finally came: I had been accepted as a "physician of rank" at the finest hospital (*Xenon*) in the City. My joy was indescribable. My father, my wife, and my siblings were proud of me. My father's business, along with that of his partner, Theodoros Vlemmydes, was flourishing, despite the fierce and often unfair competition from the Latin merchants—especially the Venetians—who controlled the sea routes and marketplaces and enjoyed extensive tax exemptions. They were forced to cooperate with the Italians, but always under burdensome terms. Unfortunately, on one hand, the behavior of the crusaders as they passed through our lands, and on the other, the greed of the Italian merchants—who were gradually taking control of all commerce—had stirred up deep resentment and hostility between the Greeks and the Latins. At that time, the City had around 450,000 Orthodox "Greek-Romans" and 60,000 Roman Catholic "Latins." The latter were Italian merchants and adventurers, mostly Venetians, but also Genoese, Pisans, and Amalfitans. The Italian merchants frequently clashed with each other, and in 1162, the Pisans and Venetians attacked the Genoese quarter, causing widespread destruction.

The Emperor ruled in favor of the Venetians, who then became uncontrollable. Two years ago, in 1171, they utterly destroyed the Genoese quarter. That act, however, crossed all boundaries. The Emperor responded by arresting the Venetians and confiscating their properties. In retaliation, Venice dispatched its war fleet against us. Manuel arrayed his troops along the battlements and outside the city walls, and the Venetians soon realized that any confrontation would be futile. They withdrew without accomplishing their aims. Nonetheless, the Latins continued to cause great turmoil for our empire. The animosity and hatred between Greeks and Latins had reached a critical level. At the time, I could not have imagined the calamity that would unfold just a few years after the death of our sovereign Kyr Manuel.

My dear friend Manuel Vlemmides, who had become my relative through Antigone, had also completed his studies in philosophy. He was about to be appointed as a teacher at a certain school and intended to devote himself to iconography and the theology behind this sacred art. Through writing treatises and deep study, his ultimate goal was to teach at the School of Magnaura—though he wouldn't admit this even to himself. But I, who knew him well, had understood it, and I believed he deserved it and would surely succeed. Nowadays, we often met and took long walks through the city, marveling at the mosaics and frescoes of the churches, which Manuel would explain to me in great detail. He himself was now working on portable icons, which he painted with both love and profound reverence. He was a deeply pious man and regarded his art as both a creative offering and a confession of his faith.

"My dear Nikiforos," he would say to me, "a true iconographer, when about to paint the image of a saint, prepares both physically and spiritually. He studies the life of the saint, and on the eve before beginning the painting, he fasts, takes a bath, and changes his clothes—so that he may dedicate himself, purified, to his sacred task."

I admired Manuel for his faith and the seriousness with which he approached his work. He, in turn, appreciated the way I viewed medicine as a vocation and a sacred service, and he would ask me many questions about my science. He was deeply concerned with the issue of decay and death, and as a philosopher, he posed to me countless questions about illnesses and their nature. I often found myself searching—his inquiries stirred in me new questions for which I, too, sought answers.

My work at the Xenon of the Pantocrator was exhilarating. Each day I came into direct contact with human suffering. The *primikērioi* and *protomēnites* phy-

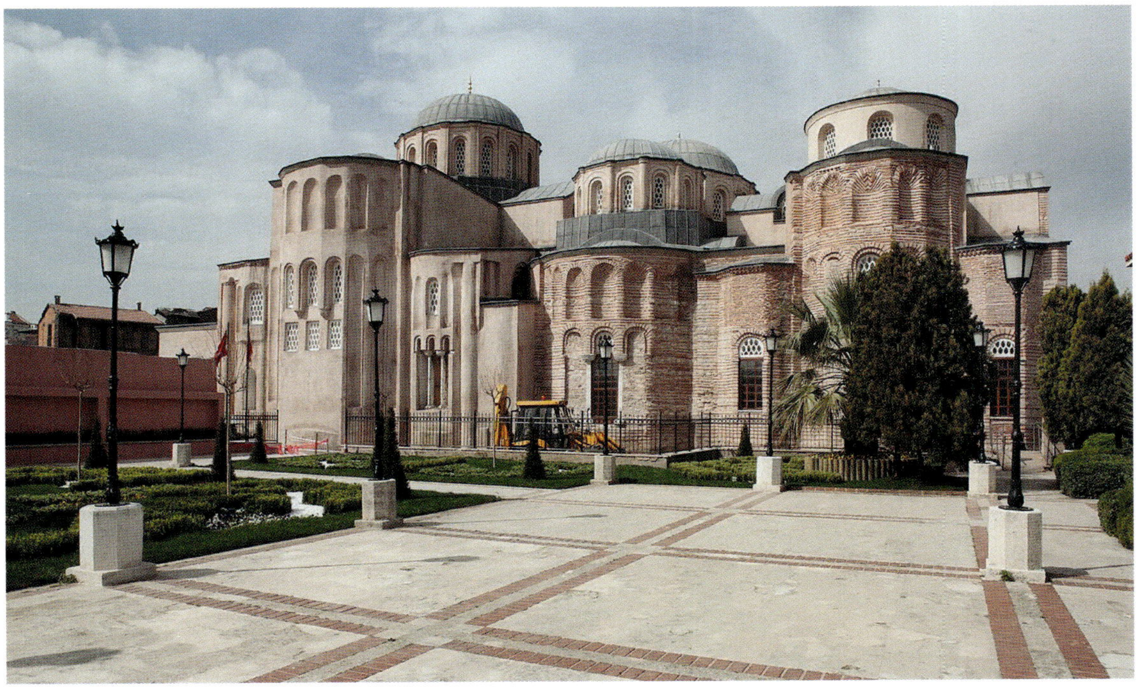

The Monastery of Christ Pantocrator in Constantinople.

Photo: Sharon Nathan, 2016.

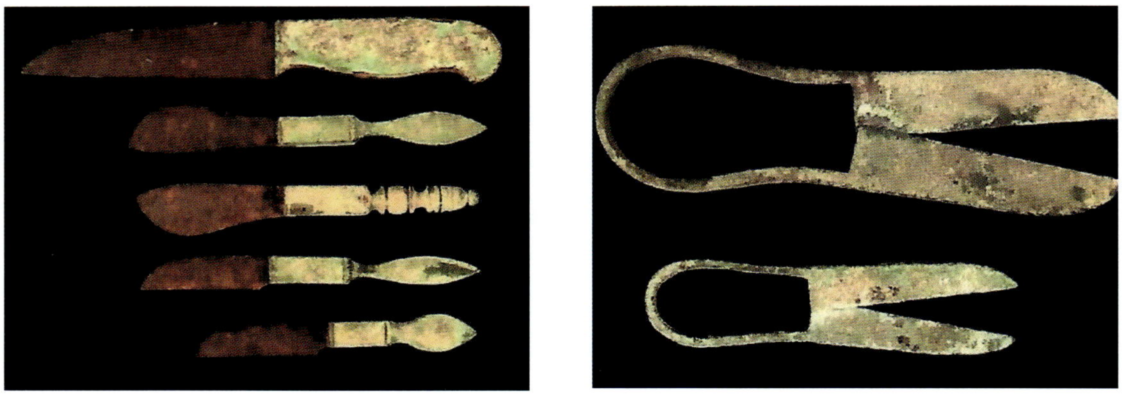

Small Knives and Scissors.
Collection of the University of Virginia, USA.

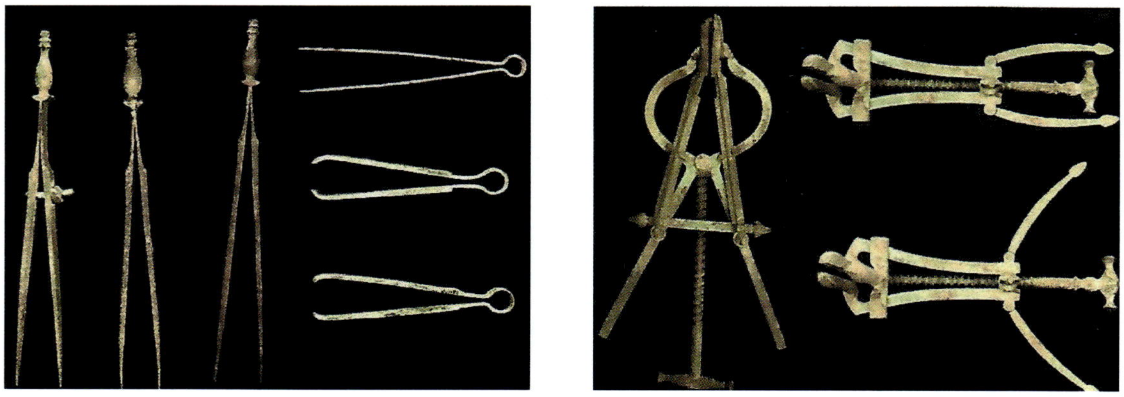

Forceps and Specula.
Collection of the University of Virginia, USA.

sicians were highly experienced and well-educated, and I learned a great deal from them every single day. Especially in the field of surgery, which interested me the most due to its immediate effectiveness, I came to understand the discipline and self-control a surgeon must possess at every moment of an operation—when everything can change in an instant. For this reason, surgery was quite literally a sacred rite. The most experienced surgeons were Nikolaos Marmarinos and Alexios Skliros. One specialized primarily in general surgeries and trauma, while the other focused on ophthalmological procedures, dental work, and reconstructive plastic surgeries. Since I was deeply interested in surgery, I participated in almost every procedure as an assistant, and as a result, I quickly gained experience. Before long, I was entrusted with simple operations, as well as the dressing of wounds, the changing of bandages, and the care of post-operative patients.

Surgery in our Eastern Empire is held in high esteem and is considered an integral part of medical science. It is taught in medical schools and practiced in hospitals by learned physicians, which has allowed it to develop greatly. In contrast, in the West it is regarded as inferior. In fact, recently in 1163, Pope Alexander issued an edict forbidding clergy from performing bloody operations, deeming them incompatible with their spiritual role—effectively banning clergy from practicing surgery. Yet in Western Europe, medicine is mainly practiced by clerics and monks, and thus surgery became separated from official "scientific" medicine. It is now carried out by practical healers, often barbers, who have taken it into their hands. It is no longer taught in formal schools and is performed in patients' homes or village squares, often as a curious spectacle rather than a respected art.

In our Eastern realm, medicine has been systematically classified into four principal specialties: *Internal Medicine, Surgery, Obstetrics–Gynecology,* and *Ophthalmology*. Each hospital has dedicated departments for these fields, staffed by different physicians. Notably, in the gynecological departments, women physicians, known as *iatrines,* and midwife-physicians, or *iatromae,* also serve. Antigone, as I mentioned earlier, would often visit the hospital along with my sister, offering her help as a volunteer. She had a deep affection for surgery, and frequently assisted me during operations, performing nursing and instrument-handling duties with dedication. By contrast, Iphigenia could not bear the sight of wounds or bloody procedures. She preferred to serve in the internal medicine division. She especially enjoyed studying pharmaceuticals—their intended and unintended effects, proper dosages, and methods of administration.

Performing surgery is the most striking and demanding activity within the hospital. For an operation to take place, the surgical room is thoroughly cleaned, and the patient is bathed head to toe the day before. The surgeons wear special aprons, and the wound along with the surrounding area is further cleaned using sponges and warm water, then surrounded with clean towels. Following this, antisepsis is performed using strong wine (*akratos oinos*), vinegar, or even sea water. In certain cases involving infected wounds, boiling oil (*zeon elaion*) is applied. When the wounds are deep, irregular, and contain hidden recesses, they are washed with strong dark wine, referred to by our teachers as "oinos austēros kai melas." The older antiseptic recipes—such as Oribasius' waxy salves or Aetius' concoction made from the milk of strychnos leaves, or even the application of pyrite stone ("pyritēs lithos")—have now largely fallen out of use. Only a few still employ them, and then only rarely.

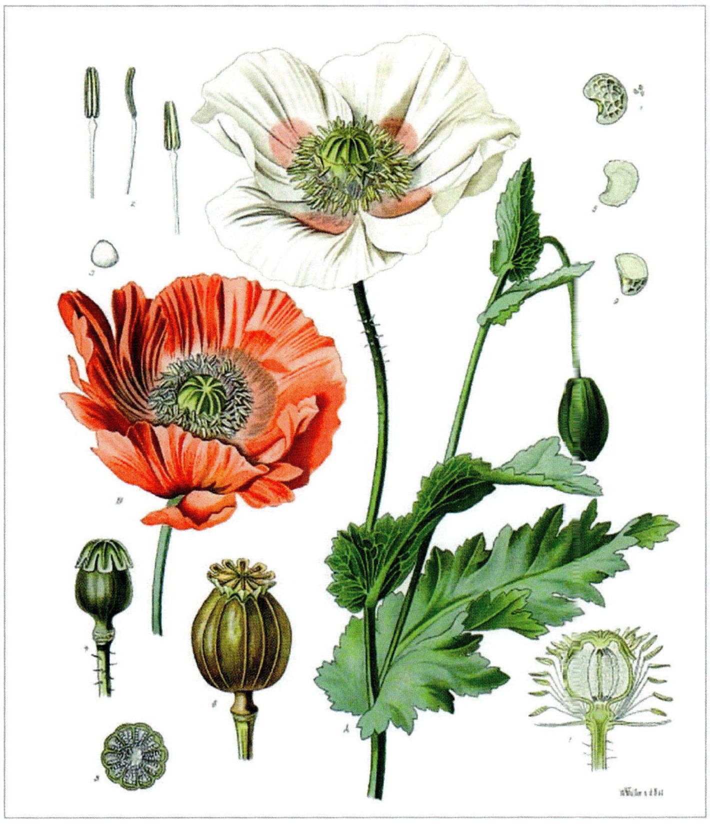

Papaver somniferum (Opium Poppy). *Eugen Köhler, Atlas of Medicinal Plants, USA, 1887.*

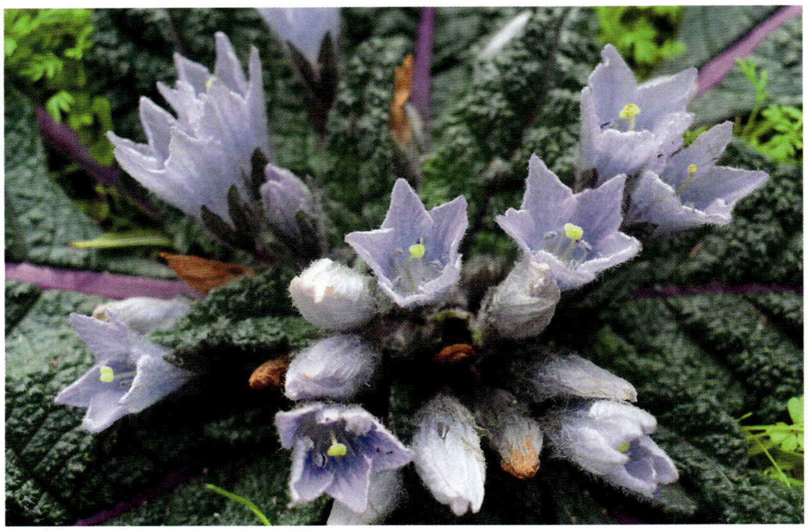

Mandrake.

The major challenges in surgery are bleeding and the pain experienced by the patient. Hemorrhage from large vessels is controlled by ligation—that is, tying them off with fine threads, usually made of silk. Smaller vessels and diffuse bleeding are managed through cauterization, performed with iron tools heated until red-hot. Surgical maneuvers are extremely painful, so strong analgesia must be administered to ensure the patient can endure the procedure. As Galen wrote, the surgeon must strive for "speed, painlessness, and safety in the operation."

The main drugs currently used in surgical anesthesia include opium, derived from the opium poppy; mandrake, whose root is boiled in wine and given to the patient; and henbane (*Hyoscyamus*), administered either as a liquid taken orally or applied to the wound as an oil. Other substances used are colchicum, hemlock, and aconite, each extracted from their respective plants. Local cooling is also applied to induce analgesia, as well as intoxication by means of strong wine. All these substances, however, must be used with great caution, as they are potent poisons in higher doses. Pharmacology is a complex science and demands great experience.

Once analgesia and antisepsis have been completed, the surgery begins. The guiding principle and model is the exhortation of Hippocrates: "*In surgery, everything must be performed nobly, properly, decorously, swiftly, rhythmically, cleanly,*

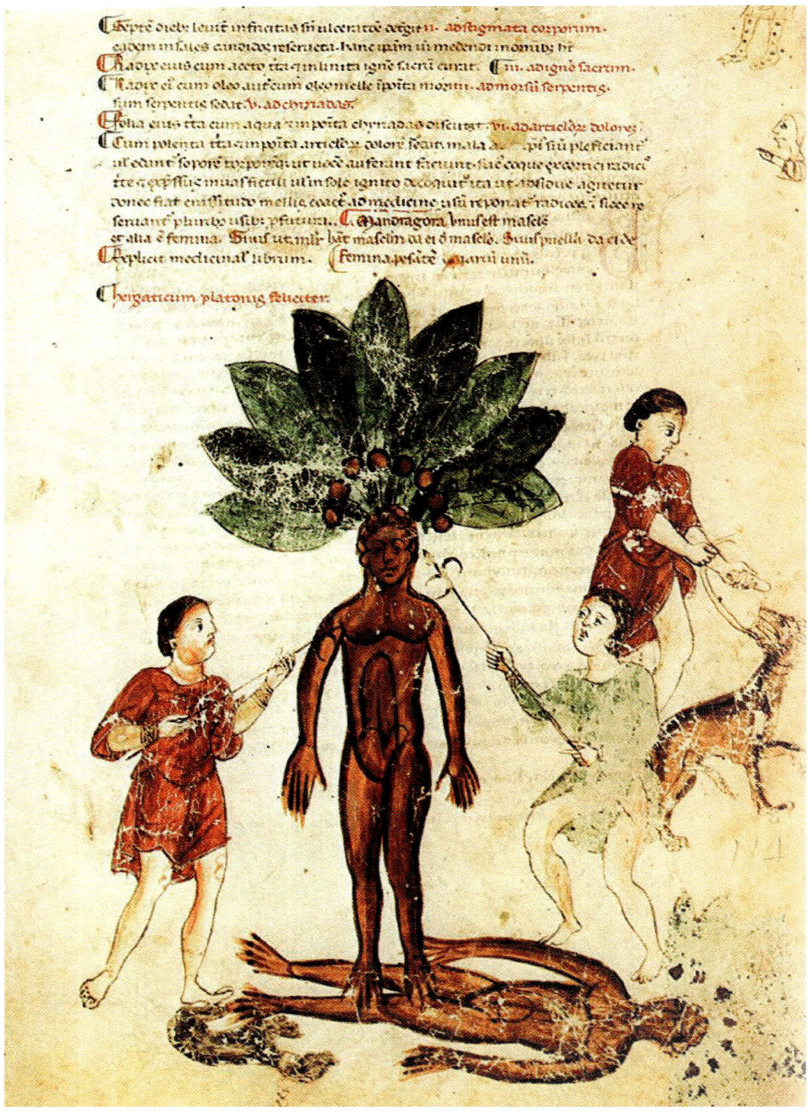

Imaginary treatment with mandrake.

Miniature, 13th century, Austrian National Library, Vienna.

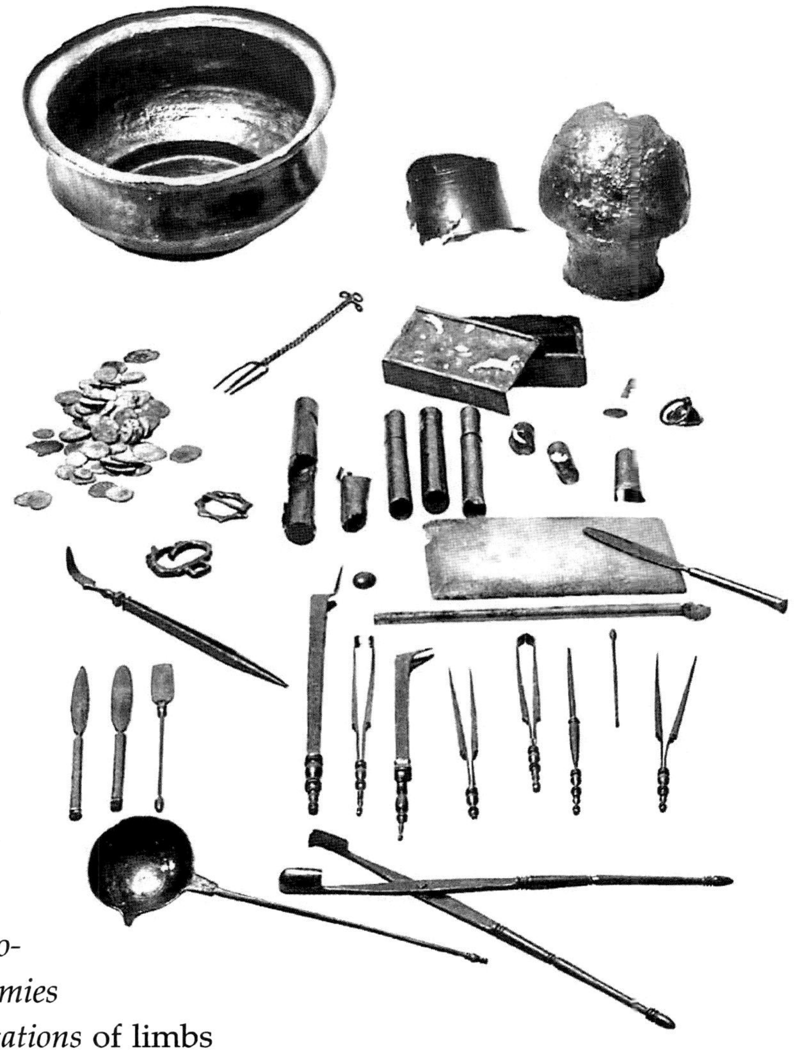

Byzantine-era surgical instruments. *Carnavalet Museum, Paris.*

and painlessly." Nikolaos Marmarinos primarily performed excisional surgeries—those in which a diseased organ or tissue is cut out and removed, or in which a pathological accumulation is drained.

Such operations include trepanations (*craniotomies*) for the drainage of hematomas formed after head injuries; *tracheostomies* in cases of obstruction of the upper respiratory tract, so that the patient can breathe; tonsillectomies (*ἀμυγδαλεκτομές*) in cases of chronic inflammation; *thyroidectomies* and *mastectomies* in cases of tumors or cancer of the neck or breast; and *pleurectomies,* as well as the drainage of pleural fluid. He also performed intra-abdominal operations, such as *drainage of liver abscesses or ascitic fluid.* Additionally, he performed *hemorrhoidectomies, lithotripsies* of the urinary bladder, *saphenectomies* for varicose veins in the legs, and *amputations* of limbs in cases of gangrene. He was very quick and precise in his movements. I admired his composure when faced with complications such as hemorrhage or the fainting of a patient. He knew the steps of the procedures extremely well and inspired trust in his assistants and collaborators.

However, I must admit that I admired Alexios Skliros even more. He performed reconstructive surgeries in cases of trauma or fractures of the facial skull. He also carried out extractions or stabilization of teeth, excision and restoration of burn scars, but most notably, he performed with remarkable skill plastic surgeries for the restoration of rhinotomy, ototomy, as well as the reconstruction of defects of the lips (cleft lip) or the eyelids. The amputation of the nose (rhinotomy) or ears was, unfortunately, a very old practice used as punishment for various crimes. Rhinotomy was a form of torment, because beyond the aesthetic disfigurement, there was an open wound on the face that was constantly prone to infection and caused respiratory problems. Skliros, with great dexterity, mobilized skin flaps and covered the gap, creating artificial nostrils, so that both the functional and aesthetic outcome would be very good. This type of surgery had been performed since ancient times, and a characteristic example is the story of Emperor Justinian II, who was overthrown by the army in 695 due to his cruelty and was punished with rhinoto-

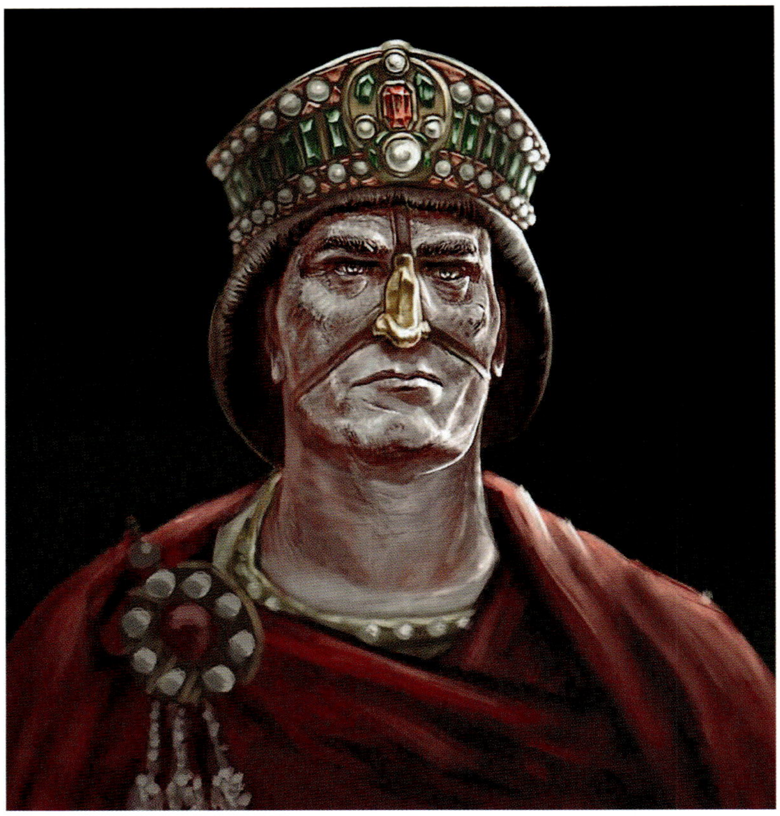

Justinian the Slit-Nosed with a golden nose prosthesis.

my and exile. He returned to the throne ten years later and went down in history as "the Slit-Nosed" (Rinotmitos). He underwent a successful reconstructive surgery, likely performed by Paul of Aegina, who was prominent at the time, and there is a bust of him where the signs of the restored rhinotomy are clearly visible.

Skliros also performed plastic surgeries for inguinal hernias, as well as reconstructive surgeries for malformations of the genital organs, such as hypospadias or certain cases of hermaphroditism, where the procedures are extremely complex. I admired his dexterity, the delicacy of his techniques, and his profound knowledge of anatomical structures, which allowed him to carry out such operations. However, the ophthalmological procedures—most notably the removal of the lens in cases of cataracts—were performed by the Head Physician of the Ophthalmology Department, Eustathios Phokitis. Naturally, for these procedures, surgeons use specialized instruments, many of which they have invented themselves. Surgical tools are highly specialized. In our hospital, there is a modern catalog listing a total of 88 instruments. Sixty of them we have inherited from the ancient authors, while the rest have been devised in our own century. Our surgical ward possesses nearly all of them.

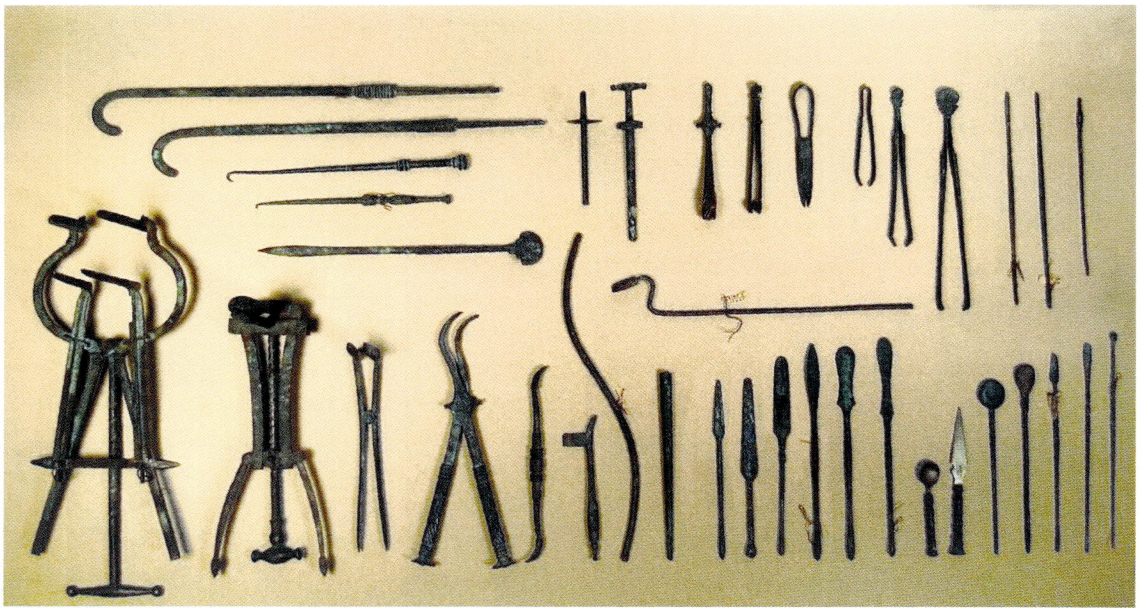

Surgical instruments.

Greek Surgery Through the Centuries, Militos Editions, Athens 2019.

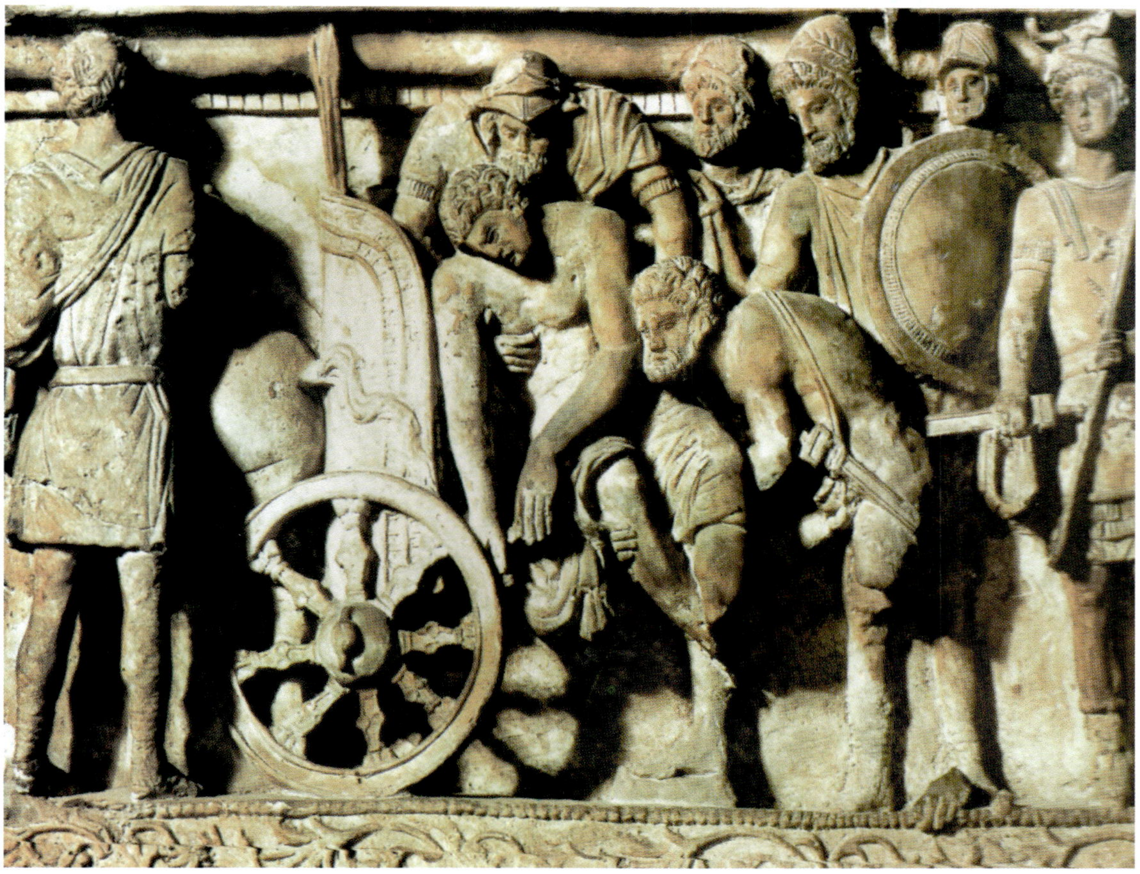

Wounded soldier being cared for.

Etruscan relief, 2nd century BC, Archaeological Museum, Florence.

I will mention selectively a few names that have been given to instruments according to their use: the various scalpels are called *smilē* (chisel), *lonchē* (lance), *spathion* (small sword), *pterygotomus* (wing-cutter); the forceps include *labis* (tongs), *mydion* (small spoon), *ankistron* (hook), *typhlangistron* (blind hook), *blepharokatochos* (eyelid retractor), and *glossokatochos* (tongue depressor). The needles of various types—straight and curved—are called *raphis, egkopeus,* or *kynorrhaphos* (dog-stitcher). Other instruments include: *psalidion* (small scissors), *trypanon* (drill), *catheter, mēlē, spathomēlē, lithoulkos* and *lithanaboleus* (instruments for extracting stones), *dioptra* (vaginal speculum), and *antioptra* (rectal dilator). There's no point in listing more—I only wish to emphasize the high level surgery had reached in our century, just before the calamity of the Fourth Crusade, which God allowed me to witness. The standard of our surgical practice was far superior to that of the West, and only the Arabs—and perhaps the Indians—could boast of comparable achievements.

Antigone supported me in all of this most positively. God did not bless us with children—a reality she faced with courage. Every event in life, whether joyful or sorrowful, depends on how we choose to handle it. From an unfortunate circumstance, one may draw forth blessings—and likewise, from a blessing, one may stumble into loss. Antigone channeled the natural maternal love she carried into care for my patients, both in the hospital and later at home. As I have often emphasized, she came voluntarily to the *xenon* (infirma-

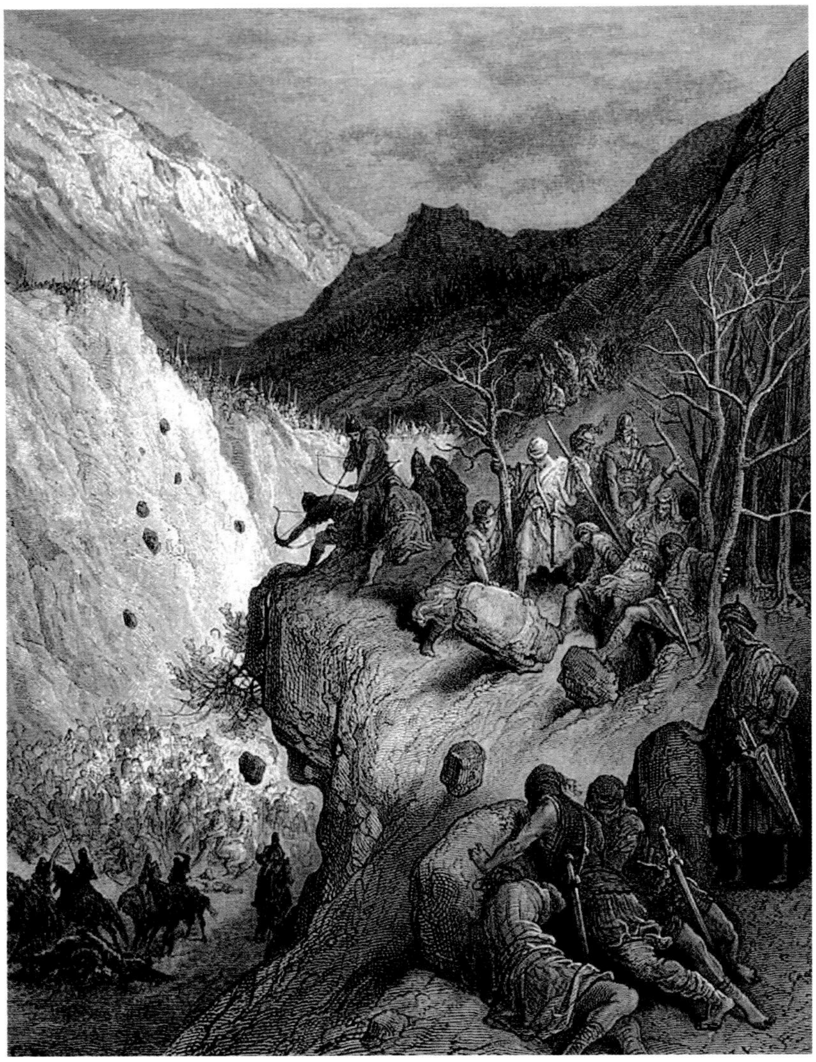

The fatal Myriokephalon.
Composition by Gustave Doré, 1877.

ry) and offered her services as a nurse, tending to the daily sufferings of the ill. At the same time, she read diligently and observed the visits and treatments, and in time, she gradually acquired the knowledge and experience of a true *iatraina*—a physician in her own right.

Yet Antigone never abandoned her role as a nurse, nor did she become conceited about her growing medical knowledge. Still, there were many occasions when her keen judgment had helped me arrive at a diagnosis. Something similar happened with my sister Iphigenia, who, after a few years and upon getting married, had to leave her nursing work and devote herself fully to her family and children.

Unfortunately, the good days of prosperity did not last long. The great military and political achievements of the Komnenoi were destined to end ingloriously. Byzantium had begun to hope that it would regain its former glory—what it once possessed before the Battle of Manzikert, when it still laid claim to being a universal empire. At that time, everyone respected the state of the Komnenoi, and especially the Emperor, Kyr Manuel. All believed that after so many victories against the Turks, he would succeed in driving them completely out of Asia Minor. Indeed, in 1176, our Emperor gathered a vast army of 35,000 men—Romans, Serbs, and Latins—along with 3,000 wagons, siege machines, and beasts of burden, and set out on a grand campaign against the Sultan of the Seljuks, Kilij Arslan. Though the Sultan had pledged vassalage, he had not remained faithful to his obligations and would, from time to time, launch raids and pillage our territories. The great army marched from Dorylaeum toward Iconium. The Turks employed a strategy of retreat and guerrilla warfare. At the narrow pass of Myriokephalon in Phrygia, the Emperor, carried away by the arrogance of his strength and past victories, advanced his forces into the defile without proper reconnaissance. When the column had become stretched out in a long, narrow line, the Turks attacked, howling from the cliffs on either side. Our soldiers fought bravely, and the Emperor himself, battling with ferocity, was wounded all over his body. The defeat was devastating. A great number of men were killed, and all the equipment fell into enemy hands. At Myriokephalon, the international prestige of the Empire collapsed. All hopes of expelling the Turks from Asia Minor were extinguished for good. It was the third major defeat of the Eastern Empire, following that at Yarmouk in 636 by the Arabs and at Manzikert in 1071 by the Seljuks.

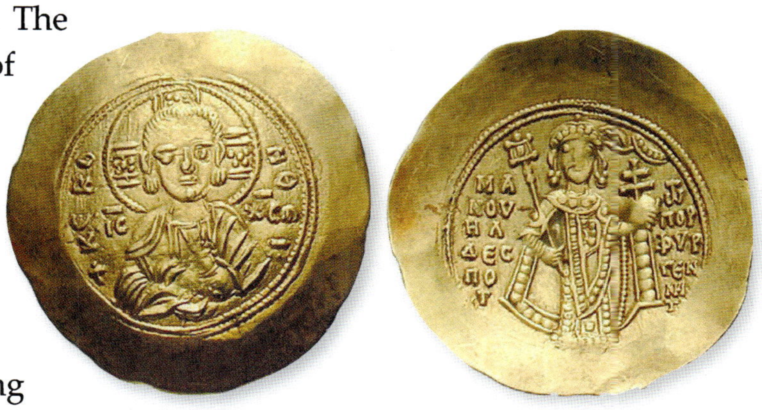

Hyperpyron of Manuel Komnenos, depicting Christ and the Emperor.

The prestige and self-confidence of Byzantium never recovered. Our Ecumenical Empire began to be regarded by others as merely one kingdom among many. Great sorrow and lamentation broke out in the Queen of Cities. The tragic warrior, the great Manuel Komnenos, fell into a state bordering on depression. So much effort, so many struggles, so many sacrifices now seemed lost. His dreams had crumbled. The Westerners, who until then had considered him the most powerful ruler in the world, ceased calling him Emperor of the Romans (*Imperator Romanorum*), and instead began referring to him merely as King of the Greeks (*Rex Graecorum*). It is worth noting that the term *rex*, which we render as *rēgas*, is far inferior to the Greek term *Basileus*, which is synonymous with the absolute monarch, the Emperor. Nevertheless, Komnenos did not cease to struggle. The territorial losses were quickly recovered, and indeed our forces once again defeated the Turks under the leadership of the Emperor himself and his brilliant general, John Vatatzes. Yet the glorious past did not return. Only four years after Myriokephalon, in 1180, Lord Manuel died at the age of 62. The people mourned him as a father and protector.

Historians and chroniclers called him *divine*, *glorious*, and *the most blessed emperor*. His heroic deeds became proverbial, as did his great courage and strong character. He was so well trained in strength and the art of war that even Raymond of Antioch, a renowned warrior, could not even hold his lance in Manuel's presence. In a great tournament, he managed to unseat two famous Italian knights, and it is said that in a single day he killed forty Turks with his own hand. In a battle against the Hungarians, he seized a banner and rode alone across the bridge that separated his army from the enemy, thus inspiring his soldiers with boldness. In another instance, he intercepted an entire force of 500 Turks and cut off their path without receiving a single wound. His death brought deep sorrow to the realm, especially because no one knew what would come next. Great uncertainty fell upon the people. The throne now passed to his underage son, Alexios II, who was only 11 years old, with the regency entrusted to his young mother, Maria of Antioch, daughter of Raymond of Poitiers—who, as a "Frankish woman," was not much loved by the people.

Manuel Komnenos

King lord Manuel Komnenos,
on a melancholy September day,
felt that death was near. The astrologers—
(the salaried ones) of the court—were chattering
that he still had many years to live.
But while they talked, he
remembered old devout customs,
and from the monks' cells he ordered
liturgical vestments to be brought,
and he wore them, rejoicing that he appeared
with a solemn air, like a priest or monk.
Happy are all they who believe,
and who, like lord King Manuel, meet their end
clothed with reverent dignity in their faith.

Constantine P. Cavafy, Poems 1905–1915

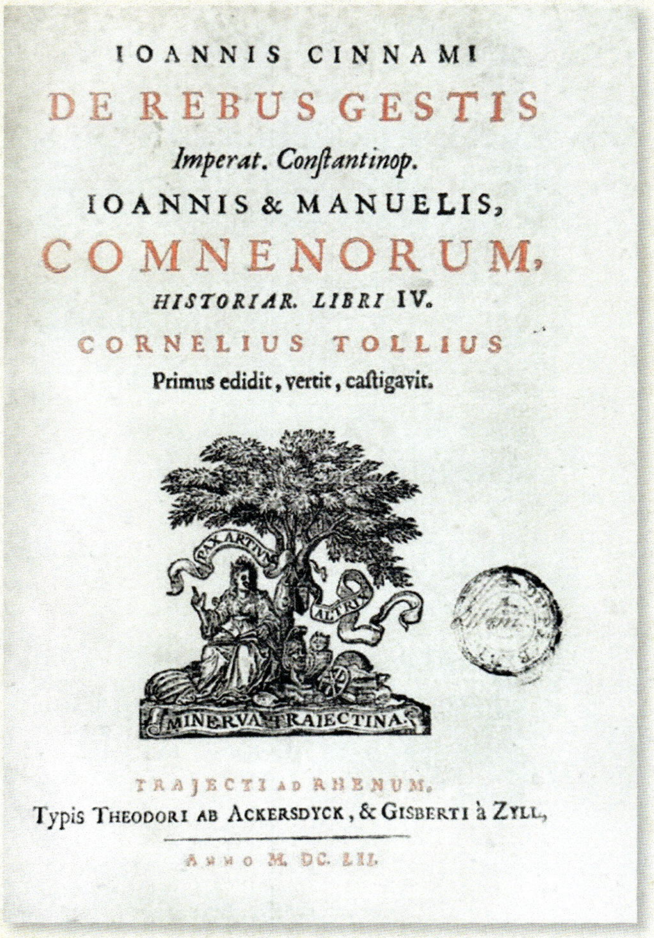

IOANNIS CINNAMI
DE REBUS GESTIS
Imperat. Constantinop.
IOANNIS & MANUELIS,
COMNENORUM,
HISTORIAR. LIBRI IV.
CORNELIUS TOLLIUS
Primus edidit, vertit, castigavit.

TRAJECTI AD RHENUM,
Typis THEODORI AB ACKERSDYCK, & GISBERTI à ZYLL,
ANNO M. DC. LII.

John Kinnamos,
On the Komnenoi.

Published by Cornelius Tollius, Trajectum (Utrecht), 1659.

Alexios was the long-awaited heir whom Manuel had fathered at the age of 51. His mother hastened to betroth him to *Agnès of France*, then only nine years old, daughter of King Louis VII of France—a friend and admirer of Emperor Manuel. The young Agnès arrived in the Queen of Cities, but the marriage never came to pass. The governance of the Empire fell to the Empress Mother, serving as regent for the young emperor. She hoped that the kinship with Louis would secure her son's hold on the throne. Naturally, opposition began to stir—first from the daughters Manuel had from his first marriage, who now laid their own claim to the throne, and then from the palace courtiers whose intrigues and machinations undermined the stability of the imperial administration. During the three-year reign of Alexios, the once-allied Hungarians seized Bosnia and Syrmia, the Venetians took Dalmatia, and the Turks captured Kütahya and Sozopolis. The once-glorious state of the Komnenoi now appeared defenseless. The people felt a growing sense of insecurity under a weak administration. Maria's policies clearly favored the Latin merchants of the City, who had grown arrogant and emboldened, provoking the people's deep resentment. It was in this time of unrest and discontent that a fateful figure emerged on the stage of history—Andronikos Komnenos.

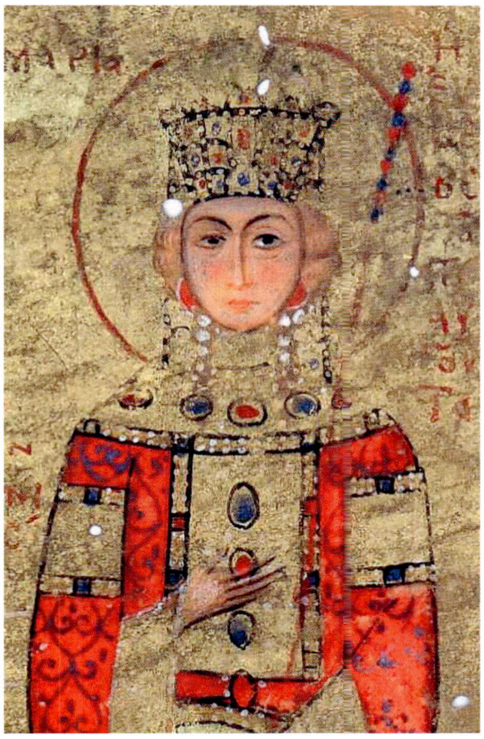

Maria of Antioch, Regent.

Miniature, 12th century, Vatican Library, Rome.

Andronikos was the beloved first cousin and peer of Manuel—born in the same year, 1118—and bore a striking resemblance to the great Emperor. He was intelligent, courageous, physically strong, charming with women, and an eloquent speaker, possessing notable administrative and military gifts. But the similarities ended there. Andronikos was supremely ambitious and arrogantly self-assured. He lacked moral restraint and was known for his cruelty, ruthlessness, and violent nature. In his relations with the opposite sex, he embodied the very definition of a playboy of his time. At the age of 21, he was captured in battle by the Seljuks, having fought bravely on the front lines. He was ransomed by our own and returned to Constantinople, where he seduced his niece, Eudokia Komnene, and took her with him on a military mission to Armenia, where

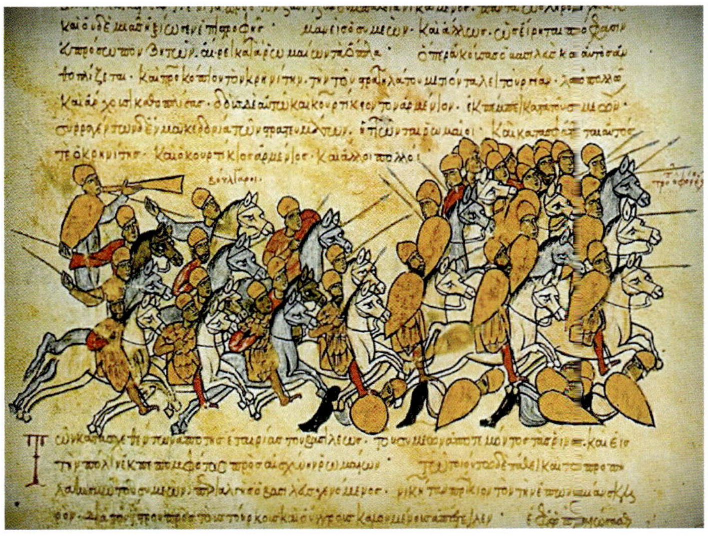

Battle between Bulgarians and Hungarians.

Miniature from Skylitzes, 12th century, National Library of Spain, Madrid.

he had been appointed governor. In 1153, he became entangled in a conspiracy against Emperor Manuel and was imprisoned. He escaped in 1165 and fled to Kiev, to the court of Prince Yaroslav. From there, the unpredictable Andronikos reversed course once again: he reconciled with Manuel, forged an alliance, and fought valiantly at his side, commanding a force of Rus' warriors from Ukraine against the Hungarians.

He returned to the City reconciled and was appointed governor in Cilicia. Yet within a few years, due to serious abuses of power, Emperor Manuel dismissed him from that post. Andronikos then sought refuge at the court of Raymond of Antioch, where he once again worked his dangerous charm—this time on the beautiful Philippa, Raymond's daughter and sister of our Empress Maria. Expelled from there as well, he found his way to the Kingdom of Jerusalem, where he was appointed governor of Beirut. But there, too, he seduced another of his own nieces—Theodora Komnene, widow of King Baldwin III—and fled with her to the court of Sultan Nur ad-Din in Damascus. Once again unwelcome, the pair sought shelter in Georgia, where Andronikos fought valiantly alongside King George III and gained his favor. At last, he was granted pardon by Emperor Manuel, who, despite Andronikos' grievous faults, always held an affection for him. And so, he settled with his beloved and loyal Theodora in Oinoë of Paphlagonia, as if destiny herself wished to give him yet another chapter in his wandering, perilous tale.

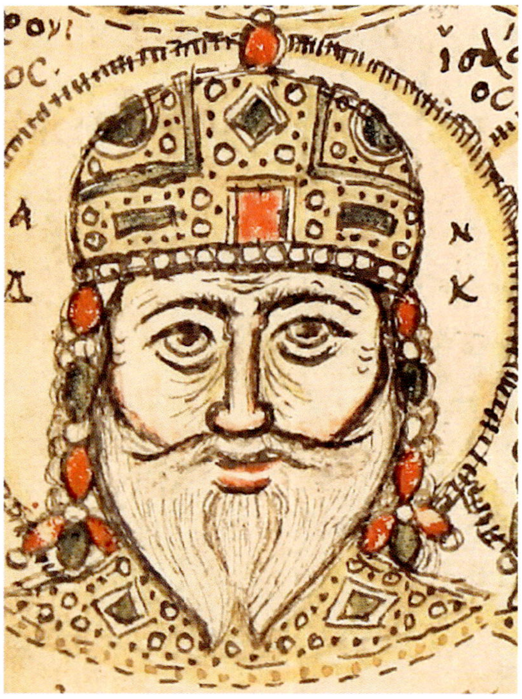

Andronikos Komnenos.

Miniature, 15th century, Zonaras, d'Este Library, Modena.

In April of 1182, two years after Emperor Manuel's death, Andronikos seized the moment. Capitalizing on the people's growing discontent toward the Latin merchants and toward Empress Maria of Antioch, he entered Constantinople at the head of a band of mercenaries, having already secured the cooperation of key military commanders. He presented himself not as a usurper, but as the protector of the realm and the rightful regent for the young Emperor Alexios II. At first, he revealed his better nature and the talents which—had they been guided by virtue—might have made him one of the most glorious rulers of the Komnenos line. He restored the city's fortifications, curtailed the excesses of the powerful aristocracy, ordered a redistribution of land to the poor, and lightened the burden of taxes. The common people, weary of neglect and exploitation, were heartened. Hope flickered again in their hearts, and they placed their trust in him.

Unfortunately, however, Andronikos was not Manuel. He quickly revealed his ruthless nature. He spread the rumor that the Latins of the capital were plotting to attack the Greeks, and so the mob, incited by his mercenaries, stormed into the Latin quarter of the city and began assaulting its inhabitants. The massacre was merciless. Homes, churches, and charitable institutions were looted. The frenzied crowd pillaged and burned everything, slaughtered clergy and laypeople, women and children—even the sick in the hospitals. Those who managed to escape fled by sea. The treatment of the Catholic clergy was especially brutal. Cardinal John, the papal legate, was beheaded, and his head was dragged through the streets tied to a dog's tail. The Massacre of the Latins remains a dark stain on our history. Their population was around 60,000; we do not know the exact number of dead, but it was immense. This populist and criminal act of Andronikos sowed an even deeper hatred between Greeks and Westerners, with disastrous consequences for the Empire.

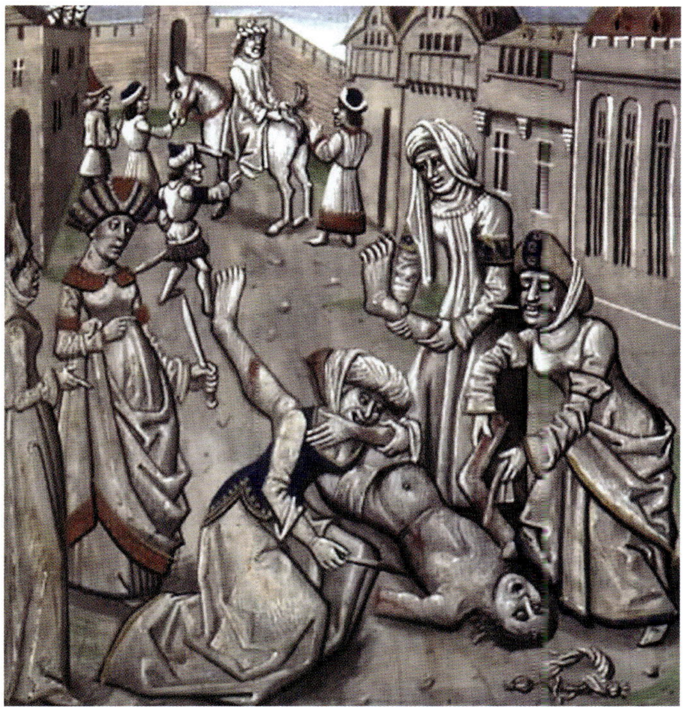

The death of Andronikos Komnenos.

15th century, National Library of France, Paris.

From that point on, Andronikos lost all control. He gave himself over to an unprecedented wave of bloodshed, targeting anyone he considered a threat to his power. He murdered or mutilated members of the Komnenos family and other nobles whom he saw as potential rivals. He had the Empress Mother Maria drowned and the young Alexios strangled at the age of 13. He proclaimed himself emperor and, in an effort to solidify his rule, married Alexios's eleven-year-old fiancée, Agnes of France—while he himself was 65 years old. He had reached the brink of madness. He ruled through sheer terror. He quickly became isolated—not only from the nobility, but also from the people who had once cheered him and placed their hopes in him in 1182. Witnessing the anarchy and collapse of the state, the Serbs declared autonomy, and the Normans invaded Macedonia, capturing Thessaloniki. The army Andronikos sent was defeated and forced to retreat. The cup had overflowed. A nobleman of the Komnenos line who had once collaborated with Andronikos—Isaac Angelos—was now deemed suspicious as well. The emperor ordered his chief minister, Stephen Hagiochristophorites, to execute him. Isaac, however, killed Hagiochristophorites instead and fled to the sanctuary of Hagia Sophia, where the people rose in revolt and proclaimed him emperor. Soon after, an enraged mob stormed the Imperial Palace and captured Andronikos. For three days, they dragged him through the streets, torturing, humiliating, and mutilating him. He died in the Hippodrome on September 11, 1185. With his tragic reign, the brilliant dynasty of the Komnenoi came to an end, and the fateful Angelos dynasty assumed power over the empire.

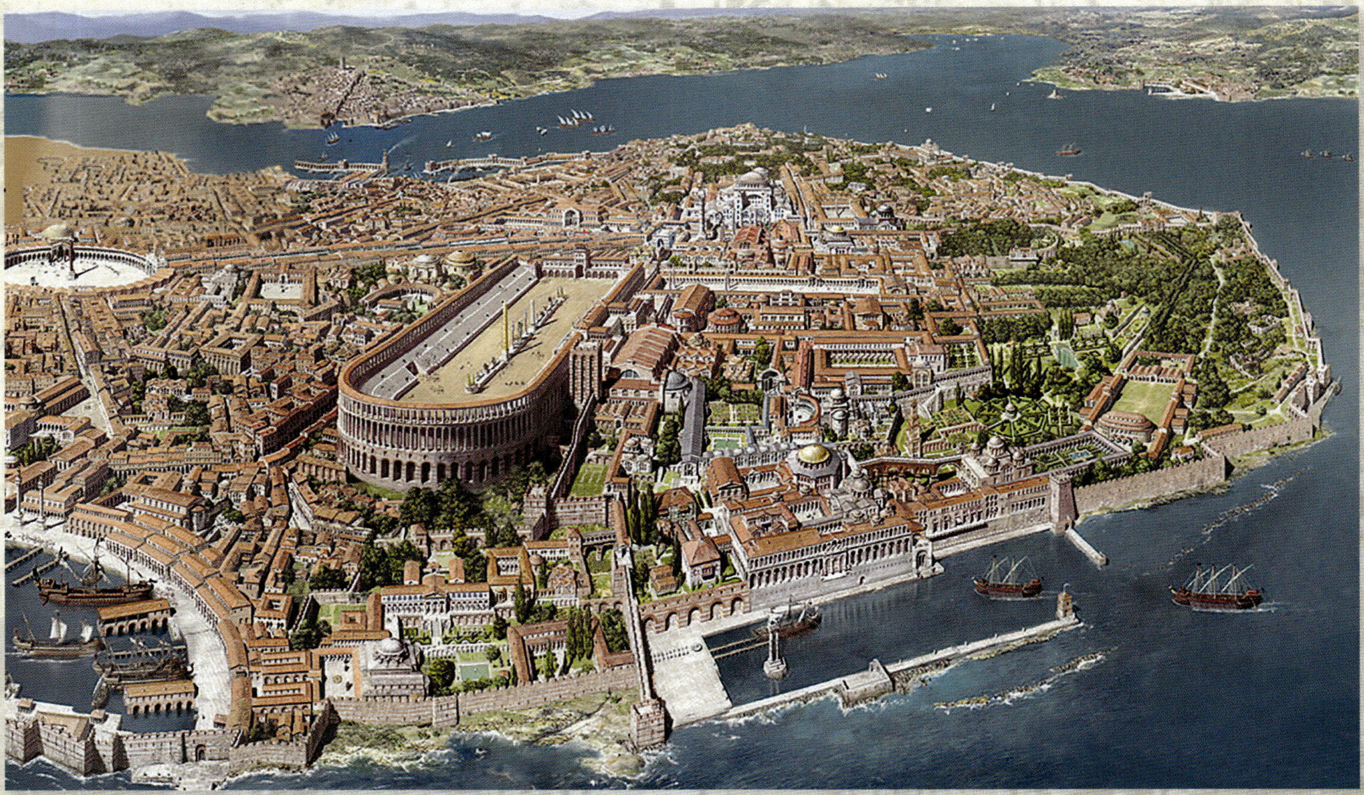

Constantinople in the 12th Century.
Reconstruction by Antoine Helbert, 1870

The Angeloi Dynasty and the Crusades

the Infirmary of the Monastery of the Pantocrator

After the reign of Andronikos, the beautiful years were gone for good. Despite my professional success—working at the Xenon (hospital) of the Pantocrator—despite the profound experiences I gained there and our relative financial comfort, we were overcome by a sense of insecurity and anxiety. Our daily life in Constantinople was not noticeably affected, at least in the beginning, but the news we kept hearing was far from pleasant.

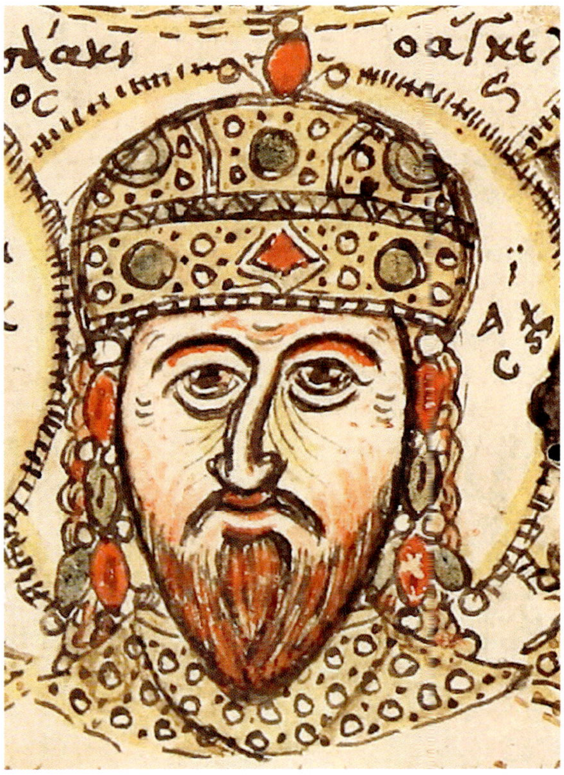

Isaac II Angelos.
Miniature from Zonaras, 15th century, Biblioteca d'Este, Modena.

From 1185, the Angeloi dynasty ruled for about twenty years, until 1204. The three Emperors—Isaac II, Alexios III, and Alexios IV—were the worst possible leaders for the Empire, exemplifying greed, irresponsibility, and incompetence. The security and prosperity that had existed during the reign of the Komnenoi vanished, giving way to insecurity, economic ruin, and military defeats and humiliations. Isaac, initially a collaborator of Andronikos Komnenos whom he overthrew and delivered to the enraged mob, made desperate attempts to establish a foothold in power, as the provincial aristocrats and local rulers did not take him seriously. The Angelos family did not belong to the old aristocracy, and the older families looked down on them, considering them inferior.

In our time, intermarriages between the prominent houses of Europe have become quite customary, often creating temporary or even lasting alliances. Isaac married Margaret, daughter of King Béla III of Hungary, and arranged for his sister Theodora to marry Conrad of Montferrat, his niece Eudokia to marry Stefan Nemanjić, son of the Grand Prince of Serbia, and his daughter Irene to marry Philip of Swabia, son of Frederick I of Germany. The first steps of his ten-year reign were positive. In November 1185, his capable general Alexios Vranas achieved a crushing victory against the Normans and expelled them permanently from the Balkan Peninsula. At the same time, however, the Bulgarians revolted and established their own state under the rule of the Asen dynasty. Isaac defeated them, they rose again, but were ultimately crushed by Vranas.

We all took heart at first, hoping for a new revival of the state. People began to feel optimistic, and the operation of the Hospital where I worked was excellent. I had been promoted to *Protomenitis*, taking on more rights and responsibilities. Now Antigone had the freedom to come daily to the hospital and was truly my right hand, offering her services selflessly and without being carried away by her new role. She maintained her modesty and grace, earning the love and respect of the entire staff. We worked together on the diagnosis and treatment of patients; she was present as support staff during surgeries, mainly ensuring that supplies were sufficient and that conditions of cleanliness and antisepsis were properly maintained. In the evenings, we would discuss the patients' problems and what we could do to improve the functioning of the hospital. The absence of the joy of children brought us even closer, and we had become almost entirely devoted to our medical mission.

But the good times ended after the first few years. Isaac was neither Kaloyannis nor Manuel. He left the administration unchecked in the hands of corrupt officials. Embezzlement, the sale of offices, bribery of officials, and extortion by tax collectors became everyday occurrences. Rumor had it that the Emperor sold public offices as if they were vegetables in the marketplace. The various aristocrats, the so-called *eupatrides* (the noble) or *dynatoi* (the powerful), considered themselves more fit to rule the country than the pitiful Isaac, and thus separatist tendencies began to emerge in

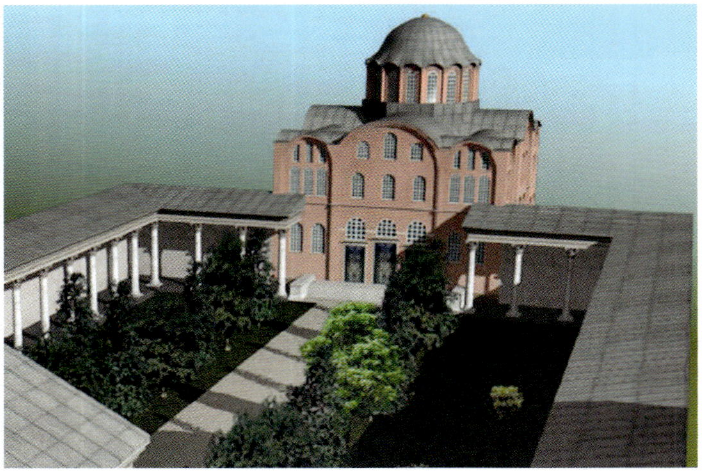

Imaginary reconstruction of the Senate building in the complex of the Great Palace, identified with the Magnaura.

byzantium1200.com

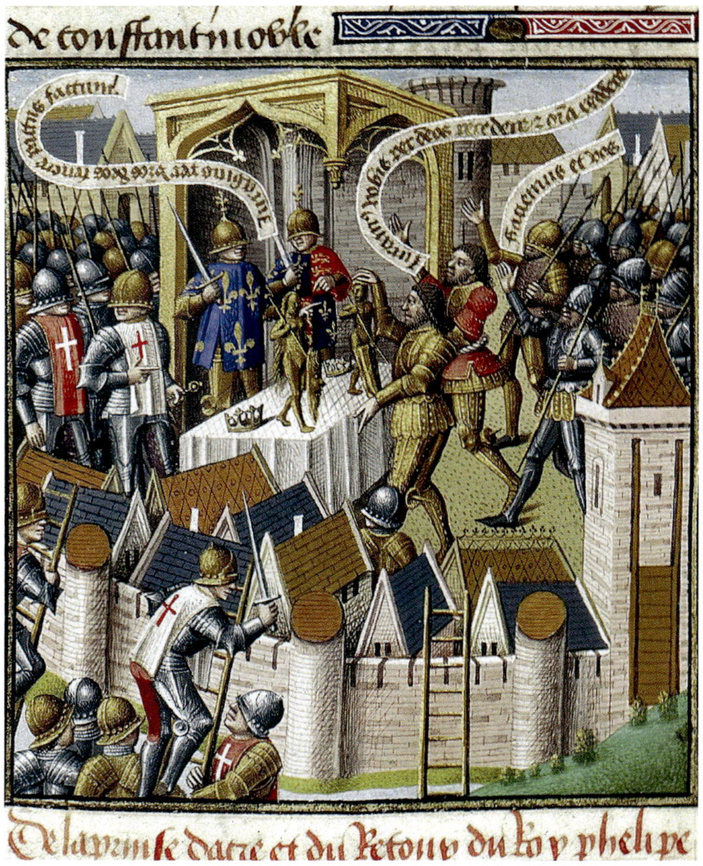

The soldiers of the Third Crusade lay siege to Acre.

Miniature, 13th century, from the Encyclopaedia Speculum Majus.

various parts of the Empire. Returning to the Capital from a military campaign, the great general Vranas rebelled against Isaac, but unfortunately, he was killed in a skirmish and the uprising failed. Had Vranas succeeded in overthrowing Isaac, the fate of the state might have been different. But God did not permit it.

In 1187, the Third Crusade was proclaimed by three kings: Frederick I of Germany, known as Barbarossa—meaning "Red Beard"; Richard of England, famed for his bravery and called the Lionheart; and Philip II of France, known as the Prudent. Their goal was to liberate Jerusalem, which had been captured by Sultan Saladin after he crushed the Christian armies of the local Latin principalities. Fortunately, the English and the French traveled by sea to Palestine. The problem, however, was Barbarossa, who requested to march his troops through our lands. And so the same story repeated itself as with the previous

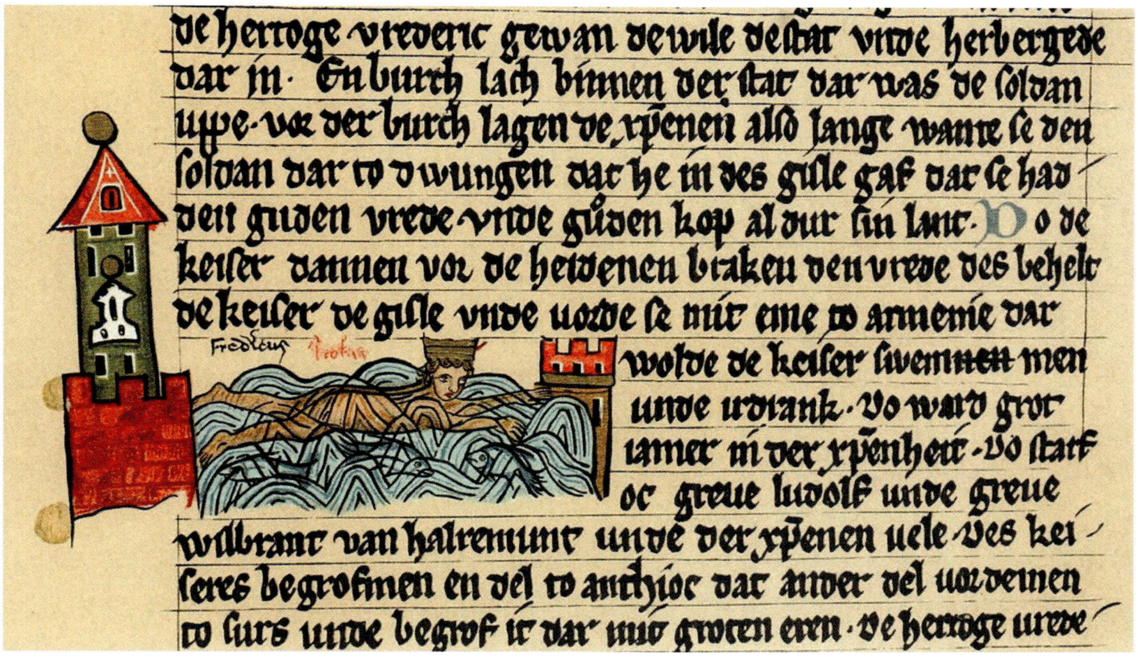

Barbarossa Drowns in the River Calycandos.

Miniature from a Saxon Chronicle, 13th century.

crusades. The Germans behaved very aggressively, pillaging the lands they passed through and occupying Philippopolis. But realizing that open conflict was not to their advantage and that their forces were simply being worn down, they reached an agreement with Isaac and crossed into Asia Minor using Byzantine ships and supplies. Barbarossa, who was a capable general, managed to defeat the Seljuks and captured Iconium. Yet divine justice punished him for his arrogance. While attempting to cross the river Calycandos on horseback—a small but swift river—he was swept away by the current and drowned. Thus, the Third Crusade ended ingloriously for the Germans, who did not continue the campaign.

Richard's voyage to Palestine brought about yet another calamity for our Roman Empire (Byzantium). After a storm, the English fleet docked in Cy-

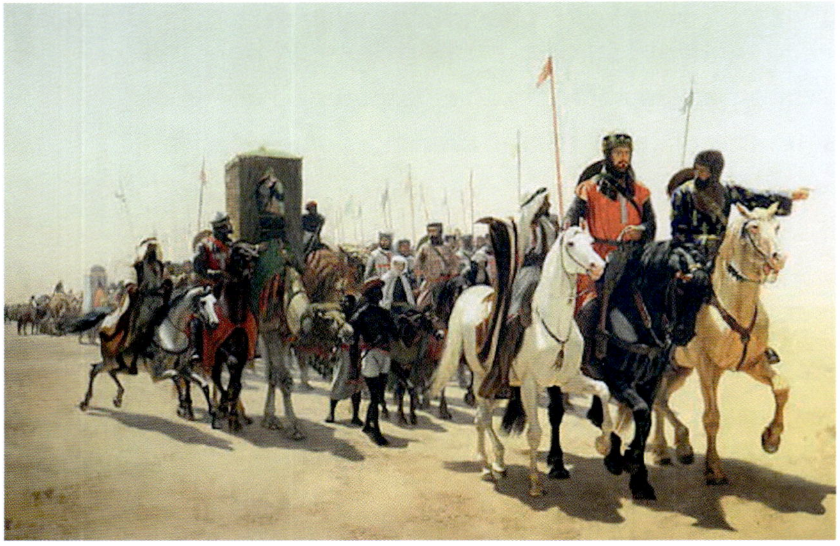

Richard the Lionheart on His Way to Jerusalem.

Painting by William Glass, 1850, Private Collection.

prus, which at the time was ruled by Isaac Komnenos Kamateros, who had partially seceded from the Empire. Richard conquered Cyprus, plundered it, and then sold it to the Knights Templar. Thus, this important island—Greek since time immemorial—was lost to us permanently. When the remaining Crusaders finally gathered in Palestine, they realized that Saladin was a far more capable adversary than they had imagined. They managed to capture the fortresses of Acre and Jaffa, but they were not even able to lay siege to Jerusalem. The only thing Richard succeeded in doing was to reach an agreement with the conciliatory Saladin to allow Christian merchants and unarmed pilgrims to enter the City. The Third Crusade ended ingloriously in 1192.

During the ten-year reign of Isaac, the administration of the state became paralyzed. Threats from neighboring powers and military failures increased. Yet, paradoxically, life in Constantinople continued as usual. The flourishing of the arts persisted, and the state's public health policy remained unchanged. In fact, Isaac founded another xenon (hospital), as was customary, within the grounds of a monastery — the Xenon of the Forty Martyrs. By this time, *xenones* (hospitals) were operating in many provincial cities: Nicaea, Nicomedia, Thessaloniki, Crete, Aenus in Thrace, and elsewhere. The Xenon of the Pantocrator, where I had the joy of serving, continued to function smoothly, just as in the time of the Komnenoi. After all, the blessed Emperor John, the founder of the complex, had provided for its financial self-sufficiency. After ten years of service as an *Embathmos* physician, I had been promoted in 1183 to *Protomenitis* (Chief Physician). Now I was working under much improved conditions, offering my services and experience to the patients and training the younger physicians. I had taken on—and continue to hold—the directorship of the surgical department. The organization of our *xenon* is truly admirable, and I shall describe it as best I can. It is based on the renowned *typikon*, the rule wisely composed by the blessed Emperor and founder.

Signature of John Komnenos, 1136.

Ed. Franz Dölger, Munich, 1931.

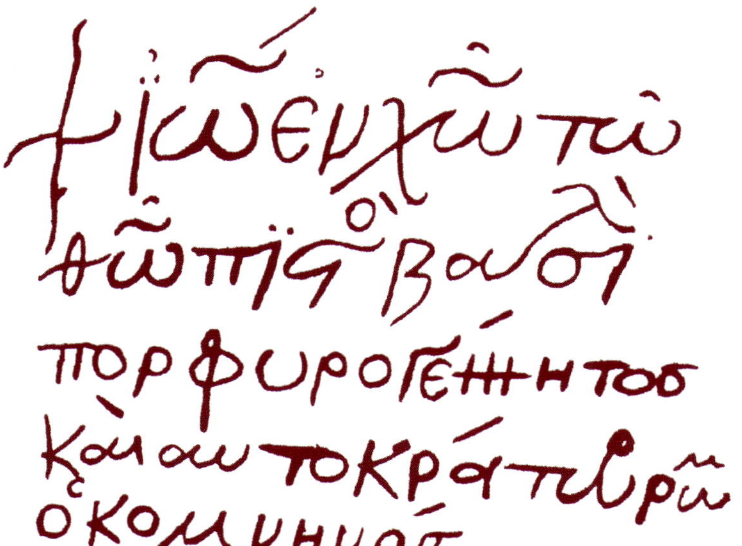

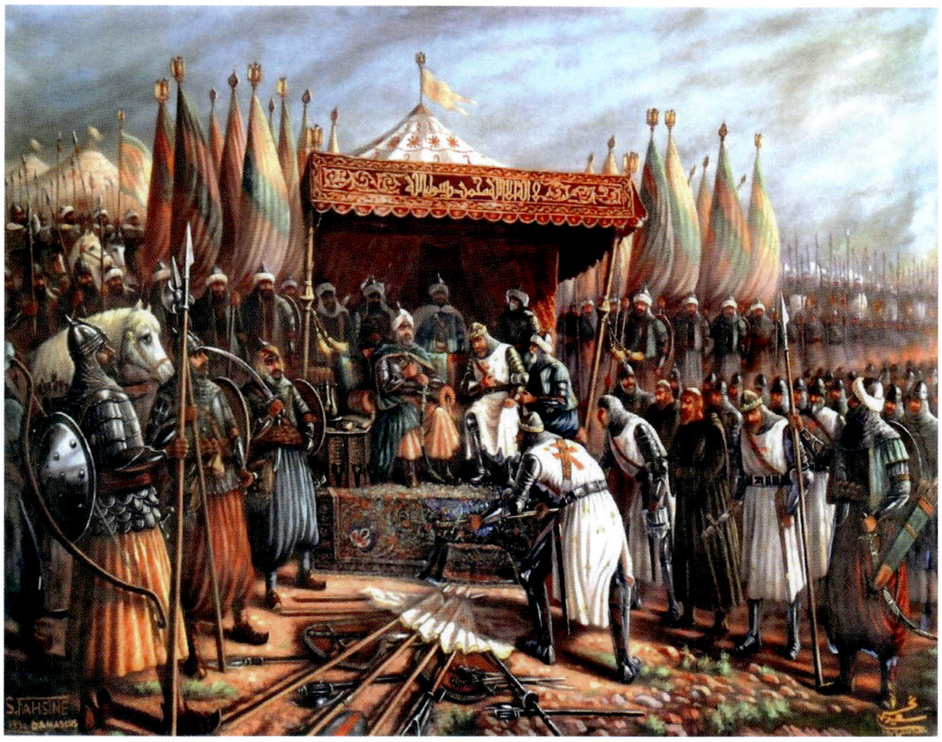

Guy de Lusignan surrenders to Saladin after the Battle of Hattin in 1187.

Painting by Said Tahseen, 1954, Syria.

In the *typikon,* John Komnenos stipulates the construction of a complex that includes the Monastery of the Pantocrator, a family mausoleum, a *xenon* (hospital), a home for the elderly, and a leprosarium—the latter, for obvious reasons, situated outside the main complex. For the operation and maintenance of the institution, he left a generous endowment, so that it would remain financially self-sufficient.

The operational expenses were overseen by an Administrative Council. Kalogiannis explained that the founding of the Monastery was a return gift (*antídoro*) for the divine favor he had received during his reign, particularly in his handling of internal and external affairs. He hoped that the care offered to the elderly, the tending of lepers, and the treatment of the sick in the associated institutions would contribute to the remission of his sins. The *typikon* specified in detail the number of clergy and monks who would serve the liturgical needs of the Monastery, as well as the functioning of its philanthropic establishments.

The *Xenon* (hospital) includes five wards with a total of fifty beds, one for each patient (unlike in the West, where it was not uncommon for two patients to share a bed). The beds are divided among five ordines, or departments: the surgical ward with 8 beds, the gynecological ward with 12 beds, the ophthalmological ward with 10, and two additional departments for other illnesses (such as internal medicine, gastroenterology, etc.).

For emergency cases, an additional *parakravaton* (extra bed) is provided in each department, along with six beds equipped with special mattresses for bedridden patients—bringing the total number of beds to sixty-one. Each bed

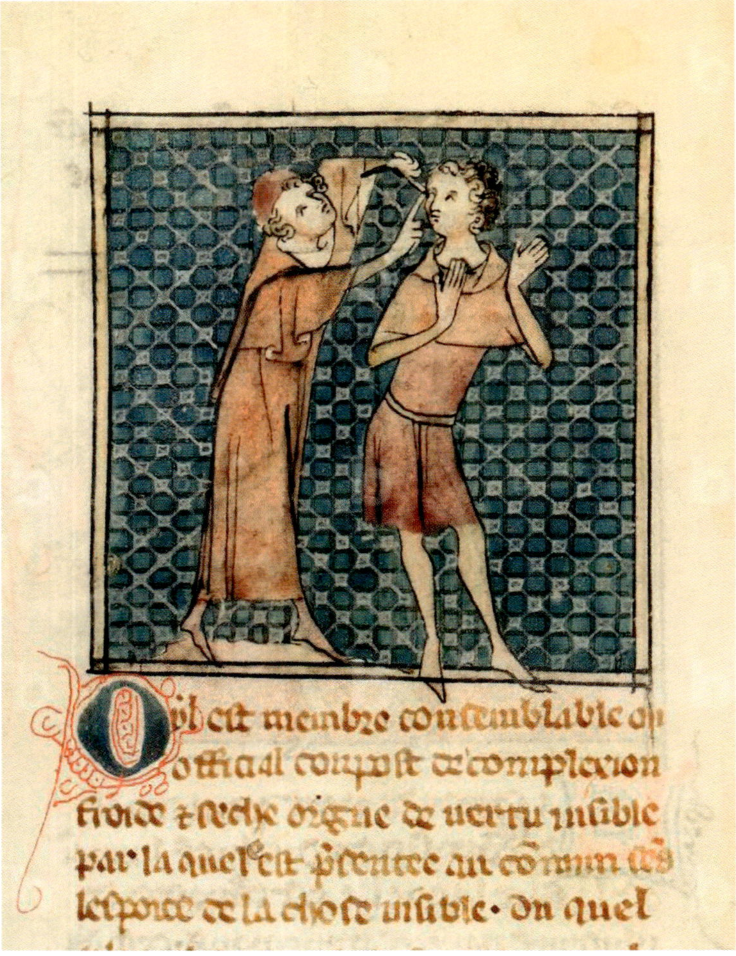

Ophthalmological examination.

Miniature, 14th century, Henri de Mondeville, National Library of France, Paris.

is furnished with a mat, a mattress, and three *iosnikia*—coverlets made from goat wool. In the winter, three *aroules* (heaters) operate: one large and two smaller ones, designated respectively for the gynecological, surgical, and internal medicine departments. Patients also have access to two latrines and bathing facilities, which they may use as frequently as the doctors deem necessary for their treatment. All of this is ensured through timely provisioning, diligent maintenance, and strict cleanliness. The hospital staff is required to supply the poorest patients or those who are gravely ill with fresh clothing for the duration of their stay. Each patient's personal garments are laundered and returned to them upon discharge. The poor are permitted to keep the hospital clothing even after their treatment has ended. Furthermore, all linens—including mattresses, coverlets, and pillows—are replaced annually with new ones. Any of the older items that are still in usable condition are stored and distributed to the poor.

The *xenon* (hospital) also includes a large pharmacy and dedicated spaces for the medical staff, where physicians can rest and study, drawing from the rich medical library available on-site. A sizeable team serves at the xenon: doctors, nurses, *pimentarioi* (pharmacists), cooks, servants, and doorkeep-

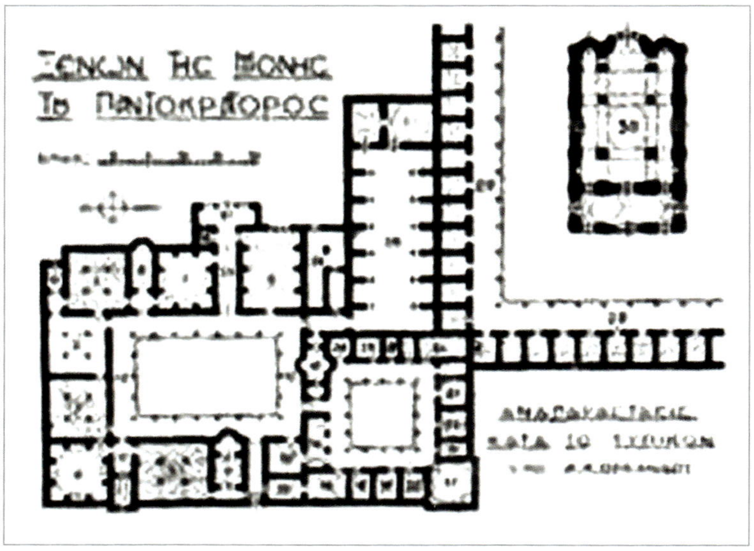

Floor plan of the Hospital of the Monastery of Pantocrator.

Reconstruction by Anastasios Orlandos.

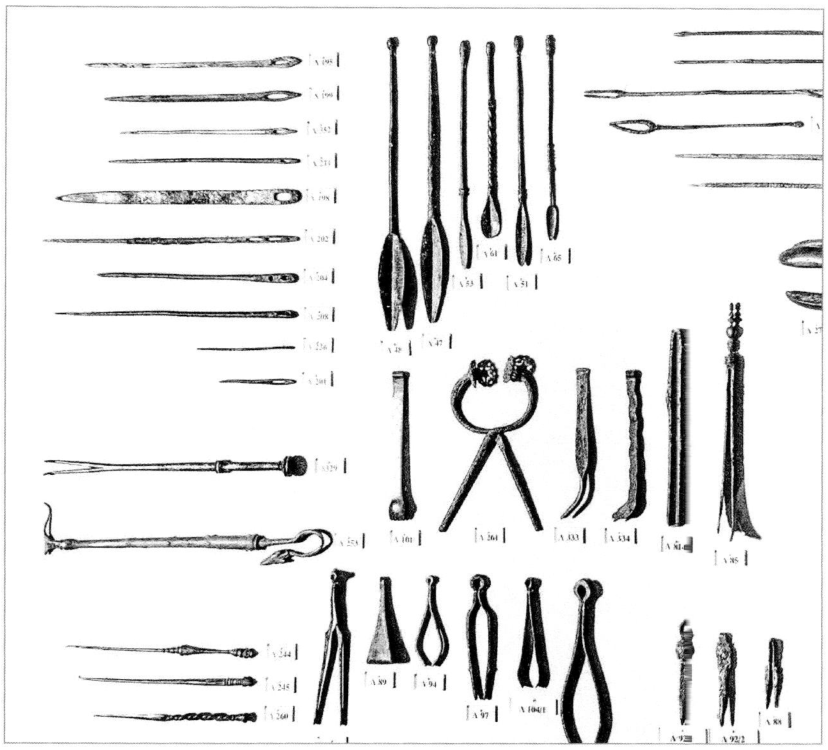

Surgical nstruments from the collection of Konstantinos Lampros.

National Archaeological Museum, Athens.

ers—all organized in a clear hierarchy according to their specialties and responsibilities. The overall scientific direction of the hospital—that is, the supervision of diagnoses and the monitoring of treatments—is entrusted to the *Primikērios* physician. There are two *Primikērioi,* who alternate in service each month.

In each men's ward, two *Protomēnítai* (senior supervising physicians) serve, alternating monthly and acting as the ward directors. There are also three certified physicians, known as *Embathmoi* (or *mesoi*), who serve as ministers (i.e., attending doctors); two resident physicians, referred to as *Perissoi Ypourgoi* (junior ministers), and two servants who perform nursing duties. For the women's ward, the staff includes three doctors—two men and one female doctor (*iatraina*)—as well as four specialized female assistants (*embathmoi ypourgissai*), two trainees (*perittai ypourgissai*), and two female nurses (*ypērettriai*). The *xenon* (hospital) also operates outpatient clinics, where patients come to be examined and receive the appropriate treatment. For these outpatient services, there are two internists and two surgeons, who are assisted by both specialized and apprentice aides. The monks of the Monastery, who contribute significantly to the nursing and auxiliary care, are provided with a separate ward within the facility should they fall ill and require hospitalization.

The *protomenites* (chief resident physicians) serve one in each ward. We bear full responsibility for our ward: we determine the diagnosis and prescribe the treatment, and we assign duties to the ministers—both the *embathmoi* (qualified doctors) and the *perissoi* (apprentice physicians). The *primikērios* (chief physician) supervises the condition of all patients daily, monitors the course of their treatment, and corrects any errors or oversights that may arise. He is also responsible for inspecting the bread, the other foodstuffs, and everything else distributed daily to the patients. When a seriously ill person is admitted, he is first taken on by the *protomenites,* who ensures his accommodation and initial care, and then provides a detailed report to the *primikērios,* who in turn assigns the patient to the ward he deems most suitable. Some of the "ministers" (junior physicians) remain at the hospital overnight to be on duty. In addition to the *primikērioi,* each ward also has nearby a "Master of the Medical Art". This mas-

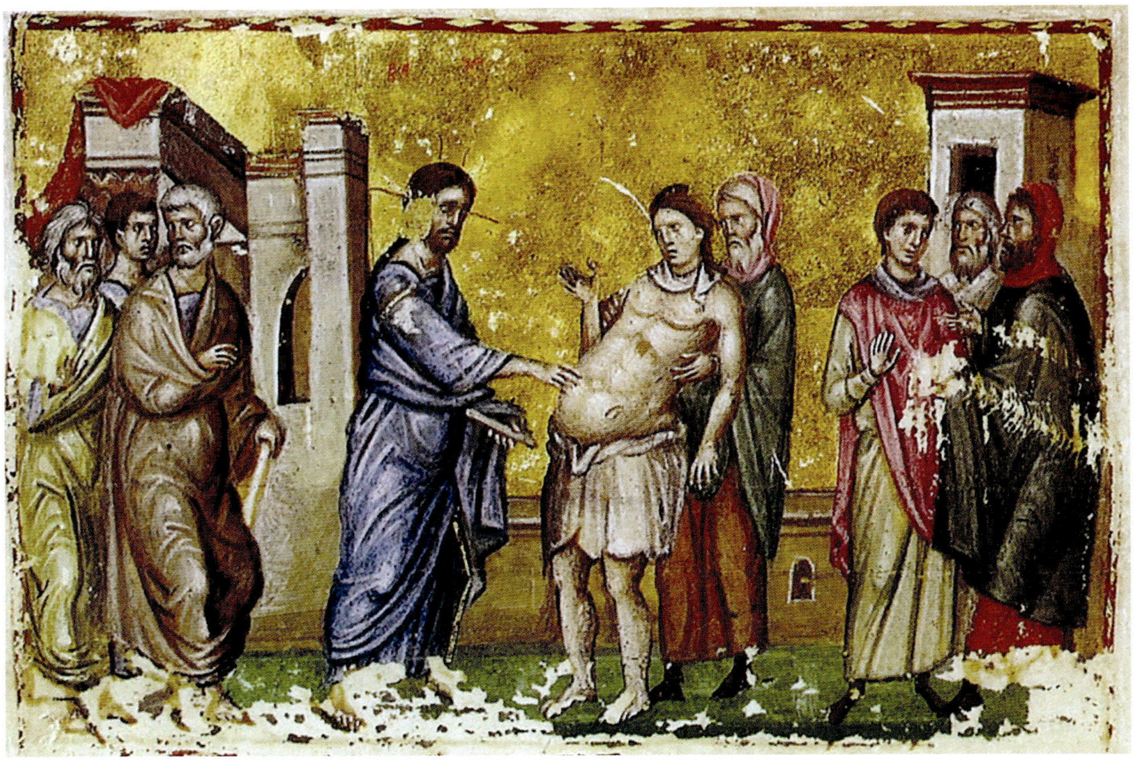

The healing of the dropsical man.
Miniature, Pemptousia, September 2020.

ter is a seasoned physician of recognized authority, whose duty is to train the young doctors in the knowledge of medical science. In our day, this position is held by the venerable and wise Gregorios Frantzis, whom we often consult and deeply honor for his invaluable service. Frantzis possesses not only medical expertise but also profound philosophical knowledge.

The *Typikon* sets forth the system of promotions and the tiered salaries for all categories of the staff, which are only slightly above the average wage level. The *primikērioi*, who are the chief physicians, are two in number and rotate monthly in their duties. During the month in which one is off duty at the hospital, he has the right to practice medicine privately, thereby increasing his earnings while also benefiting from the prestige conferred by his service at the *xenon* (hospital). This alternation also applies to the protomēnitai and the ministers, so that each month only half of the total medical staff is actively serving in the hospital. This is a very clever arrangement, for it is strictly forbidden for physicians, during their term of service at the *xenon*, to undertake any duty outside the hospital—even if such a duty involves the Emperor himself. In general, they are prohibited from performing their functions in any external assignments beyond the hospital, and from accepting gifts or payments from the hospital's patients—commonly known as "blessings." Thus, through rotational service, the economic gap between private and public physicians is reduced, and public doctors are better enabled to fulfill their obligations during their period of service within the hospital.

The Administrative Director of the Xenon is called the *Nosokomos* (Hospital Steward), previously known as the *Xenodochos* (Host of the Xenon). The *Noso-*

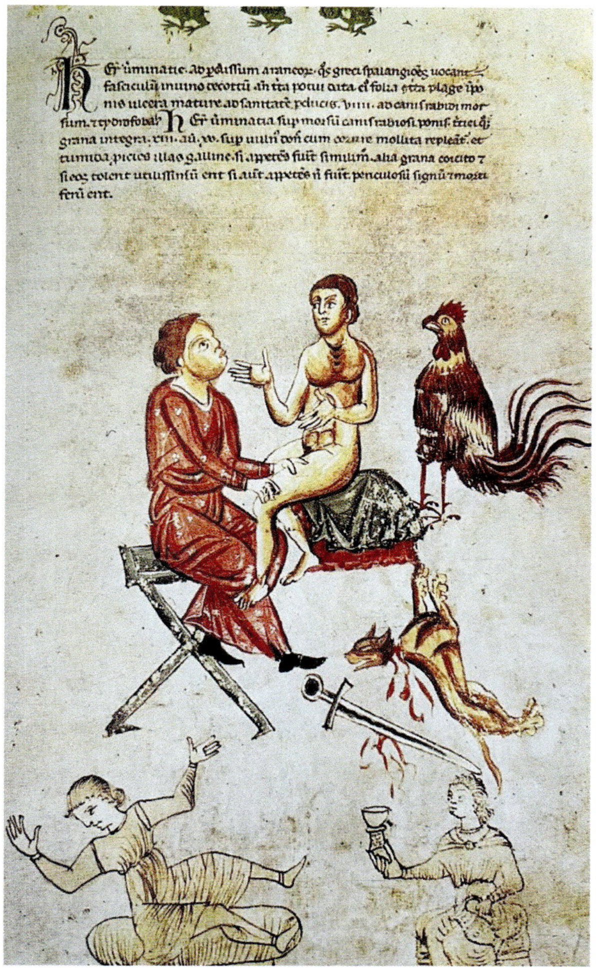

The sacred herb,
an antidote to poisons.

Pseudo-Apuleius Herbarium, 13th century.

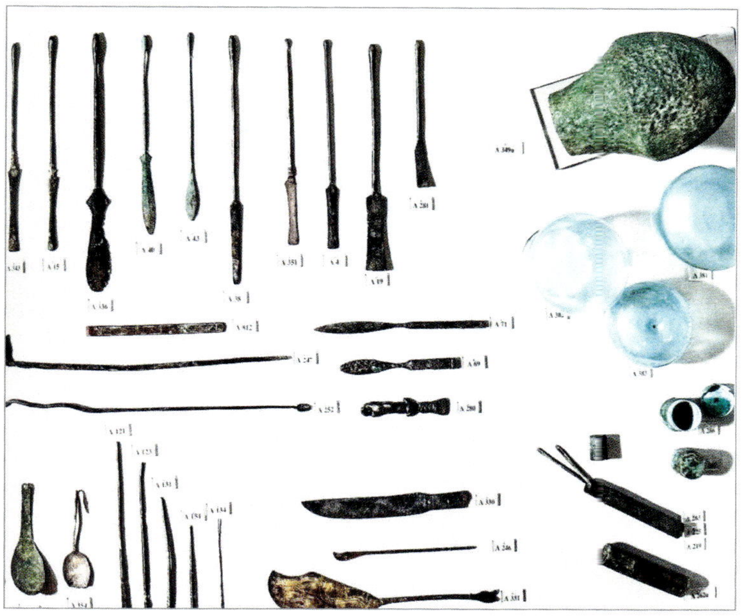

Surgical instruments
from the collection
of Konstantinos Lampros.

National Archaeological Museum, Athens.

komos, together with the *Epistates* (Overseer), is entrusted with funds and is responsible for securing all necessary supplies for the hospital in sufficient quantities, ensuring that all needs of the patients are met abundantly. They also oversee the timely payment of the staff's salaries, which is carried out without delay. The management of the pharmacy is entrusted to four certified *pimentarioi* (pharmacists): one serves as the *Epistikon* (chief pharmacist), one as the regular pharmacist (*takticos*), and two as assistant or junior pharmacists (*perissoi*). There is also a "mylocharaktis" (grinder-sharpener), responsible for ensuring that all surgical instruments are clean and sharp; an *ostiarios*, who serves as a porter or herald; five women *saponistriai* working in the laundries; a man assigned to maintain a constant supply of hot water; two cooks, two *mangipes* (bakers), a miller, and a stablekeeper (*stavlitis*), who tends to the doctors' horses and also assists in the mill. There is an *opsoniator*, in charge of purchasing all necessary provisions, a *pyloros* who guards the gate, and finally a *kanaloplyntis*, who maintains and cleans the drainage system. For the spiritual needs of the patients, the staff includes three priests, who provide confession and conduct funerals, two readers of ecclesiastical texts, and four gravediggers.

The monastery's *typikon* (rule or charter) meticulously defines the food rations allocated to both the hospital staff and the patients. Each patient receives daily: two and a half litrai of bread (approximately 850 grams), typically two dishes of vegetables prepared with olive oil, and two heads of onions. From time to time, meat or fish is also served. Additionally, each patient is granted a small monetary allowance, one *rough coin* per day, to purchase supplementary food or a bit of wine—provided the doctors approve its use for their condition. The *typikon* also provides for the care of the patients' personal hygiene, which is the responsibility of the hospital staff, as well as the availability of hygiene supplies (such as towels and washbasins) and cooking utensils. I would go so far as to say that, although other hospitals in the City are of a similarly high standard, the Xenon of the Pantocrator is the most complete and rationally organized medical institution in the empire. And judging from the condition of Western hospitals that I came to know a little later, it is without a doubt the finest in all of Europe.

A distinctive feature of medical care in the Empire is that women participate equally with men in the operation of hospitals (*xenones*) and other philanthropic institutions. In our hospitals, women—mainly nuns, but also laywomen, even from the higher social and economic classes—are actively involved, most often serving as nurses. Of course, there are also female doctors (*iatraines*) and midwife-physicians (*iatromaiai*), who now receive full medical training and serve on equal footing with us men. Because the care provided in the hospitals is of a very high standard, beds are considered precious. Thus, when a patient reaches a desperate and terminal condition, they are moved from the hospital to free the bed for another patient. They are transferred to a separate building, where they are cared for by the nurses so that they may pass away peacefully.

Care for the sick, however, does not end with medical treatment alone. In the operation of the hospitals, there are also the *parabolani*, who serve as social workers. They care for the patients and the poor from the perspective of state welfare, ensuring that some assistance is provided to them once they leave the institution. At the same time, the state has established the office of the "Investigator" (*Ereunitēs*)—a public official whose task is to find public employment for healthy but unemployed and impoverished citizens. On this occasion, I should also note that under the Komnenian emperors, even in prisons, where conditions were naturally far from ideal, there were special "Inspectors" who visited every Sunday and asked the inmates whether they were being given the food allocated to them.

I worked in the *xenon* (hospital) for another ten years as a *protomenites* (senior ward physician), until the year 1193. During these years, I had the opportunity to perform many surgeries and to perfect my skill in the art of surgery. I studied extensively the writings of the great physicians, but above all, I acquired my own experience by practicing medicine broadly within the hospital setting—encountering many different cases, listening to colleagues, engaging

Metrodora the Athenian

She lived in Athens during the 3rd or 4th century AD. She was a physician and the author of the work "On the Diseases of Women's Wombs", which is the oldest known medical text written by a woman. The work is preserved in two volumes, comprising a total of 63 chapters, and it covers several areas of medicine and gynecology, though not obstetrics. Metrodora was particularly influenced by the writings of Hippocrates, as were most physicians of her time. She presents strong positions on controversial topics of symptomatology and etiology—for example, regarding inflammation of the uterus. Her work includes original contributions to the advancement of medical theory and causation. It was cited by many other medical authors and was even translated into Latin, circulating widely in medieval Europe. Beyond her name, no other details are known about Metrodora's identity. It is known that there were several female physicians in the ancient Greco-Roman world, and Metrodora is considered the first woman to have authored a medical book.

Sharon James, & Sheila Dillon

in discussions with them, and learning from both my successes and my mistakes. I observed my teachers with reverence, but at the same time I evaluated their actions, constantly learning. Yet, above all, what I truly learned was respect and love for the patient, and a deep concern for their full recovery—not just the isolated treatment of a medical issue, but the restoration of the person as a whole.

All of us who have been engaged in the medical art have come to realize that the human organism is extraordinarily complex, and its functions are extremely difficult to understand and interpret. The disruption of the balance of humors, which brings about illness, is not easily restored. Our medicines and interventions are often powerless in the face of disease. That is why we stand in awe before the mystery of life and death, fully aware that it surpasses both our knowledge and our capabilities. Thus, the physician must understand that he should not act with arrogance, thinking himself important, but rather should approach each case with humility, summoning all the knowledge he has acquired to correctly diagnose the illness and to choose the proper treat-

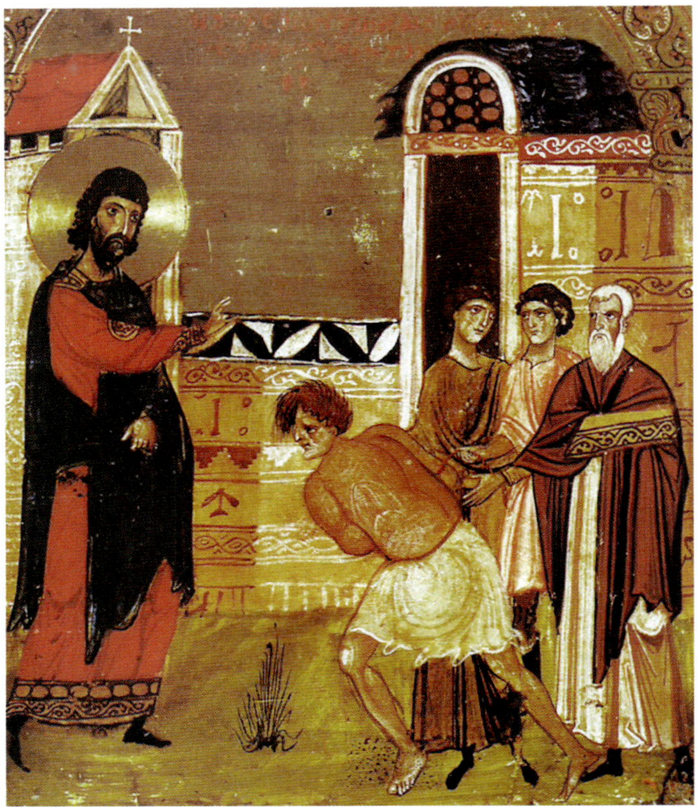

Saint Eustratius healing a sick man.

12th-century icon, Sinai Monastery.

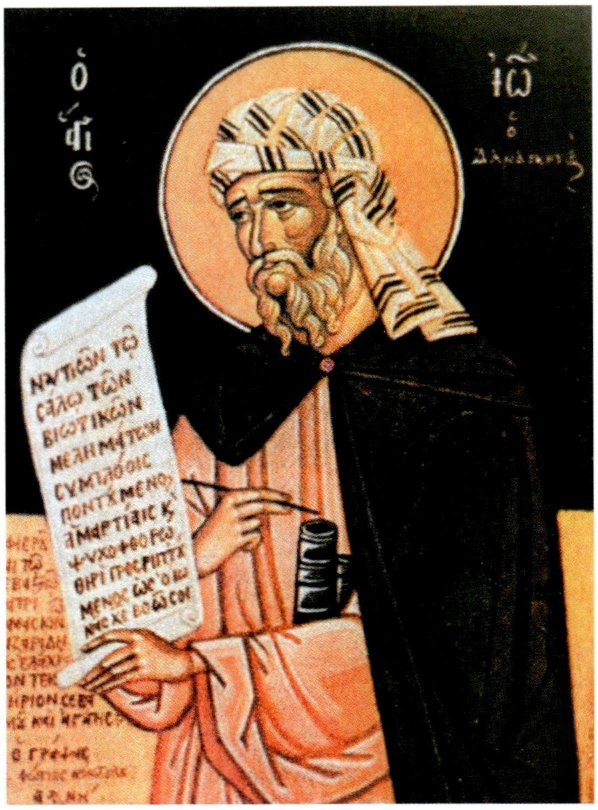

Saint John of Damascus. He primarily dealt with neurological and mental illnesses.

Icon by Fotis Kontoglou.

ment. And he must be ready, in the course of the illness's progression, to revise both diagnosis and treatment, if new evidence demands it. He must acknowledge his mistakes and correct them. Above all, he must recognize that there is always an imponderable factor that can overturn the situation at any moment. We, the physicians of our God-protected Empire, acknowledge the power of faith, prayer, and the invocation of divine help—whether from God Himself or from His Saints. Without dismissing the value of science, after exhausting every effort with the knowledge granted to us through study and experience, we always call upon the aid of God and His Saints. And we know well that the faith of the patient and of the doctor can make the impossible possible. And we encourage our patients to have faith and to invoke the Divine. Naturally, we must draw a clear line between true faith and superstition. Among the people—and regrettably even among the educated—there remains a widespread reliance on amulets, exorcisms, incantations, and all manner of nonsense: the so-called *"iatrosófia"*, which are remnants of pagan magical rites. These we fight against with resolve—not only we physicians, but also the enlightened hierarchs of the Church—because they often do harm rather than good.

Our medicine is founded on reason, observation, experimentation, and the adjustment of various treatments and remedies. It is aided by faith and prayer, for we know how inadequate and incomplete we are before the mystery of life.

Nevertheless, there are always physicians who are incompetent or greedy, just as there are always patients who are dissatisfied, whether justly or unjustly. Many complaints have been voiced—especially concerning avaricious doctors—though at times, these grievances may be exaggerated.

As it seems, not everyone had good experiences with doctors.
From an 11th-century writer, we learn:

Pray that you do not fall into the hands of a doctor, even if he is very learned. For he will tell you things that are not necessary. And if your illness is minor, he will greatly exaggerate it and say you need herbs of great cost—'but I shall heal you,' he says. Then, having taken coins from you, he claims, 'This is not enough for the market,' and takes more. Wanting to milk you dry, he tells you to eat what is contrary to your illness, thereby worsening it. And again he will tend to you, and once more the pain will flare up. And thus, having done this many times, he will take from you all that he needs and scarcely ever truly treat you.

From another writer of the 7th century,
we hear the sick man say to his doctor:

You have not healed me, and I have given you a six-nummus coin, a three-nummus coin, and four keratia, and so many tokens of kindness—and I have gained nothing from you. But as many times as you did something to me, just as many times I had a worse day, growing worse each time. Get out of my house

There is, however, also the positive side:

The Byzantine State, in recognition of the services provided by physicians for the health of its citizens, honored them—according to Roman and ancient Greek custom—and granted them privileges, as we learn from the laws. Thus, it exempted them, especially professors of medicine, from burdensome public duties, guardianship, and curatorship, as well as from council responsibilities and supervision of weights and measures, as stated by Julian in the law "On Physicians," which is "in accordance with the ordinances established by the emperors above."

Phaedon Koukoules, Byzantine Life and Civilization

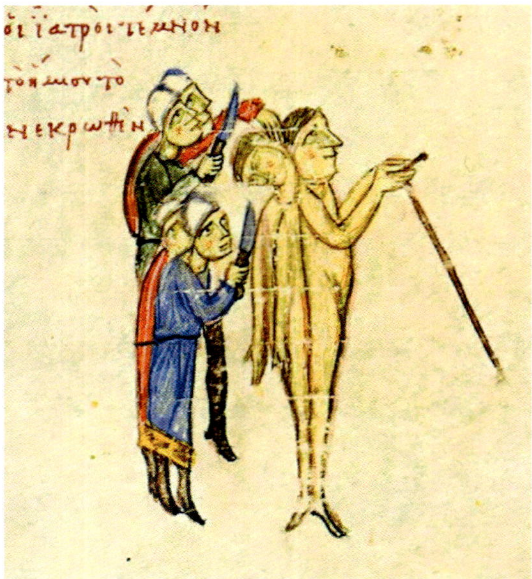

Separation surgery of conjoined twins.

Miniature, 12th century. The Skylitzes Matritensis, National Library, Madrid.

After ten years of service as *protomēnites* (chief ward physician), I was promoted to the position of *primikērios* (head physician). It was a vindication for the labors I had undertaken. I have written a number of notes on diagnosis and treatment for the benefit of young doctors, in which I lay out my personal views and therapies for many illnesses, along with a clear and accessible description of various fundamental surgical procedures. This book has become very well-loved among physicians and played a significant role in my promotion. As *primikērios*, I now have the opportunity to carry out my work with greater freedom, performing many surgeries—particularly restorative ones, which I greatly enjoy—and I quickly became well known. During the months when I practiced privately, I had the opportunity to treat some prominent individuals and form connections with them. These acquaintances proved to be life-saving when the catastrophe of the Fourth Crusade struck.

Meanwhile, matters in the Empire were going from bad to worse. Not so much because of external enemies—this time the Bulgarians—who constantly engaged our armies and with whom we were locked in frequent skirmishes, sometimes victorious, sometimes defeated, in a veritable display of incompetence and blunders on the part of our generals. The true calamity was that the state was steadily losing its prestige, both abroad and at home. The various nobles paid less and less heed to the Emperor, and the many officials who had undeservedly gained their posts had lost the respect and trust of the people. Nevertheless, Emperor Isaac tried as best he could to assert his authority. In 1195, he organized a major military campaign against the Bulgarians. He al-

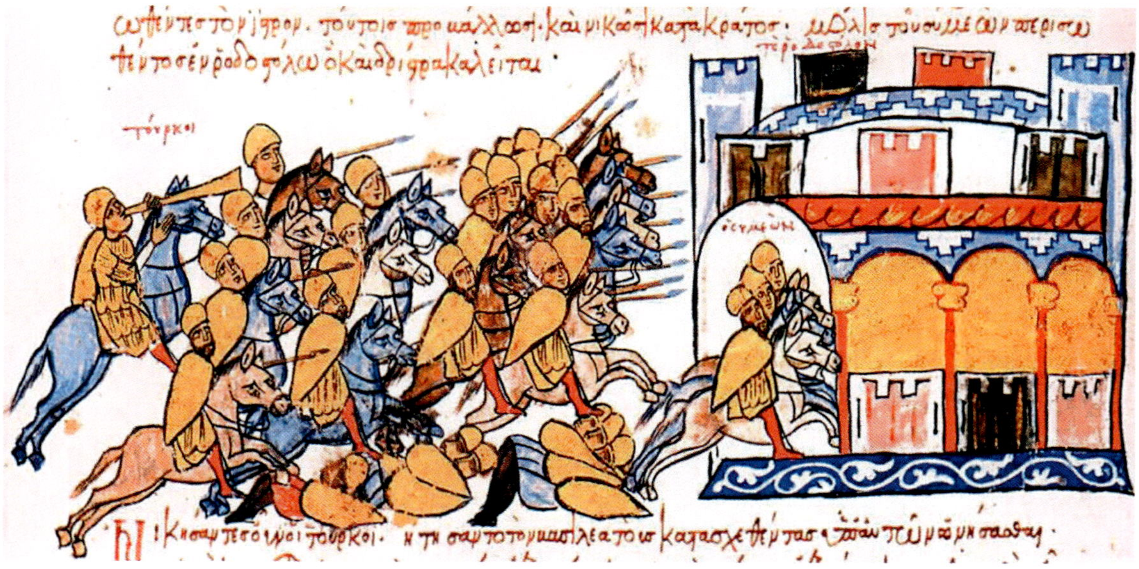

The Hungarians (referred to as Turks) pursue the Bulgarian Tsar Symeon.

Miniature, Skylitzes Matritensis, 12th century, National Library of Spain, Madrid.

lied himself with his relative, the king of Hungary, and assembled a respectable army.

In May of 1195, during the preparations for his military campaign, he went on a hunting excursion in Thrace. That hunt proved to be fateful—both for him personally and for the Empire.

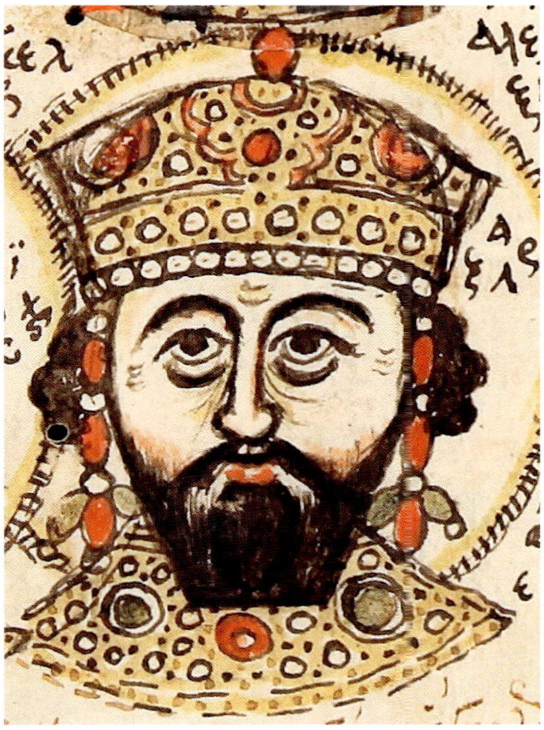
Alexios III Angelos.
Miniature, Zonaras, 15th century, Library d'Este, Modena.

Isaac had an older brother, Alexios, whom he loved and trusted deeply. When Alexios had been taken captive by the Latins of Acre, it was Isaac, then Emperor, who paid a large ransom to the Franks to secure his release. He welcomed him into the palace, bestowed upon him the high title of *sebastocrator*, and arranged his marriage to Euphrosyne Doukaina Kamatera, from the illustrious Kamateros family—part of his effort to ally his dynasty with the aristocratic houses of Constantinople. Alexios, however, "repaid" his brother's affection all too well. He took advantage of the growing discontent with Isaac's poor governance and the powerful connections his wife had, thanks to her noble lineage, within both the military and political leadership. He won over the commanders of the army, and in 1195, during his brother's absence, he proclaimed himself Emperor under the name Alexios III Komnenos, shedding the surname Angelos and usurping the name of his grandmother, Theodora Komnene—seeking, of course, to bolster his legitimacy through association with the more prestigious Komnenian dynasty. The rebel generals found Isaac in Stagira, in the region of Chalkidiki, captured him, and brought him in chains back to Constantinople. There, Alexios III—who would forever disgrace the name of the Komnenoi—had his own brother and benefactor blinded and thrown into prison, alongside his only son, also named Alexios. With this heinous and treacherous act, he began his reign, laying bare the depths of his immorality and ruthless ambition.

He ruled the Empire for eight years (1195–1203), leading it to the brink of destruction. It quickly became evident that he was far worse than his brother. He began squandering enormous sums from the state treasury on extravagances, dismantling the economy. He cared only for pleasures and idle pursuits. Empress Euphrosyne, though herself fond of luxurious living and the very one whose ambition had brought her husband to the throne, nevertheless tried in every way to maintain the loyalty of the court. She implemented some positive reforms through trusted associates, issuing imperial decrees herself—and even going so far as to amend or overturn Alexios' own decrees at will. In effect, she served as co-ruler. However, she was accused by her enemies of adultery, and Alexios confined her to a monastery for some time. Although she was later reinstated, her influence had waned and her authority was shattered. The Empire drifted steadily toward collapse. Matters reached such a low that, at Christmas of 1196, Emperor Henry VI of Germany demanded tribute from us under threat of invasion.

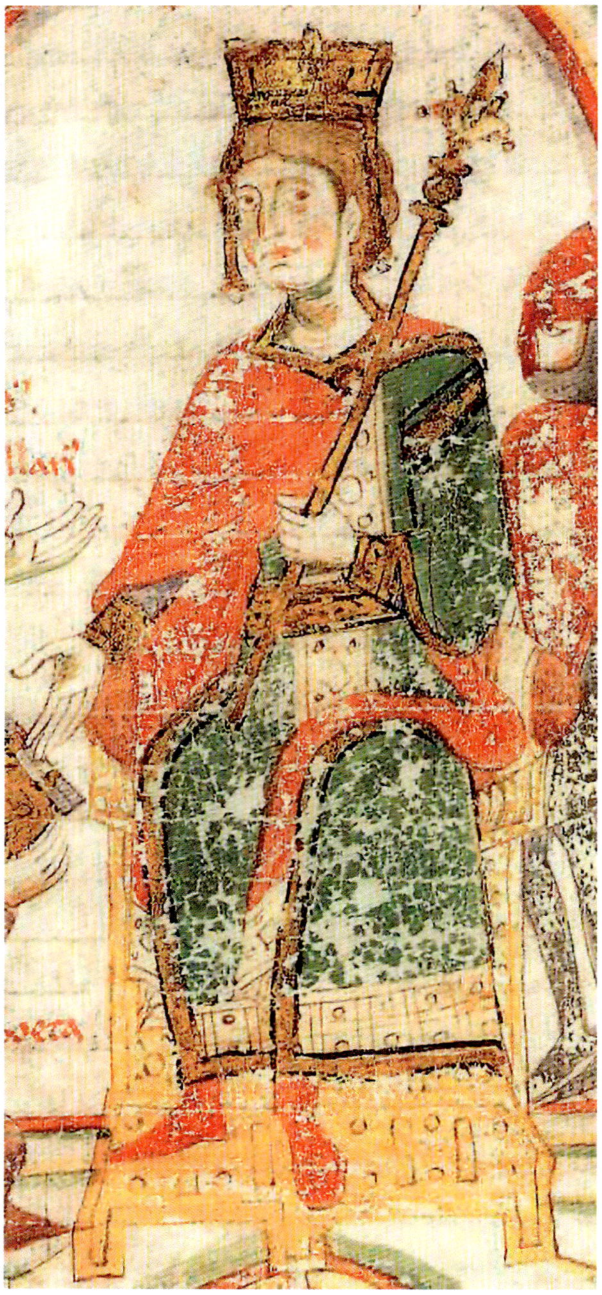

Henry VI
Emperor of
Germany.

Miniature from Peter of Eboli's Liber ad Honorem Augusti, 12th century, Municipal Library, Bern.

Alexios, seized with terror, plundered the imperial tombs in the Church of the Holy Apostles and imposed enormous taxes on the people to meet the German emperor's demands. Fortunately, Henry died and his threat never materialized. Yet the situation continued to worsen. The imperial court spent recklessly, disbursing large sums to foreign monarchs in hopes of gaining their favor—but instead reaped only disdain and contempt. The tax collectors abused their authority, and the excessive taxation exhausted the populace. While Isaac II had ruled, the Empire—though weakened—had managed to maintain some of its positions. But under the reign of Alexios III, it lost even its final defensive strength. Our relations with the neighboring Bulgarians and Serbs, once marked by imperial authority, had now become merely equal—on level terms, not by choice but by weakness. The administration and the ties between the provinces and the capital collapsed entirely. Every local governor, once he gained sufficient power, refused to acknowledge the authority of Alexios—a man who embodied the perfect blend of unrestrained lust for power and cowardly ineptitude. Despite all these negative traits, Alexios did possess one advantage: he made strategic marital alliances for his relatives to bolster his political standing. He married his daughter Eudokia to Stefan Nemanja, the Grand Prince of Serbia. Though the marriage itself was unsuccessful, Serbia remained under the cultural influence of Byzantium. Later, Eudokia married a distinguished nobleman, Alexios Doukas, who would briefly ascend the throne as Emperor of the Romans. His other daughter, Irene, married Alexios Palaiologos, a noble who protected his father-in-law from numerous assassination attempts. Lastly, his third daughter, Anna, married Theodore Laskaris—a noble and admirable man, utterly unmatched with the corrupt Angelos family—who would later preserve the honor and continuity of the Roman State in Nicaea after the fall of Constantinople to the Crusaders in 1204.

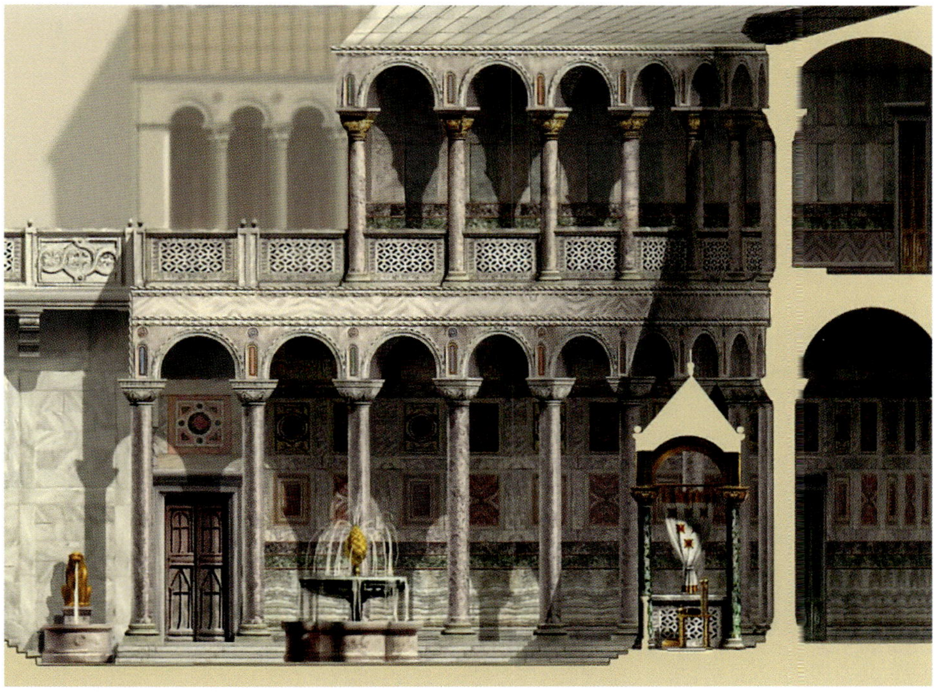

The Palace of Theophilos (Section View).

Reconstruction by Antoine Helbert, 1876.

I had the good fortune to meet Theodore Laskaris as a patient of mine at the xenon in 1199, when he was a 24-year-old young man hospitalized with a severe case of gastroenteritis. The Laskaris family was a prominent household in Constantinople, held in high esteem within the capital's circles. Young Theodore was already known for his military prowess and bravery in battle. He would later be considered a warrior equal to Lord Manuel Komnenos. I was deeply impressed by his composed character, his breadth of knowledge, and his courage in the face of illness. But what struck me most was his thirst for knowledge. He asked me countless questions about the human body, the nature of illnesses, and the available treatments. His greatest interest lay in systems of care—the operation of hospitals, the challenges of medical provision. Even then, one could see his concern for public affairs, which would later shine forth in Nicaea. Despite the age difference—I was already 49—we formed a strong bond of friendship. I became the personal physician of his family, as well as of the Emperor's other sons-in-law, whom I also came to know more intimately.

Theodore had a deep interest in the arts—particularly in theatre and painting, which in our time finds its most noble expression in the sacred iconography of our churches. He was delighted when I introduced him to Manuel Vlemmydes, already a professor at the *Pandidakterion,* whose acquaintance I had arranged precisely because I knew how much Theodore would appreciate such a mind. The three of us became a close circle, engaged in endless conversations. In those exchanges, Theodore's innate gift for leadership revealed itself. He saw the health care system as a true means of tending to the people's needs; the iconography of the churches as a gentle way to teach the faith to the unlettered; and good theatre as a public path to moral cultivation and education.

It is worth recounting a very memorable gathering that took place a year after his recovery, at the Laskaris family estate. He invited me to a dinner as a gesture of gratitude, since it was not permitted for him to offer any monetary reward. Manuel Vlemmydes was also invited to the meal. What made the occasion even more interesting was the presence of the emperor's other two sons-in-law—both named Alexios: Palaiologos and Doukas—men who would

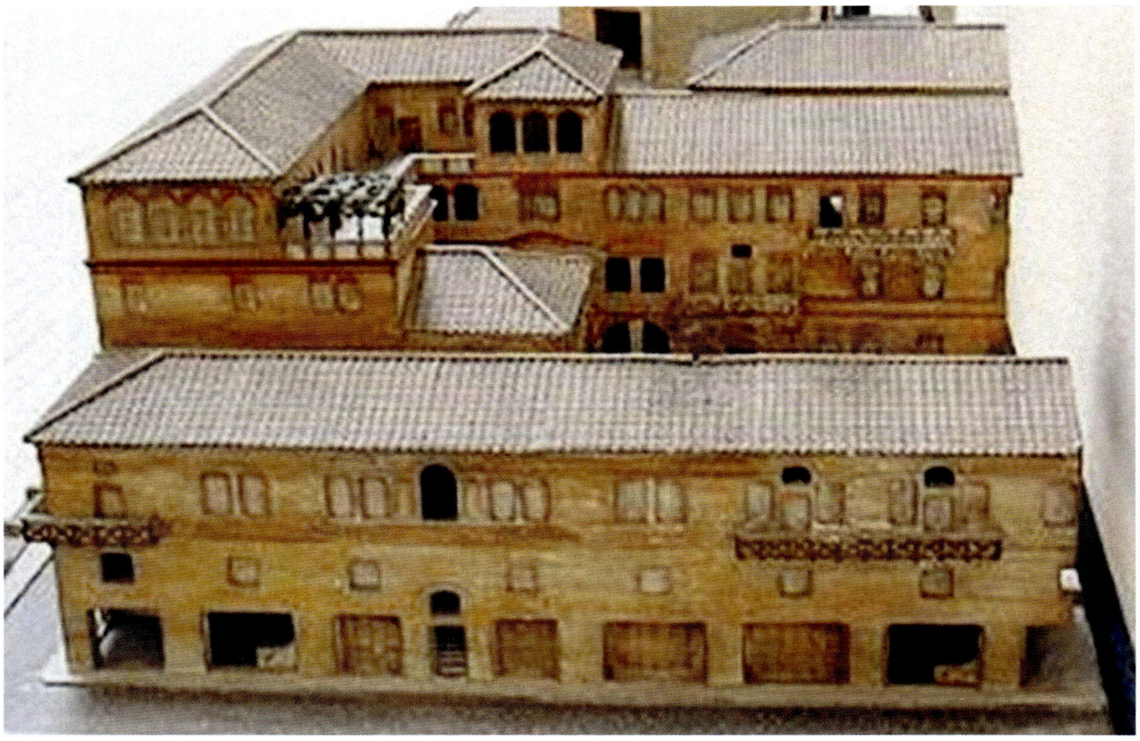

Byzantine Mansion.

digitalzoot.weebly.com

later play significant roles in the political history of our land. The Laskaris residence was situated near the Augustaion, in the area of the old imperial center, where the Sacred Palace (To Hieron Palation) and the Pandidakterion stood. That district was traditionally home to the old aristocracy, while the newer noble families had settled in the Vlachernae quarter, on the far side of the Capital, where the emperors had taken residence after the Komnenoi.

The house, built of brick and stone, is two-storied and situated on a street lined with elegant arcades near the Imperial Road. Its façade is adorned with delicate decorations of colorful marble plasterwork, embellishing the cornices that divide the floors and the border beneath the roofline. The windows are covered with so-called *kaitia*—small square panes set within wooden frames—and are protected by iron grilles. The upper floor is graced with small balconies, where the residents would often sit during the warm summer evenings. The entrance, centrally located on the façade, is guarded by a large double-leaf iron door, richly adorned with large bronze studs. When we arrived on time, the door stood wide open, watched over by a servant. We entered the vestibule with a touch of unease—entry into such homes was not easily granted. Yet there, to welcome us, stood the master of the house himself and his wife, Anna Komnene Angelina, a graceful lady just one year his junior. Theodore was a sturdy and handsome young man, dressed with elegance—splendidly yet modestly, without excess. The young Anna, as the Emperor's daughter, was clad in rather luxurious attire. He addressed Vlemmydes as "most illustrious teacher," and me as "Lord Actuarios," while we, in turn, greeted them as "most noble and exalted."

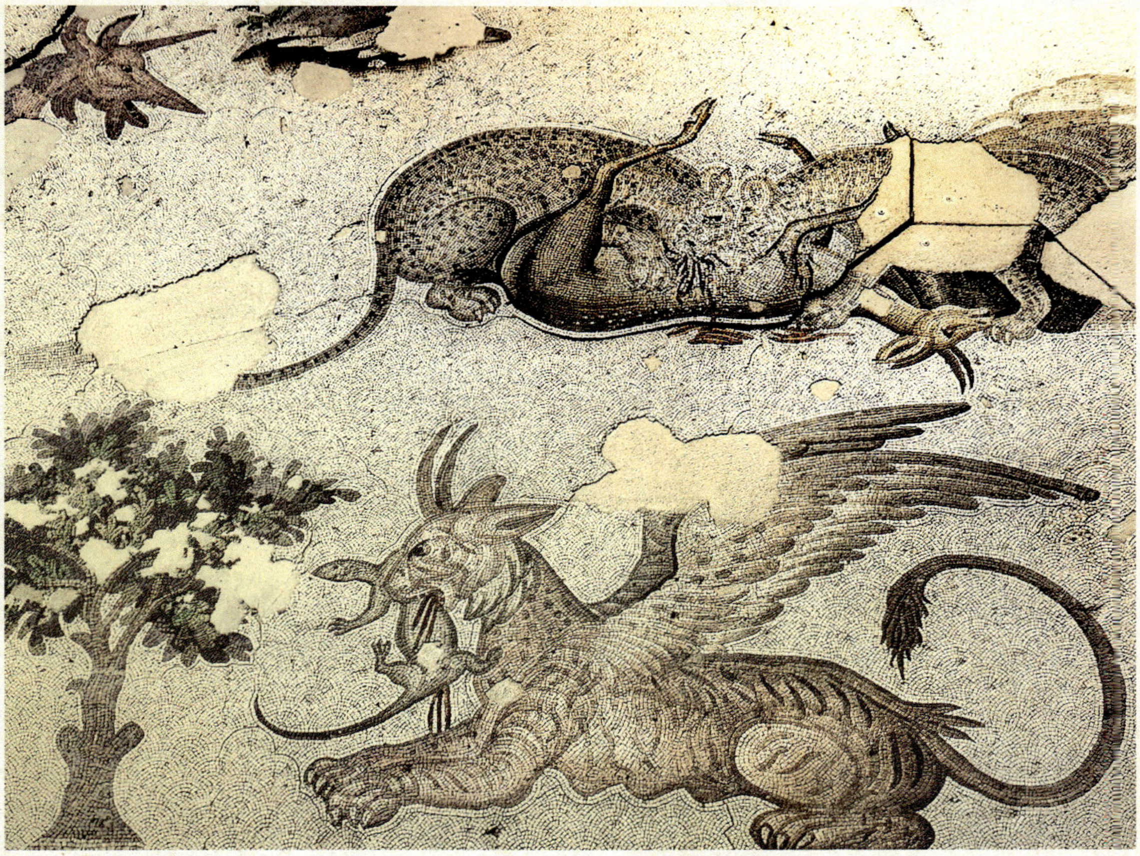

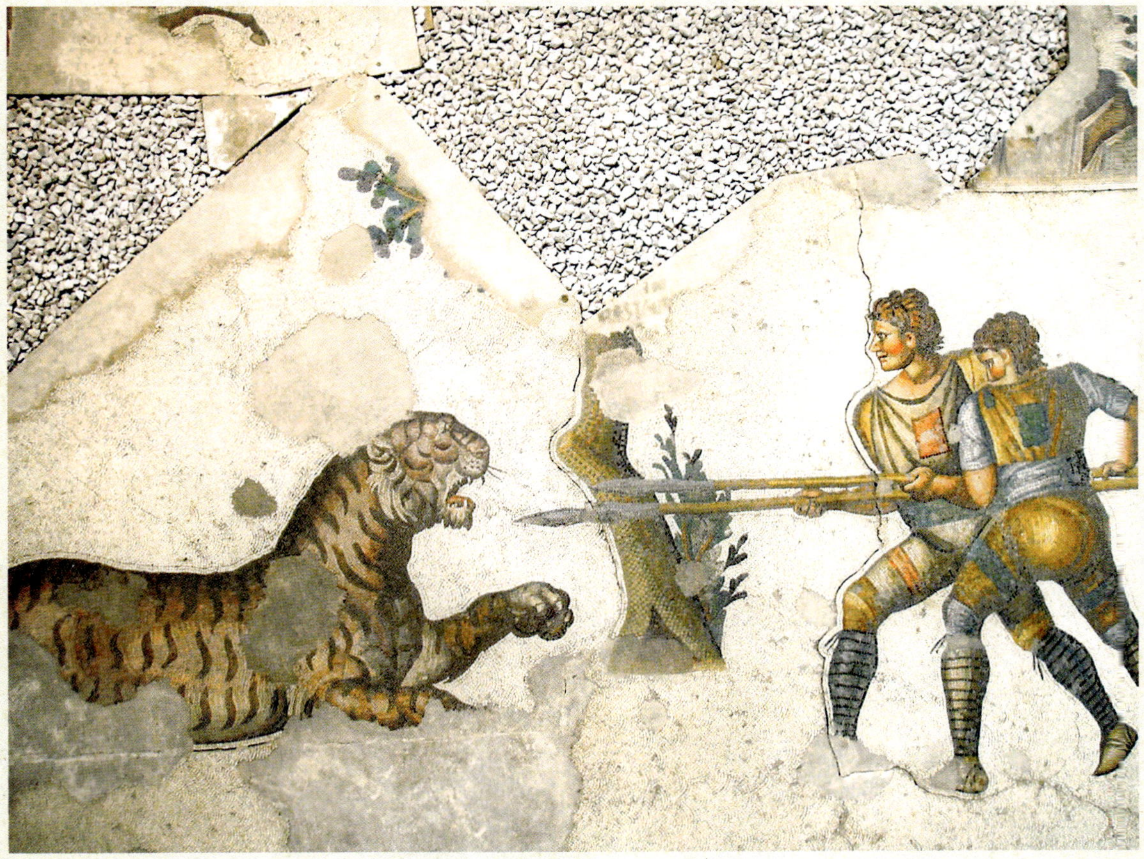

Mosaics from the Great Palace, 450–550 A.D.
Museum of the Great Palace Mosaics, Constantinople (Istanbul).

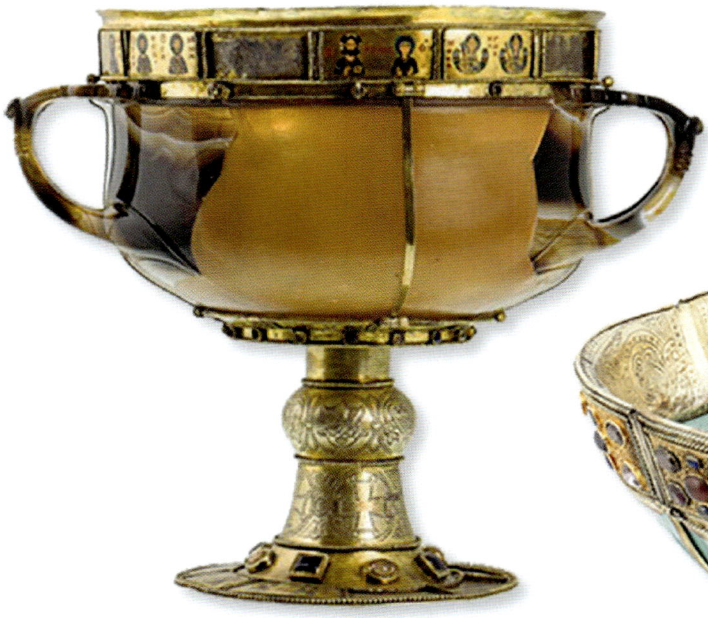

Chalice of Emperor Romanos.

Gold, silver, and enamel. 10th century. Saint Mark's Museum, Venice.

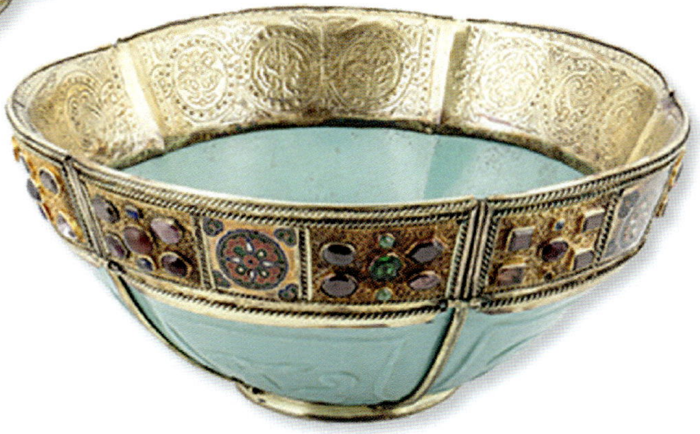

Cup made of turquoise, glass, gold, and precious stones.

10th century, Saint Mark's Museum, Venice.

They led us into a large hall, its floor adorned with mosaics, and its walls beautifully painted with scenes from nature. This central hall spanned the entire height of the house. All around it stood columns supporting the upper floor, where the family's chambers—both small and large—were located, separated by partitions or walls. At the center of the hall hung a bronze chandelier, holding many oil lamps, and beneath it stood a large round table. Around the room stood candle stands with additional lamps, bathing the space in ample light. The table was laid with a white tablecloth, and around it were large high-backed chairs, comfortable for seating. In front of each place setting lay a napkin and a *chernibon*, a small basin for washing one's hands.

In the hall, the other two daughters of the Emperor awaited us with their husbands: Irene with Alexios Palaiologos, and Eudokia with Alexios Doukas. Palaiologos was around thirty years old, sharp-witted, with a gaze that revealed a strong personality. He was somewhat slender and frail, but already had a reputation as a capable general, and he would soon prove his worth. Doukas was considerably older, around sixty, courteous and talkative. However, he was very dark-complexioned, with thick, unruly black eyebrows that gave him a fierce appearance—so much so that the people mockingly called him *Mourtzouphlos*. The two Angelinas, daughters of the Emperor, were courteous enough, but their arrogance was not well concealed. A rivalry simmered between the two Alexioi, as both sought to claim the succession of their father-in-law.

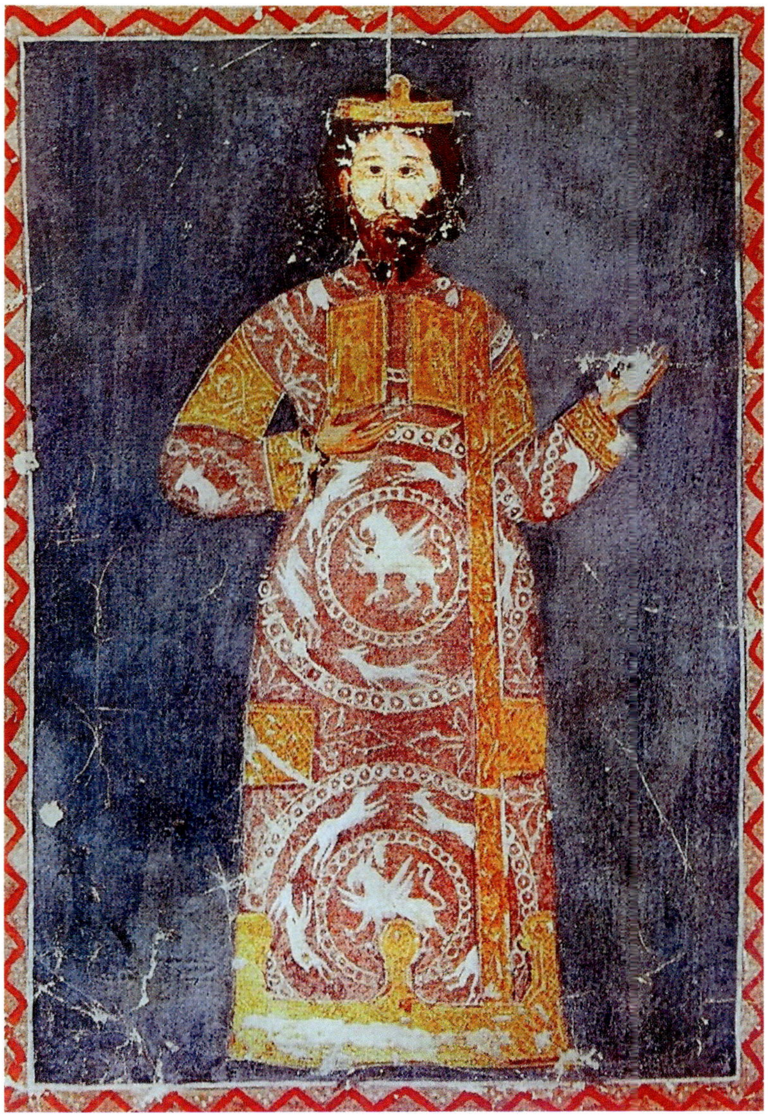

Alexios Doukas Mourtzouphlos.

Miniature, Niketas Choniates, Chronikai Diēgēseis, 13th century, Austrian National Library, Vienna.

We sat at the table. Before us were ceramic plates of exceptionally fine quality, imported from the East. They were adorned with elaborate decorations—animals, plants, flowers, and other intricate motifs. The drinking glasses were made of glass set on golden bases. At the center of the table stood a large *kantharos* filled with red wine, surrounded by small rolls made from the finest flour. The host began the meal with the opening prayer: "Lord, bless the food and drink of Your servants…", and the servants began to bring in the dishes. Theodoros wished to host a banquet worthy of his imperial rank. First came the appetizers: soft-boiled eggs served in egg cups, which we ate with spoons that had golden handles. These were followed by artichokes in a white sauce and fried fish sprinkled with mustard powder, accompanied by a sauce made with nard and coriander. We ate slowly, and only began to drink the splendid wine when our host gave the signal, striking a small bell, at the sound of which the servants came and poured our cups. The traditional blessing at the raising of the glass, directed toward the hosts, was "Blessings upon you," or "Bless, O master." Soon the main course arrived: a stuffed kid goat, filled with garlic, onions, and leeks, bathed in a savory sauce. We "blessed" the wine several times alongside the delicious goat dish, and at last came the dessert—an assortment of fruits: grapes, pears, pomegranates, dates, and sweets made of biscuits, cream, and honey. When the meal concluded, the host, carefully observing that everyone was content, rang the little bell to signal the end of the banquet, and the servants began clearing the dishes. We all rose for the thanksgiving prayer: "Lord, bless the remnants of this table and multiply them in this house and throughout Your world."

We sat again in our chairs and, after praising the meal and the hospitality of our host, the conversation began—just like in the ancient symposia. Theodore had thoughtfully ensured that the wine cups and the large *kantharos* remained on the table. The conversation, in which the noble ladies also took part, avoid-

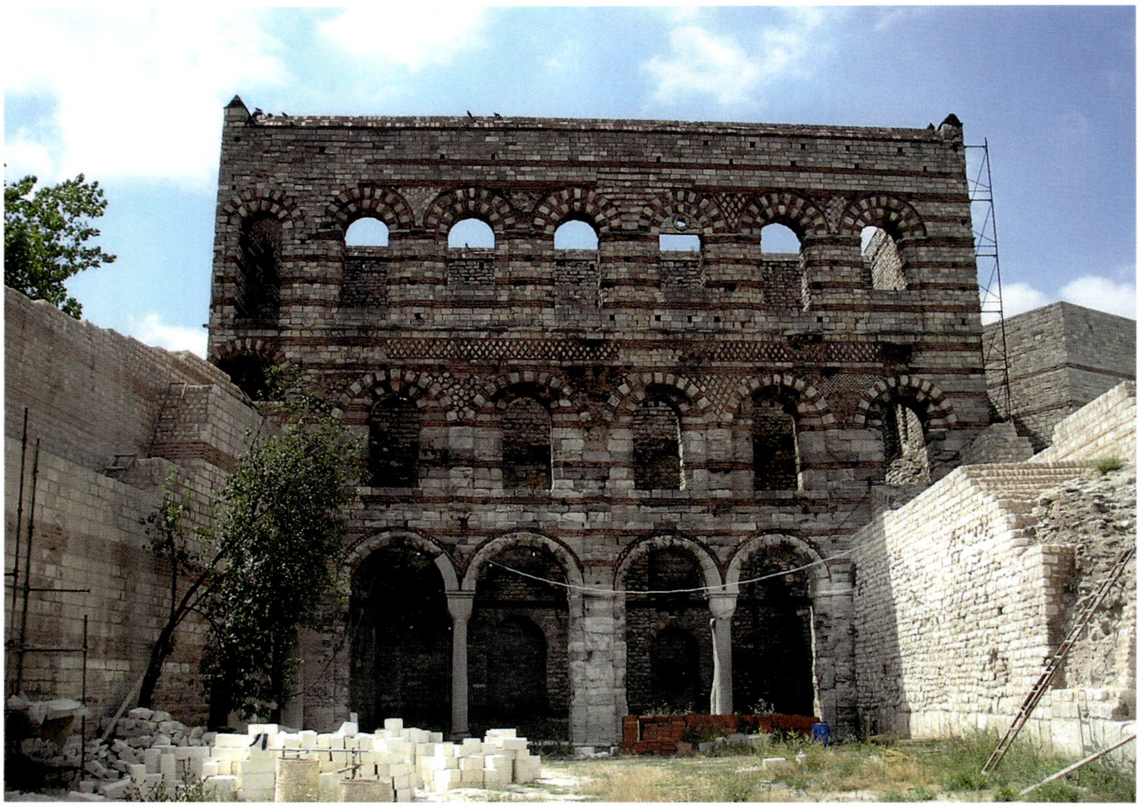

The Palace of the Porphyrogennetos: Reconstruction.

Byzantium 1200.

ed the sensitive matters of politics and warfare, and instead revolved around the operation of the hospitals (*xenones*), the overall public health policy—which, surprisingly, was still functioning quite well—and the arts, especially the role of theatre in the cultivation of the people. These were the subjects that preoccupied Theodore, but also Anna, as I came to realize. She distinguished herself from her sisters by her intelligence and the breadth of her interests. Theodore, a devoted admirer of Hellenic culture, expressed his frustration with the decline of the theatre, which had once been a powerful instrument for educating the people through sublime tragedies, but had now degenerated into a venue for tasteless satire, charlatans and mimes, and even prostitution and moral decay. In our time, there were four theatres in the City. The Great Theatre, located in the old center and existing even before the time of Constantine the Great, and three smaller ones—one near the Church of Hagia Eirene, one in the district of Vlachernae, and another in Syka, in the northern part of the city. All of them were open-air venues. Except for the first, the others had a rather poor reputation—and not without reason. They served as outlets for the suppressed frustrations of the people, a kind of social release valve, especially through satire aimed at those in power, often expressed with surprising boldness. Even Anna Komnene, the learned daughter of the great Emperor Alexios I and author of the *Alexiad*, writes that she was deeply disturbed by the unfair mockery directed at her father in those performances. The Great Theatre still hosted serious plays, and even within the churches during great feasts, dramatic reenactments were performed—depictions of

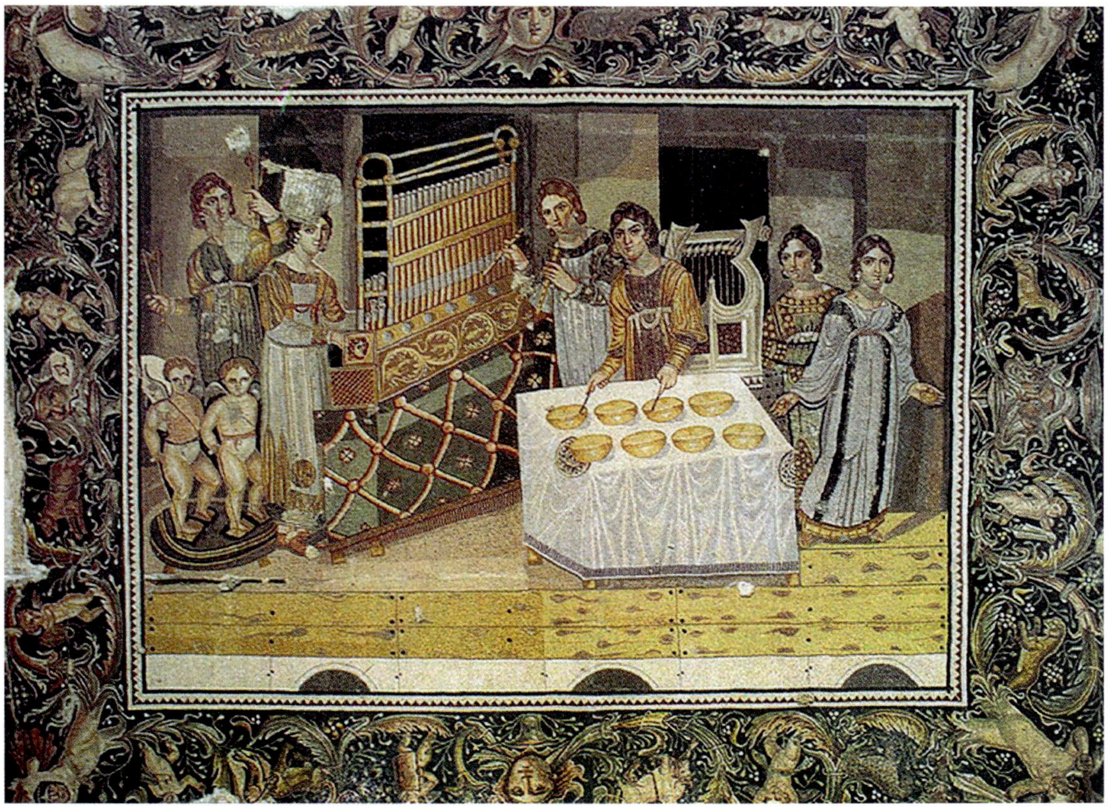

Women's dance with musical instruments.

Mosaic from a Byzantine villa in Maryamin, 4th–6th century, Archaeological Museum of Hama, Syria.

miracles or the Passion of the Lord—with the participation of professional actors. Theodore dreamed of restoring the ancient tragedy to its rightful place in the theatre.

Here I must note that the Laskaris couple stood in stark contrast to the other two. Devoted to the ideal of prudent governance and genuine care for the people, they were a shining exception amid a sea of corruption and greed that had come to dominate the imperial court. Palaiologos gave me the impression of being loyal to his unworthy father-in-law merely out of ambition, hoping to preserve the privileges his proximity to the throne afforded him. Murtzuflos, on the other hand, seemed to have completely rejected the emperor, and may even have aspired to the succession—something I did not find entirely unjustified, for anyone in power would surely have been better than the wretched Alexios III. What struck me most was the affection he showed toward his much younger wife. That meal drew us closer to the Laskaris household, beside whom we would soon live through the stormy events that were to follow.

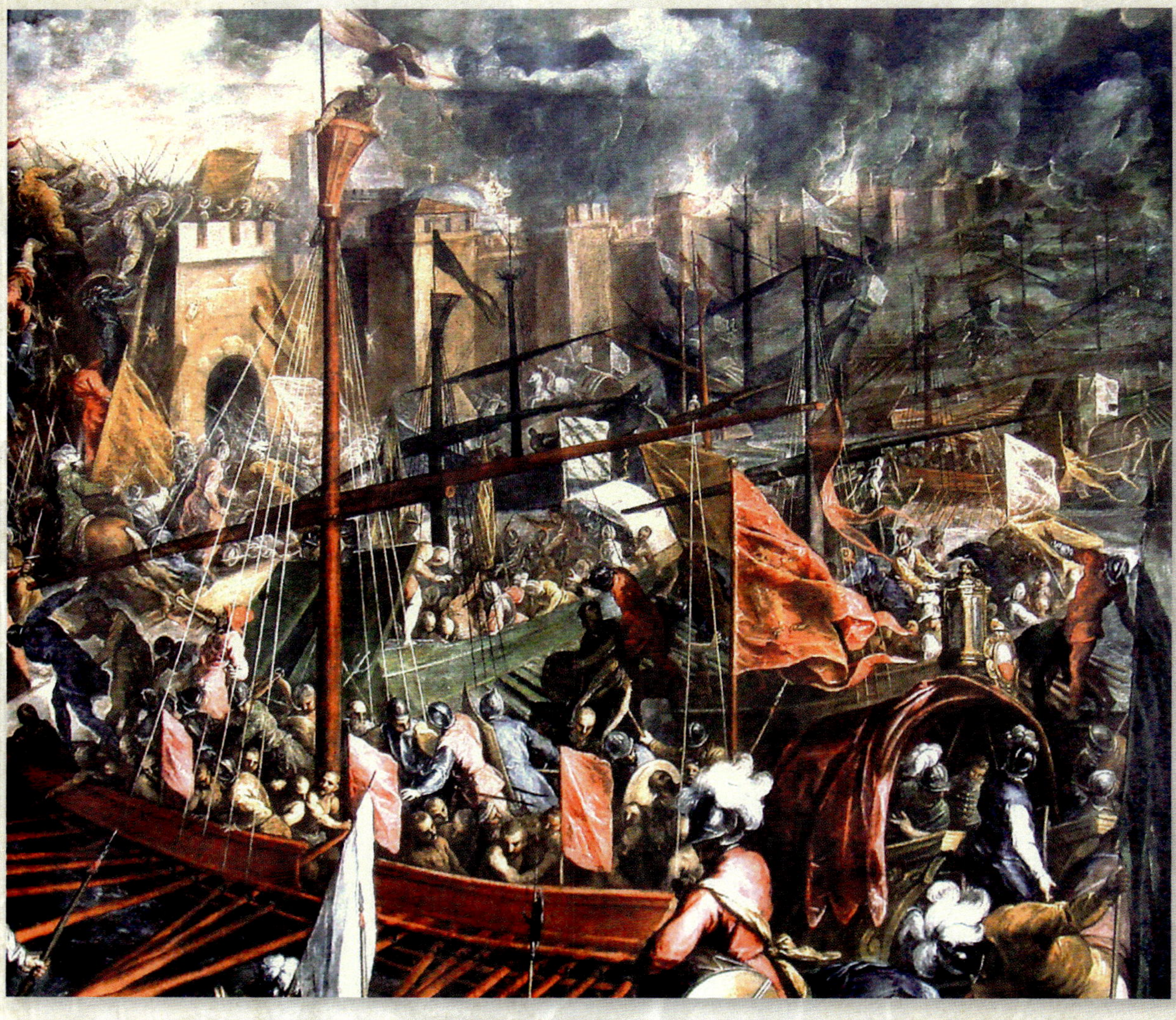

The Fall of Constantinople in 1204.

Painting by Palma il Giovane, 1587, Doge's Palace, Venice.

The Fourth Crusade and the Sack of Constantinople – the Flight to Nicaea

Life often reserves for us great surprises, and our experiences are so numerous and varied that we cannot foresee them before they unfold. Who would have expected that the mighty Empire of the Komnenoi would collapse within such a short span of time? Yet, beyond our own disastrous conduct—especially that of certain powerful families—the international circumstances were, quite literally, catastrophic.

The years that followed as we entered the thirteenth century were marked by a succession of dramatic and unsettling events. The governance of Alexios was so poor that two separate attempts were made to overthrow him—the second, in July of 1201, was instigated by his own son-in-law, Alexios Mourtzouphlos. Yet both revolts were suppressed by the capable Alexios Palaiologos. Mourtzouphlos was imprisoned, and Palaiologos appeared to be the likely successor to the throne, but he died a few years later from a sudden illness.

At the hospital, work continued without interruption. Fortunately, the foresight of its founder to secure its financial independence spared it from the grim condition to which other institutions—and indeed the entire population—were driven by the unacceptable administration of Alexios. Our lives went on as usual, yet we felt the dark clouds gathering in the sky, as though some great misfortune would inevitably follow from this situation. There was little more I could do beyond remaining diligent in my duties, striving to maintain my composure, and dispelling the fears and anxieties of my loved ones. Antigone visited the hospice less frequently; her forebodings led her to retreat somewhat into herself. Iphigenia had devoted herself to her family, and my father was trying to secure whatever funds he had by entrusting them to his Venetian friends with whom he conducted business. At that time, Venice was the dominant naval power in the eastern Mediterranean and possessed the most stable economy, governed by an original system of aristocratic democracy.

The following year, in 1202, Pope Innocent III convened the fateful Fourth Crusade. This time, the crusaders' plan was to assemble in Venice and from

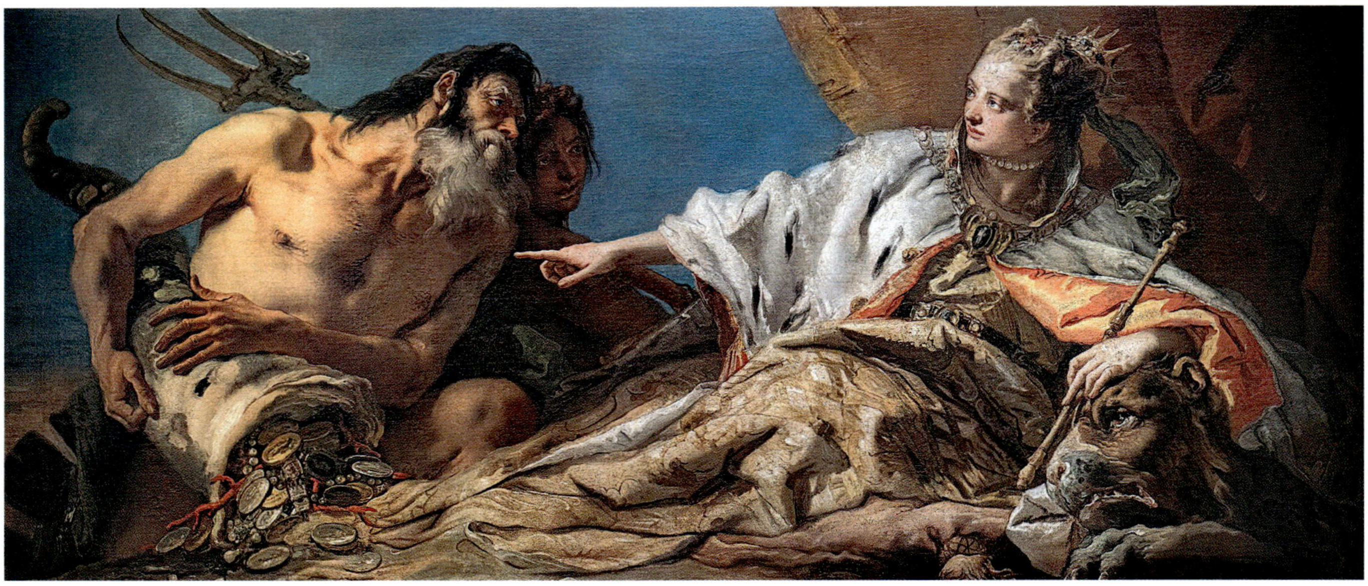

Poseidon offers Venice the riches of the sea.

Painting by Giovanni Battista Tiepolo, c. 1740–1745, Doge's Palace, Venice.

there be transported by Venetian ships to Egypt, from which point they would begin their campaign to liberate the Holy Lands—thus avoiding the long and debilitating overland route. By the end of the year, they expected to gather in Venice 4,500 knights, 9,000 retainers, and 20,000 infantry soldiers. The Crusade's leader was elected to be the brave and capable Boniface of Montferrat. Yet in the end, control passed to the shrewd Doge of Venice, Enrico Dandolo, who would prove to be fatal for our Empire. The aged Dandolo—then already 92 years old and nearly blind (presumably from cataract), yet still vigorous—demanded for the transportation, provisioning of the army for one year, and the support of fifty war galleys, the exorbitant sum of 85,000 silver marks. This amount was overwhelming for the primitive agrarian economies of the Western European kingdoms.

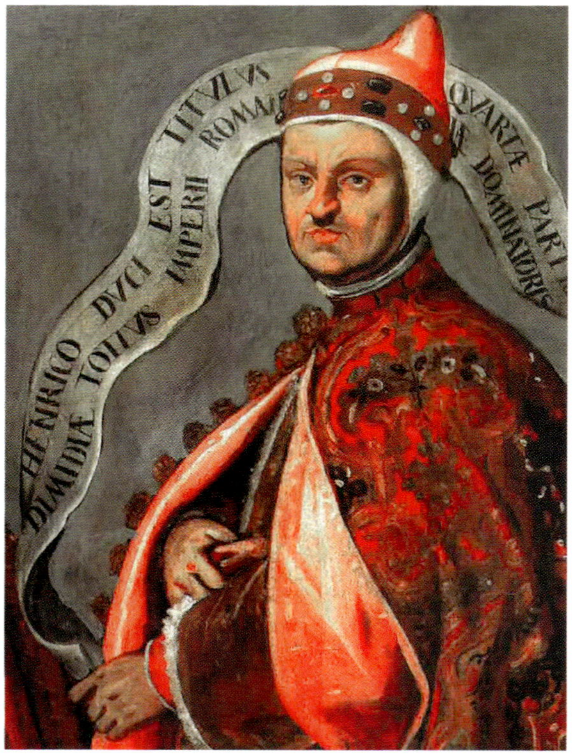

The crusaders who ultimately assembled in Venice were far fewer than anticipated, yet the Venetians remained inflexible, demanding the full amount previously agreed upon. The Frankish crusaders found themselves at an impasse when, as if sent by divine intervention, a ruthless adventurer appeared in their camp: the twenty-year-old Alexios Angelos, son of the deposed and blinded Emperor Isaac, who had been overthrown and mutilated by his own brother. Alexios had been imprisoned alongside his father but managed to escape and, with the help of two Pisan merchants, fled to the West. He then presented himself before the Pope and the crusaders,

Enrico Dandolo.

Painting by Domenico Tintoretto, c. 1600, Doge's Palace, Venice.

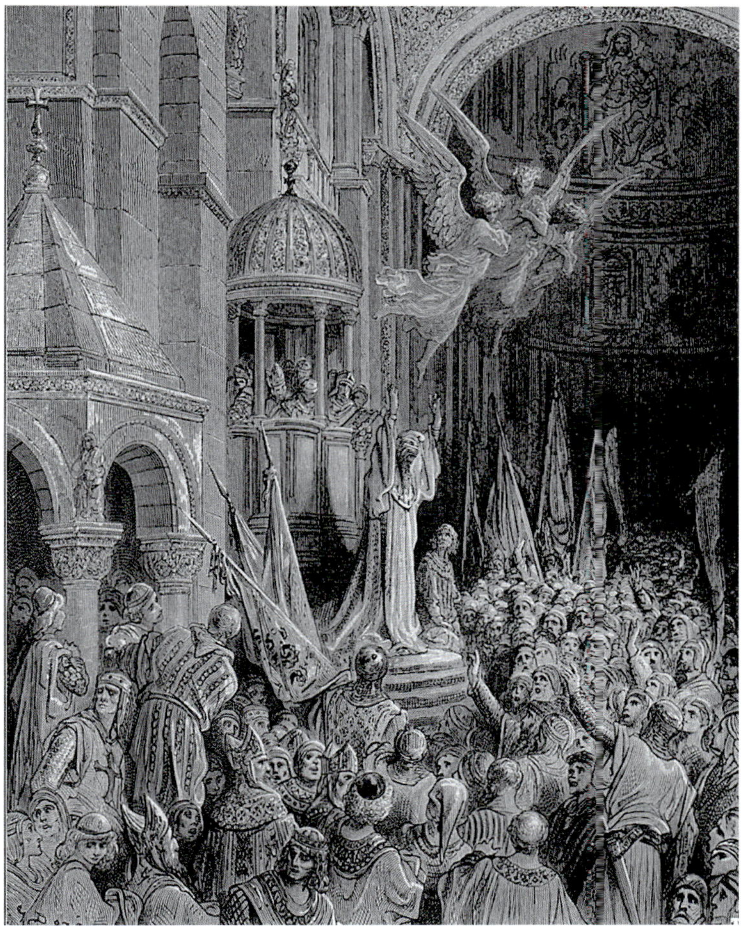

Dandolo Proclaims the Fourth Crusade.

Composition by Gustave Doré, Hachette edition, 1877.

offering a bold proposal: if they would depose the usurper—his uncle, Alexios III—and restore his father to the throne of Constantinople, he would pay 100,000 silver marks to the Venetians, another 100,000 to the crusaders, maintain 10,000 soldiers for a year, and support five hundred men for life in the defense of Palestine. Most significantly, he pledged to bring the Eastern Orthodox Church into submission to the Papal throne.

The sums promised by the reckless Alexios might have been attainable during the Komnenian era of Byzantine prosperity, but in the state to which his father and uncle had reduced the Empire, they were nearly impossible to procure. The Latins, for their part, needed no further encouragement. The agreement was ratified in the spring of 1203, and by summer, 200 Venetian ships bearing the crusaders arrived—under papal sanction—at the walls of the City. Geoffrey of Villehardouin, a nobleman from Champagne who took part in the campaign, recorded the history of the Fourth Crusade and the siege and eventual sack of Constantinople—though, of course, from his own perspective. His account was written in his native French, but some years later, while I was in Nicaea, a Frankish merchant from the Peloponnese brought me a copy and translated for me several significant chapters. Villehardouin described in vivid terms the astonishment the crusaders felt upon beholding the Queen of Cities. They had never imagined a city so vast, with walls so high and formidable, with build-

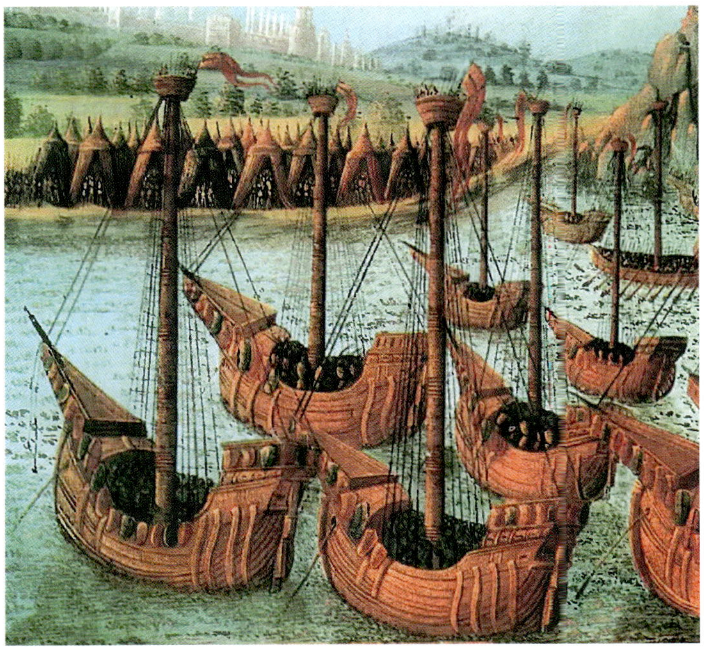

The Venetian fleet arrives in Constantinople.

Miniature by Sébastien Mamerot, 15th century, National Library of France, Paris.

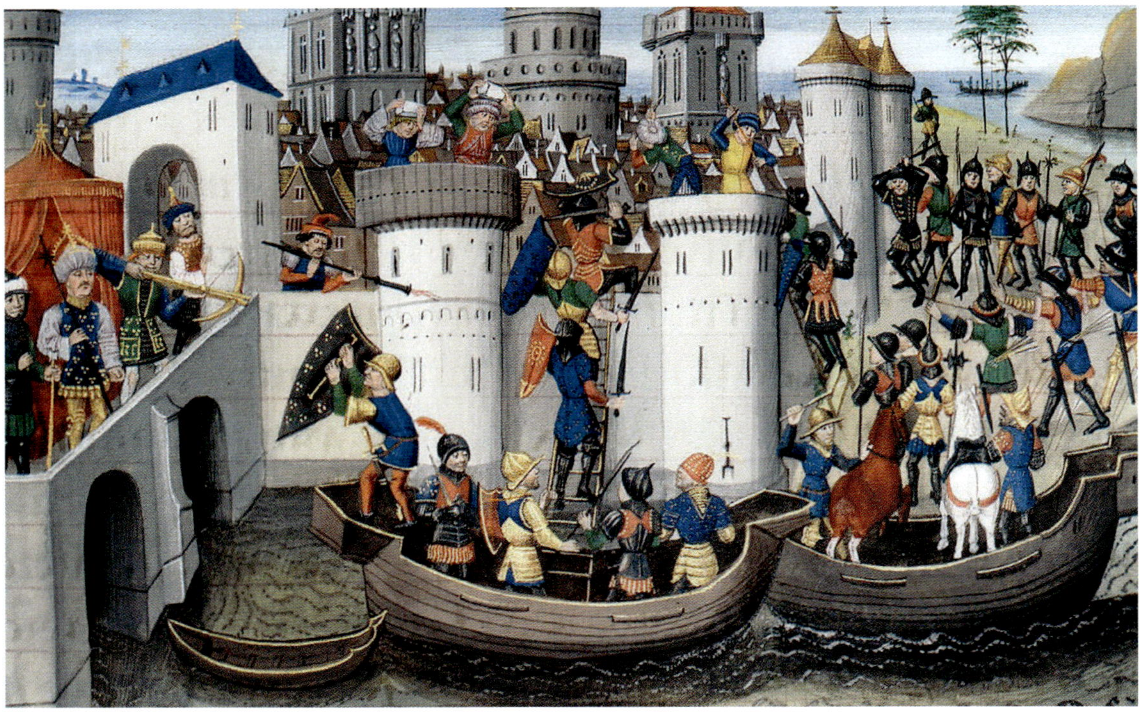

The siege of Constantinople by the Crusaders in 1204.
Miniature by David d'Aubert, 15th century.

ings and churches of such magnificence. The shock of seeing Constantinople stirred in them awe—but also a deep desire for plunder.

When the enemy ships reached the City, we were all seized with alarm. The total neglect of the military and naval forces during the two-decade rule of the Angeloi had dire consequences. The imperial fleet could muster no more than fifty poorly maintained vessels. The morale of the people had collapsed, and so had that of the army—even though it still numbered around 50,000 men. The Queen of Cities still possessed the strength to resist and expel the invaders. Had there been competent leadership, and the army been inspired by the spirit of a Kaloyannis or a Manuel Komnenos, the Latins could have been easily routed. Yet we continued to trust in the City's impregnability, as the centuries had seemed to confirm. Theodore Laskaris made several sorties from the land walls with detachments of troops, and each time he succeeded in repelling the besiegers. They were not as invincible as their heavy armor and fierce reputation suggested. He concluded that if the entire army were drawn up before the walls, they could defeat and scatter the enemy. He pleaded in vain with the terrified emperor to authorize a decisive battle on land. At last, Alexios brought the army out before the land walls, hoping the enemy would be intimidated and retreat. But when he saw their ranks unmoved, he lost heart and shamefully withdrew—along with his bewildered and disheartened soldiers—without engaging in combat. The next day, he fled like a coward and a wretch, taking with him as much money and as many precious objects from the royal treasury as he could carry.

Great embarrassment and shame fell upon the City. In order to appease the besiegers, the nobles and the people saw no other option but to proclaim the blind Isaac as Emperor. He immediately summoned the leaders of the crusaders for negotiations. They, however, insisted that his son—who had made the agreement to reward them—also be declared Emperor. Thus, yet another Alexios was crowned Emperor of the Romans, this time Alexios IV. The two hapless emperors, father and son, made desperate efforts to gather the sum demanded—without negotiation—by the cunning Dandolo and the crusaders. They plundered everything the previous regime had left in the state treasury, ransacked the churches and all they could find, and still managed to raise only half the amount. The "allies," however, remained unyielding. After much pleading, they agreed to wait until spring, when tax revenues were expected. In a state of panic, Alexios IV turned his hopes toward Pope Innocent III. He sent him a declaration of faith and compelled Patriarch John Kamateros to proclaim, in Hagia Sophia, the Pope as the first hierarch and representative of Christ the Savior.

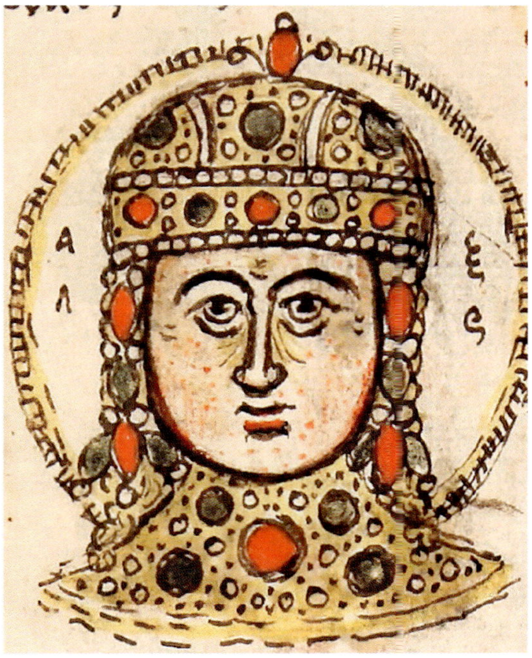

Alexios IV Angelos.

Miniature, Zonaras, 15th century, d'Este Library, Modena.

The result was even worse. The people grew indignant at the subjugation to the Pope, while the Latins, of course, remained unsatisfied. In the City, people roamed about in anger and despair. Rumors circulated wildly—of vast armies arriving from the West to destroy Byzantium—along with other fantastical tales. The morale of both the populace and the military was in a dire state. Some placed their hopes in God, yet did nothing themselves; others waited passively for what they believed would be just punishment for our sins, especially for the submission of Orthodoxy to the Pope. Fear of the invaders and a sharp rise in food prices—caused by opportunists—drove the people to desperation, while the leadership proved entirely inadequate for the gravity of the moment. The crusaders did not wait until spring. In December 1203, hostilities began. The cowardly Alexios IV did not dare to fight and watched events unfold as a passive spectator. The army was leaderless, and local commanders defended the walls in despair. It was then that Alexios Mourtzouphlos—recently released from prison following the disgraceful flight of his father-in-law and known for his particular hatred of the Latins—took the initiative to defend the City. Mourtzouphlos demonstrated remarkable energy and courage. He launched desperate sorties with the army and attempted to set fire to the Venetian fleet, fighting on the front lines himself. Yet despite his efforts, he failed to revive the morale of the demoralized soldiers. The Roman camp was overcome by defeatism and fear. Around this time, the blind Isaac died, and the people—disillusioned with his unworthy son—proclaimed Mourtzouphlos emperor at the end of January 1204. The chief cause of the catastrophe, the wretched Alex-

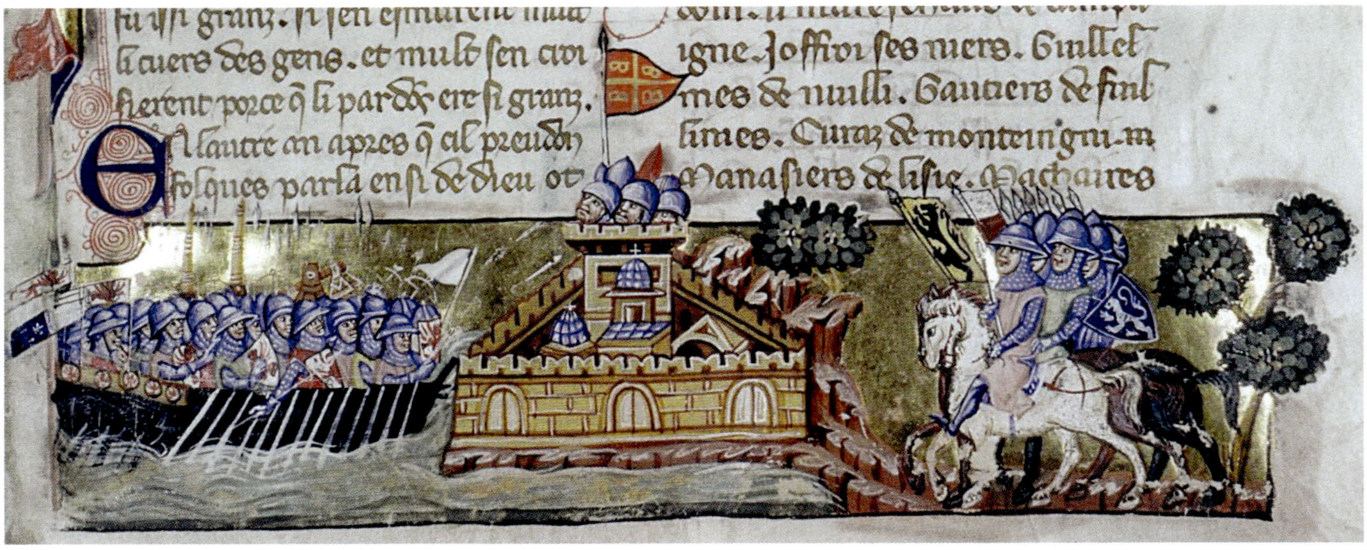

Siege of Constantinople by the Crusaders.

Miniature, 14th century, from Geoffrey of Villehardouin, The Conquest of Constantinople, Biblioteca Nazionale Marciana, Venice.

ios IV, was secretly executed, though the act was soon discovered by the crusaders. The change in leadership became, unfortunately, the pretext for the crusaders to launch their final assault. In truth, the decision to conquer the City had already been made; they had even agreed in advance how to "divide the garments" of the Empire. But now they had their justification.

Since the land walls were nearly impregnable, the Latins concentrated their attacks on the northern sea walls along the Golden Horn, where the Venetian ships had broken through the great chain that blocked the passage. These ships were designed for siege warfare: they could disembark troops and horses, fire arrows and projectiles at the walls, and raise ladders onto them, playing an active role in the assaults. On April 12, 1204—year 6712 "from the creation of the world"—during one of their repeated offensives, the crusaders succeeded in toppling a tower, setting a fire that, fanned by strong winds, spread rapidly through nearby buildings, and they managed to breach the City. Mourtzouphlos fought desperately, but it was too late. When the Franks captured the sacred banner of the Theotokos Nikopoios, his

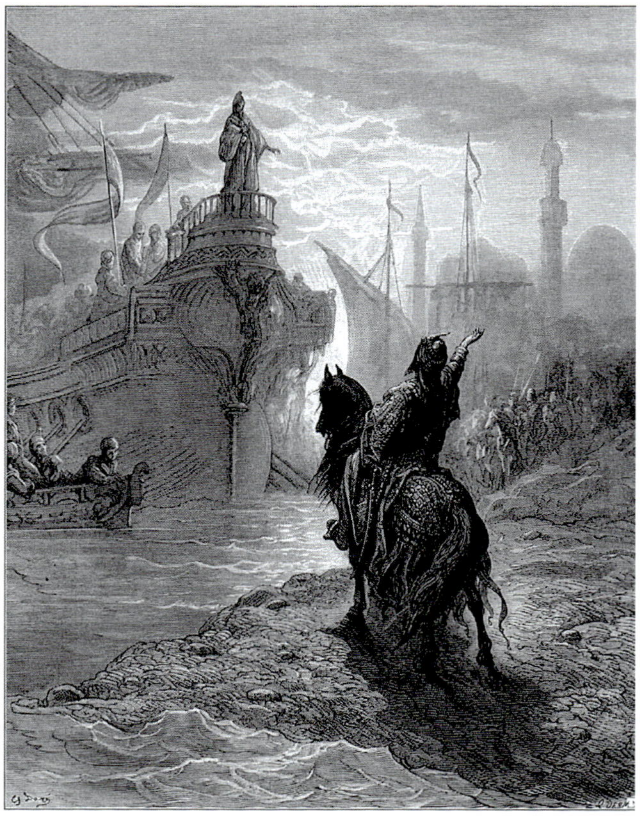

Alexios V (Mourtzouphlos) negotiating with Enrico Dandolo.

Composition by Gustave Doré, Hachette edition, 1877.

soldiers—believing this to be a sign from heaven—abandoned their positions in panic and fled.

The Franks consolidated their hold on the northeastern wall. In despair, Mourtzouphlos fled as well, taking his wife and a few companions with him toward Macedonia. As the city burned and those who could escape did so, some nobles and citizens gathered in Hagia Sophia to elect a new leader. Amid the collapse and chaos, the only ones who remained faithful to the homeland were the brothers Constantine and Theodore Laskaris. Constantine, being the elder, was proclaimed "Emperor of the Romans," though no coronation ceremony took place—there was no time for such formalities. The energetic Theodore attempted to rally and organize the people and the famed Varangian Guard, who were still present. With endless pleading, exhortations, and threats, he managed to array them before the Sacred Palace as a last line of defense. But when, after some hesitation, the hordes of Germans and French charged with fire and bloodshed, even the Varangians broke and fled. The brave Laskaris was forced to retreat as well, crossing to the Asian shore of the Bosphorus with his brother, the rest of his family, and a few loyal friends—where he would go on to found a new Greek Empire, this time on the soil of Asia Minor.

We experienced these events in an atmosphere thick with anxiety for our fate, and with sorrow and shame at the degradation of the City and the Empire, which only a few years earlier had been the jewel of the Ecumene. My family, along with that of Vlemmydes, fled to Asia Minor with the followers of Laskaris. I, however, could not bring myself to abandon my patients and remained behind with a few other physicians at the Hospice of the Pantocrator, awaiting whatever was to come. I faced a serious dilemma with Antigone, who had come with me to the hospital and refused to leave me behind. My pleading and threats did not sway her. Fortunately, she was persuaded when all the women physicians and nurses were evacuated, for the behavior of the enraged conquerors toward women was well known. She finally departed with the others for Asia Minor, after solemnly imploring me to join them in Nicaea as soon as I could. At least I was comforted by the

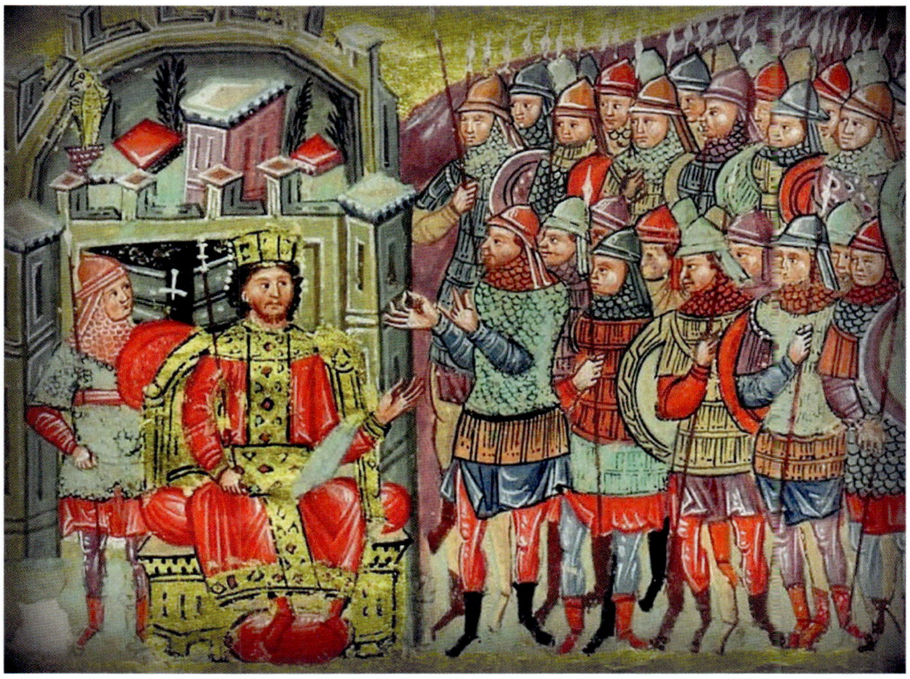

The Varangian Guard of the Emperor.

knowledge that my family and friends were safe. In the beginning, the crusaders were hesitant as they moved slowly through the vast city, wary of pockets of resistance. This allowed many who had prepared for such an eventuality the chance to escape.

After their initial hesitation, the mob of crusaders descended upon the City like carrion beasts upon a wounded animal. The pillaging of churches, palaces, the Hippodrome, and every public edifice was ruthless. Naturally, the leaders hurried to seize the grand buildings and imperial residences for themselves. Boniface of Montferrat, the commander of the Crusade, took possession of the Boukoleon Palace, where many high-ranking officials and former imperial consorts had sought refuge, including Anna, sister of King Philip of France, and Margaret, sister of the King of Hungary. The wealth discovered in the palace was described as immeasurable. The Blachernae Palace was seized by Henry of Champagne, brother of Count Baldwin, after he guaranteed the safety of those within. Villehardouin paints a vivid picture of the shock experienced by his fellow countrymen—the "pilgrims," as he calls them—who stood speechless before the wonders they encountered in the palaces. The silver and gold vessels, the precious stones, the silks and garments, the furs of ermine and other animals—such treasures existed nowhere else in the world. "I bear true witness," writes the astonished Frenchman, "that since the world was created, never has there been in any city such great wealth." Immediately, the Marquis of Montferrat, the barons, and the Doge of Venice proclaimed to the entire army that the spoils were to be gathered in three locations and distributed "justly," as they had sworn. Those who disobeyed would be punished and excommunicated.

The Crusaders Enter Constantinople.

Painting by Eugène Delacroix, 1840, Louvre Museum, Paris.

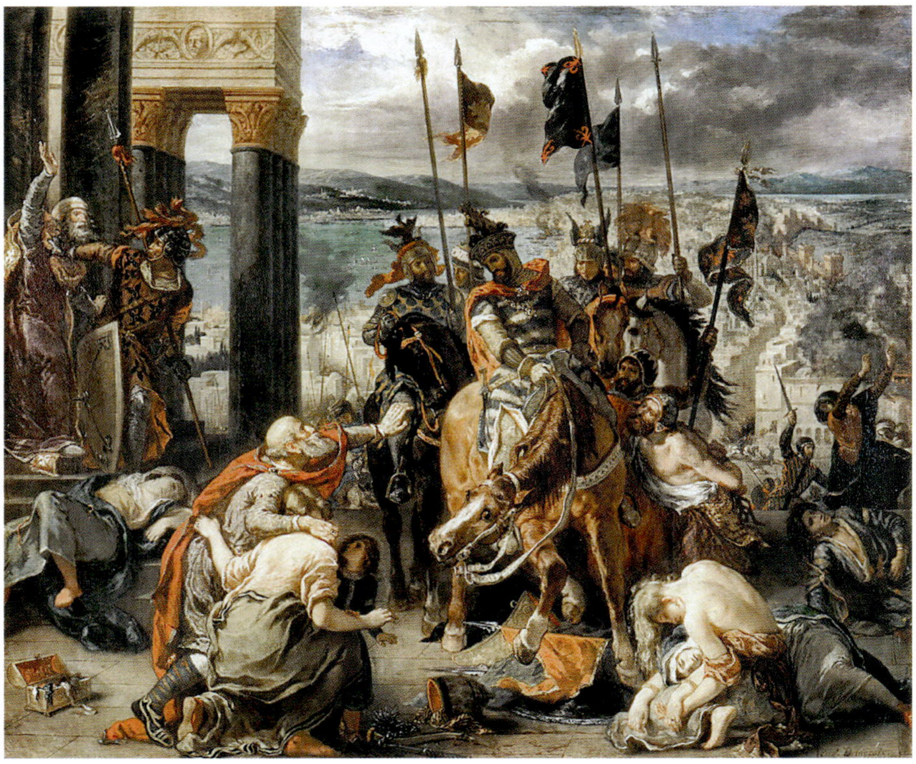

The soldiers, however—eager to seize whatever they could before it was taken from them—acted with great brutality. They showed no respect for the churches, the sacred spaces, or the works of art. Fires were set in various parts of the City, and the number of homes that burned, according to Villehardouin, "exceeded those of the three largest cities in France combined." The killings and rapes that took place in the streets surpassed all bounds. Of course, these

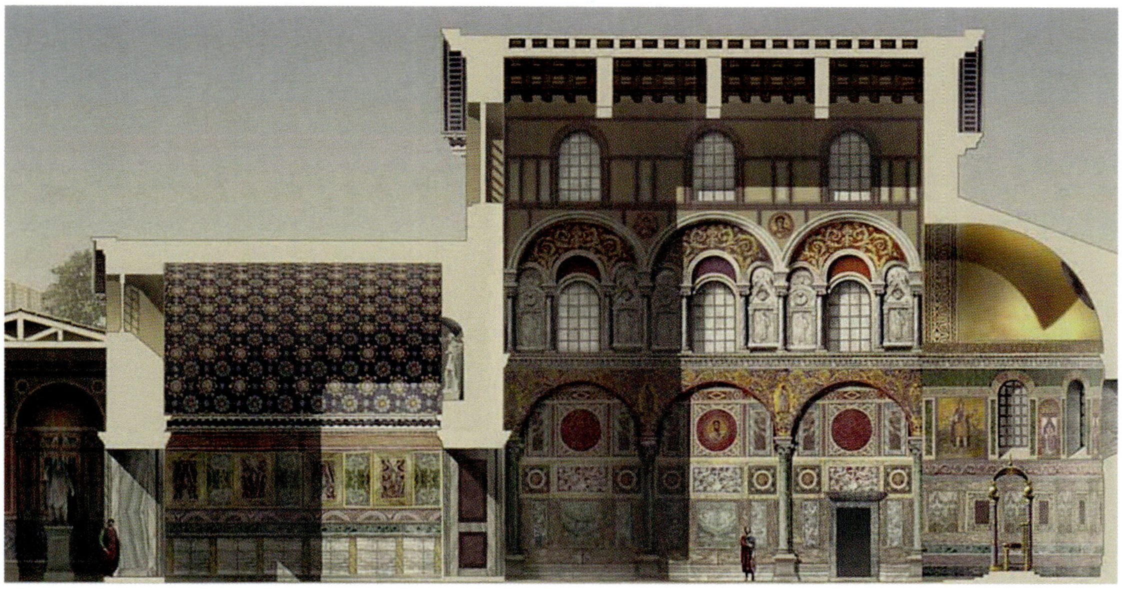

The Arched Hall of the Great Peristyle (longitudinal section).

Reconstruction by Antoine Helbert, 1870.

were considered "collateral damage," for the crusaders were not primarily intent on slaughter, but on looting. The justification that the Greeks were schismatics and in decline—as their religious and political leaders had convinced them—had stripped away any moral restraint. Their commanders, of course, who were quick to install themselves in the vacated palaces and mansions, had no desire for the City's destruction, hoping instead to claim the lion's share of its wealth. But threats of excommunication and punishment were useless against a frenzied mob. The Venetians, under the capable leadership of Dandolo, behaved with more restraint. Many priceless works of art and sacred relics were not destroyed but transported to Venice, where they now adorn that city's churches. Fortunately, the Venetians were the first to enter the Hippodrome, which meant that the magnificent work of Lysippos—the four bronze horses that once pulled a chariot—was preserved. They now stand in the Basilica of St. Mark in Venice, along with other treasured relics.

The Franks—especially the French and Germans—who followed were utterly uncontrollable. The looting lasted for three full days, until, providentially, a lunar eclipse occurred, frightening this uneducated and superstitious mob. Yet by then, countless ancient Greek and Roman works of art had been destroyed—masterpieces that these barbarians were seeing for the first time in their lives. The colossal bronze statue of Heracles in the Hippodrome, another creation of Lysippos, was melted down for its metal. The same fate befell the immense statue of Hera at the Forum of Constantine, as well as a bronze mechanical device filled with birds and animals of all kinds that produced various sounds. In the Forum of the Ox, there once stood an equestrian statue of Bellerophon, which was smashed to pieces—just like dozens of other masterpieces of art preserved through the centuries. The targets of the assault were the churches, the monasteries, the mansions, the bronze sculptures—even the tombs of the emperors. Everything was plundered and desecrated. Thou-

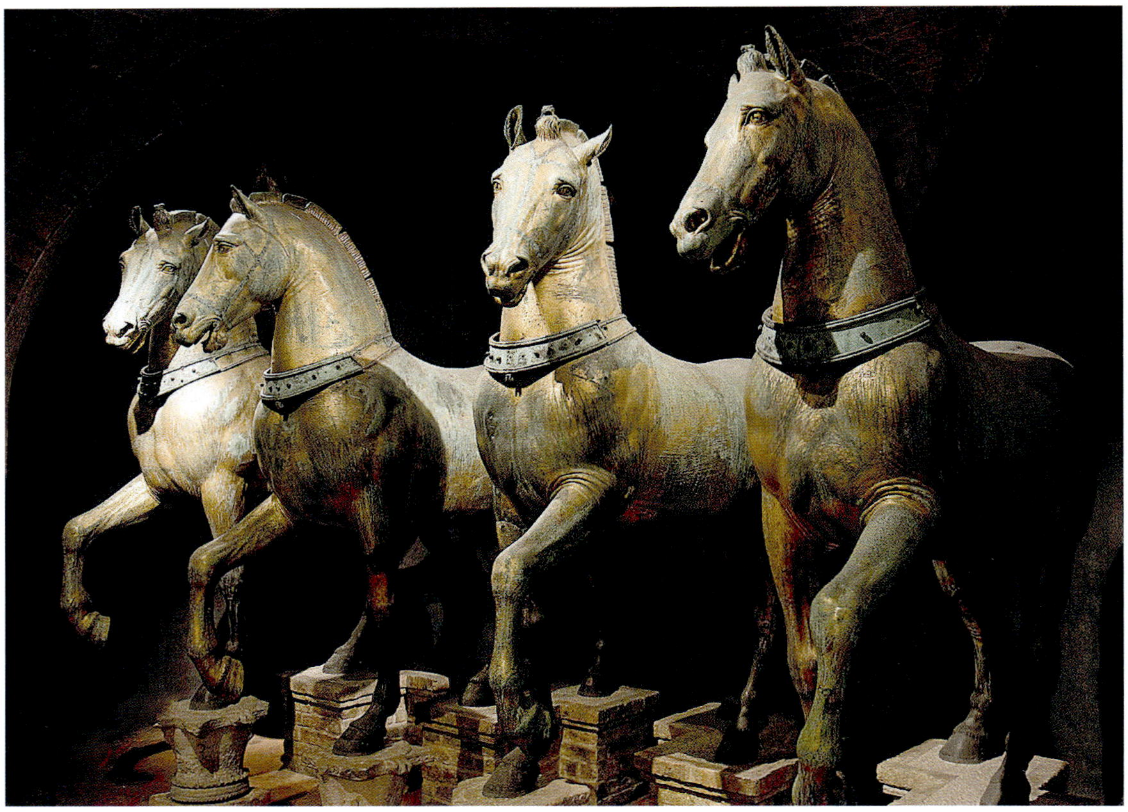

The Original Horses of Lysippos.
St. Mark's Basilica, Venice.

sands were murdered in cold blood, without cause, and thousands of women—both laywomen and nuns—were raped in the streets and in their homes. Yet perhaps, beyond the murders and rapes, the greatest and most irreparable crime was the destruction of thousands of books—burned in the fires that consumed public buildings and imperial palaces.

A vast portion of ancient wisdom—and not only that—preserved until then, was destroyed and lost forever to humanity. The total value of the plunder has been estimated at 900,000 silver marks—an astronomical sum for the economy of the Franks. From the official spoils, excluding what the soldiers secretly stole, the lion's share went, fittingly, to the Lion of the Most Serene Republic of Venice. Even the Latin residents of Constantinople were compensated for the massacre committed against them twenty-two years earlier.

It is impossible for me to describe the scale of the destruction, the grief, and the anguish I felt as I watched the events unfold from the Hospice of the Pantocrator over the course of three days. My mind could not comprehend that the very beauty of the world—the City of cities, which we believed to be impregnable and divinely protected—could be so irreparably destroyed. I lived almost in another reality, as though these events were not truly happening, as if they were a delusion, a nightmare. I was overwhelmed by fear, uncertainty, and sorrow. Lacking the literary talent to express all that took place, I must borrow the words of my friend and later colleague in Nicaea, Niketas Choniates, who both witnessed and recorded these events in his invaluable historical work. Niketas Akominatos Choniates, nearly my contemporary, was a

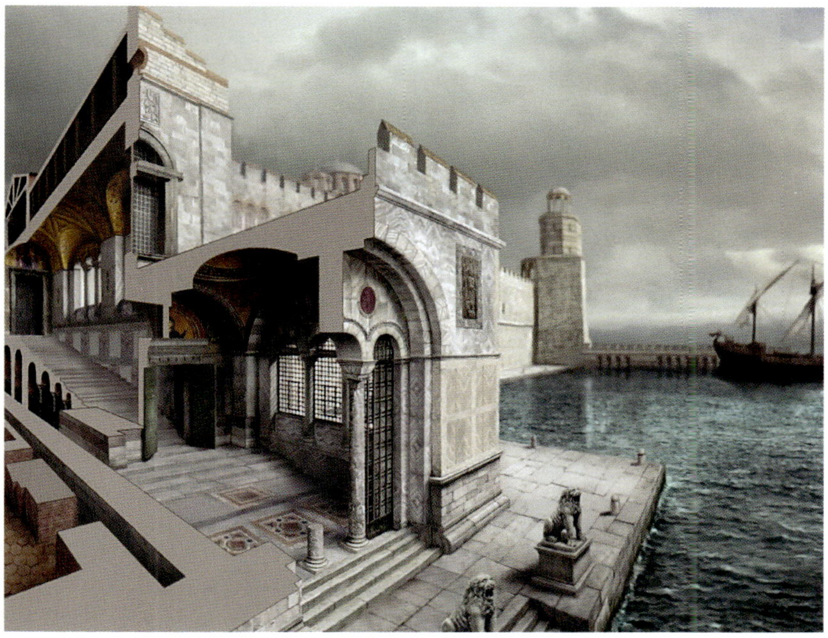

scholar who served the Empire for many years as Grand Logothete (=foreign minister). When the City fell, he saw the devastation and killings up close. He and his family escaped extermination thanks to the help of a Venetian merchant who disguised himself as a crusader and smuggled them out, pretending they were his captives, to a safe location from which they eventually fled to Nicaea.

Choniates laments the desecration of the Church of Hagia Sophia, where, in order to carry off the golden vessels and the fragments of the Holy Altar—which they had hacked to pieces—the invaders brought horses and mules into the very sanctuary, defiling everything with dung and the blood of the animals. Throughout the city, there resounded "wailing, weeping, and lamentation; the groans of men and the howls of women; enslavement, dispersal, and rapes." The so-called soldiers of Christ showed no reverence for what was sacred and holy. Choniates depicts them in the darkest hues: "a neck of bronze, an arrogant mind, haughty brows, cheeks always shaved and groomed like youths, a hand greedy for blood, eyes ever lifted in pride, jaws insatiable, hearts without pity, speech sharp and unruly"—like wild beasts in truth. And finally, he cries out: "O City, queen and eye of all cities, renowned throughout the civilized world, vision beyond this world, leader of the faith, guide of Orthodoxy, cradle of the spirit, dwelling place of all that is good—who will save you? Who will comfort you? Who will pity you and mourn for you? Who has torn us from you, like children from their mother? What shall we become? Where shall we go? What consolation will we find, naked and exhausted, abandoned and despised, eating bitter bread and drinking gall instead of water?"

Section of the Boukoleon Palace.

Reconstruction by Antoine Helbert.

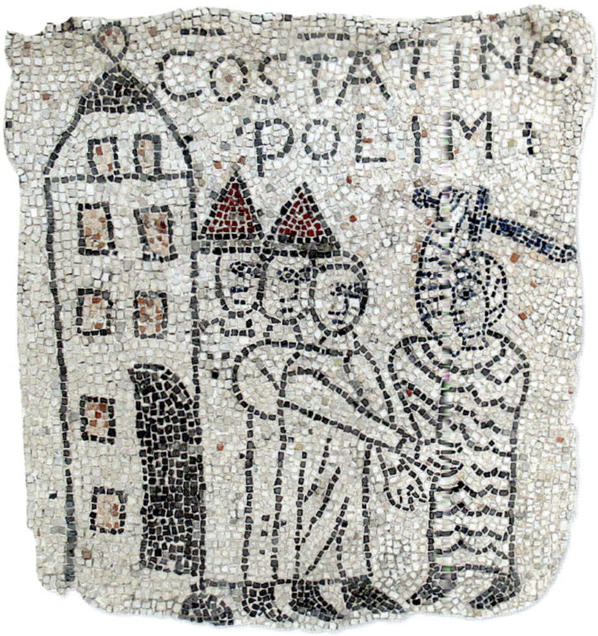

The Fall of Constantinople.

Venetian Mosaic, 13th century, San Giovanni Evangelista, Ravenna.

The hospitals were not at the eye of the storm, as the "pilgrims" did not expect to find significant plunder there. Thus, we faced no immediate danger—at least not directly. The real challenge, however, was how to continue operating and maintaining the institutions. I did not know what to do with the patients; those who were able to walk had fled in fear to check on their homes. Those of us

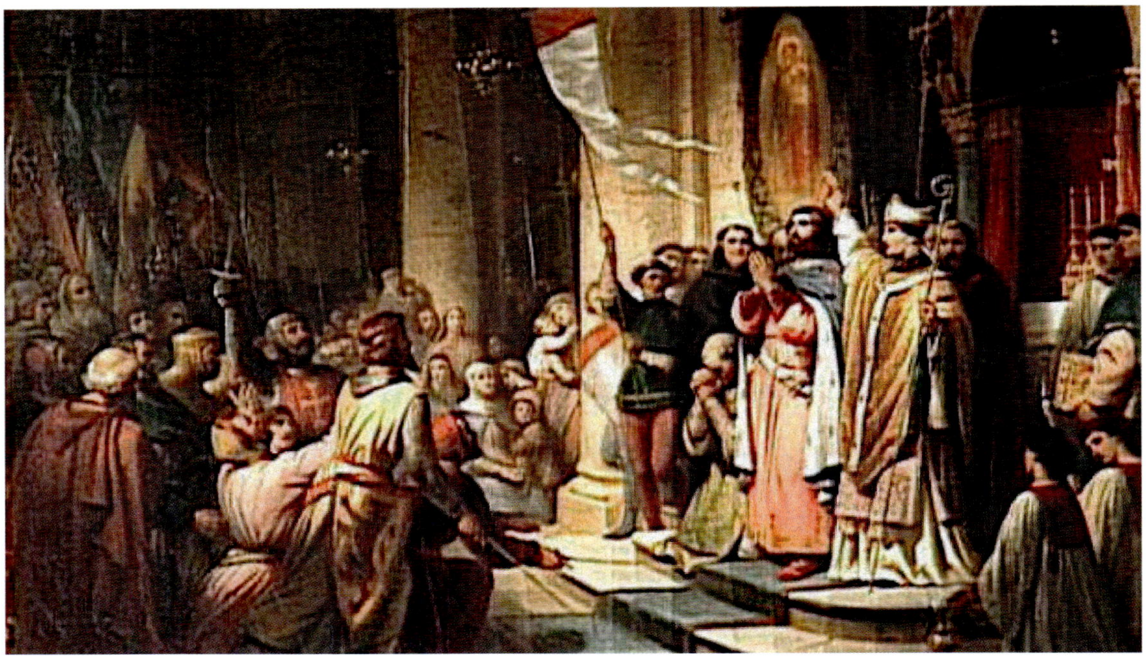

Boniface of Montferrat.

Painting by Henri Decaisne, c. 1840, Palace of Versailles, France.

who remained waited anxiously for what would come next, doing our best to manage the growing shortages of food and medicine.

Once things had somewhat calmed, I attempted to make contact and negotiate with the new leadership. I wished to continue my work—at least for a time—and not abandon the people, who, regardless of how responsible they may have been for the catastrophe, were now paying the highest price. The Eastern Roman Empire was partitioned among the crusaders. The absurdity lay in the fact that these greedy and historically ignorant men divided among themselves not only territories they had conquered, but even regions that had long since been lost to us—such as eastern Asia Minor, Egypt, and the northern Balkans. Thus was established the Latin Empire of Constantinople, with Baldwin of Flanders—brave soldier though he was, yet a mediocre leader—crowned emperor, largely because Dandolo wanted someone he could easily manipulate. According to their agreement, if the emperor were to be a Frank, then the (Latin) patriarch had to be a Venetian. The country was fragmented, in typical feudal fashion, into vassal kingdoms, principalities, and duchies.

The most prominent of the Frankish leaders, Boniface of Montferrat, established the Kingdom of Thessalonica, while the Venetians founded the Duchy of the Archipelago in the Cyclades. In addition, the Venetians seized control of Euboea, Crete, the Ionian Islands, numerous Aegean islands, and several important ports. The rest of Greece was divided among lesser-known leaders. Geoffrey of Villehardouin—a relative and namesake of the chronicler—conquered the Peloponnese, where he founded the Principality of Achaea, and Othon de la Roche took possession of the Duchy of Athens. The Patriarchal Throne was claimed by the Venetian Thomas Morosini, who immediately proclaimed the subjection of the Church of Constantinople to the Pope. The

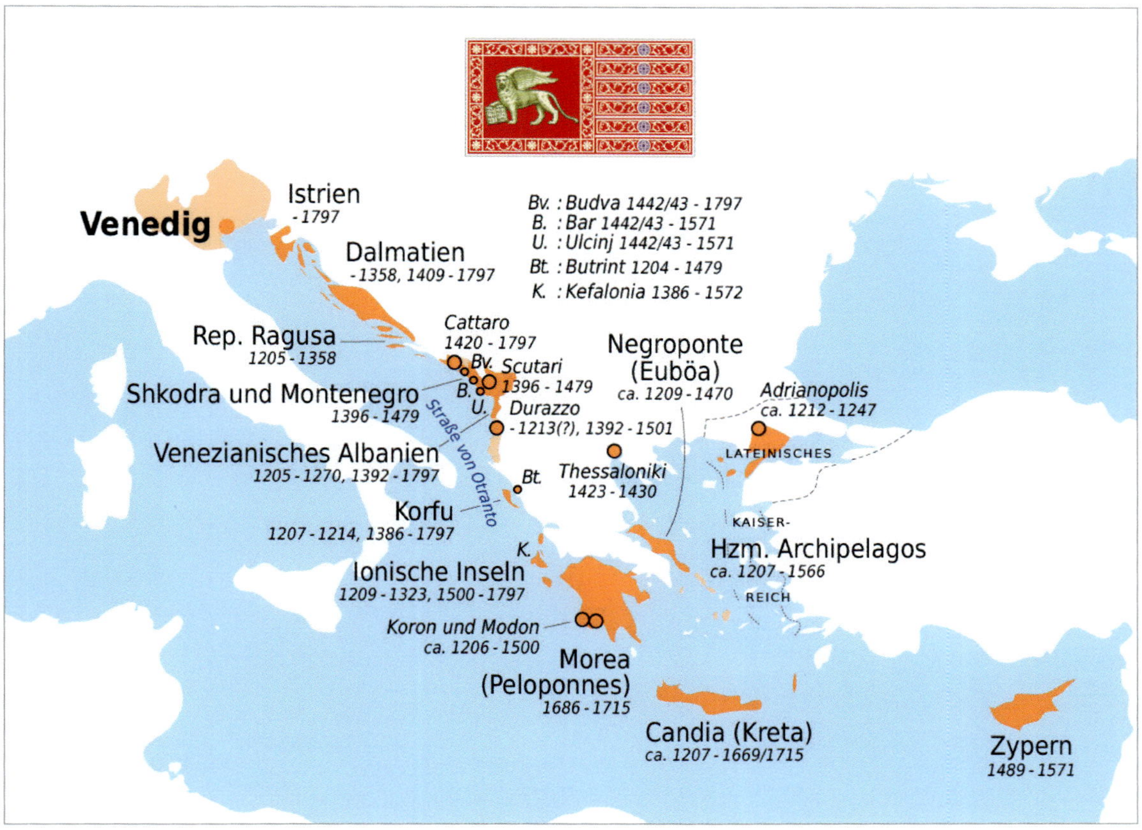

The Colonial State of Venice.

Map by Maximilian Dörrbecker, Kartenwerkstatt, 2022.

Orthodox Patriarch, John Kamateros, proved unequal to the moment. He fled hastily to Didymoteicho, which lay within the jurisdiction of the Bulgarian state.

As so often happens, it was the ordinary, poor people who paid the highest price. Yet they, too, were by no means blameless for the City's downfall. The population of Constantinople—both civilians and soldiers—was widely accused of cowardice, indecision, and a fatalistic attitude in the face of these world-shaping events. They were also blamed for outbreaks of destruction and looting of their own.

But alas for any human community that falls prey to the psychology of the mob. The inhabitants of Constantinople were among the most cultured and educated people in Europe—or rather, of the entire civilized world. Education and social welfare within the Empire, and especially in the capital, were at a remarkably high level. This same people had demonstrated great endurance and courage in other critical moments—when they had capable leaders and were treated justly. Yet after more than two decades of incompetence, misrule, lawlessness, and ruthless exploitation by rulers concerned only with maintaining and enjoying power, the cosmopolitan citizens of the Queen of Cities were reduced to a mob.

These mobs, skillfully incited by demagogues, slaughtered the Latins of the city like wild beasts—killing, mutilating, plundering churches and palaces during each transition between the wretched final emperors. And in the end,

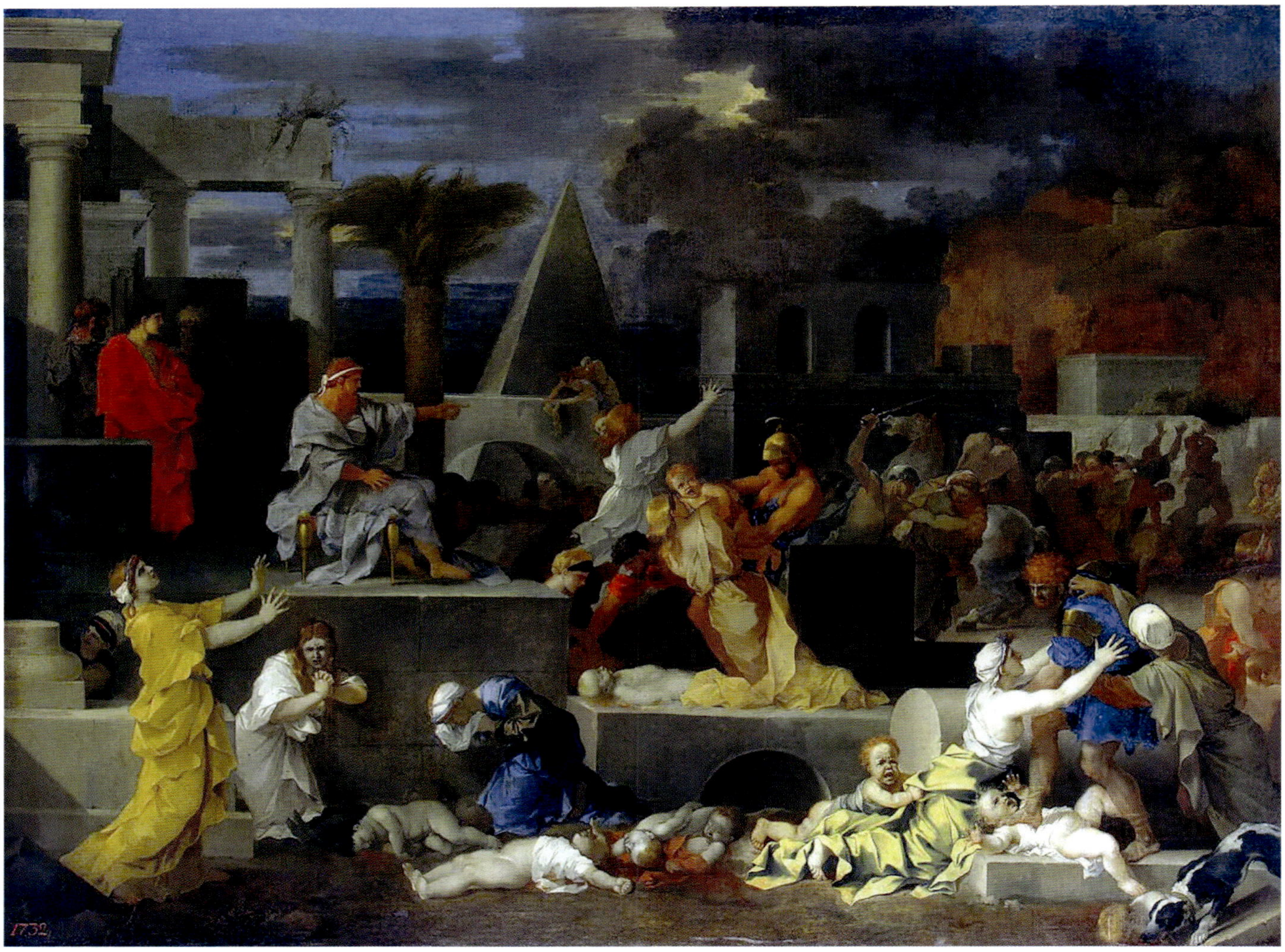

The Massacre of the Innocents. Such was the fate of the inhabitants of Constantinople.

Painting by Sébastien Bourdon, 1640, Hermitage Museum, St. Petersburg.

they succumbed to a superstitious panic and scattered in fear when the banner of the Nikopoios Theotokos fell into enemy hands. I would say that something similar applies to the crusaders as well. Certainly, among them were thieves and plunderers. Yet we cannot deny that many of them initially set out with the sincere intention of liberating the Holy Places. But when their leaders convinced them that the Greeks were heretics, traitors to Christ, corrupt thieves hoarding unimaginable wealth they did not deserve—they, too, were transformed into beasts who killed and humiliated without reason, destroying the monuments of one of the greatest civilizations the world has ever known.

A few weeks after the fall of the City, the assistant of a Venetian merchant—who had previously collaborated with my brother—brought me a letter from Nicaea. Commerce, of course, continued despite the hostilities, for the enterprising Venetians never missed an opportunity for profit, just as our own people seldom did. Constantinople relied on agricultural and other goods from the plains of Bithynia, which our countrymen transported to the ports along the Propontis, where the Venetians received them by ship. The letter was from Antigone, and it read as follows:

My beloved husband and lord, Three weeks have passed since I was compelled—following the urging of everyone, but above all your own wish—to leave Constantinople, leaving you there alone, guarding, like Leonidas at Thermopylae. How deeply I admired your decision, even though it pains me greatly, for I cannot even bear the thought that some misfortune might befall you. But that is precisely what I expected of you: to choose the unreasonable path of service and sacrifice, rather than the path of "reason" and safety. How I wish I could be with you during this most difficult period of your life. The only thing that consoles me is the thought that my presence beside you might have added to your anxiety and made your decisions and stance more difficult. Stay there, my dearest—remain where you have chosen to stand in life: beside the suffering and the powerless, without regard for consequences. I understand that you could not flee, abandoning your patients to their fate. You could not disappoint them, even though leaving would have been entirely reasonable and prudent. But the most glorious moments in history are not written by the prudent and cautious—but by the unreasonable, the strange, and the blessedly reckless. All of us here are praying for you—that the Theotokos may protect you from the wrath and murderous rage of the Latins. I have heard that Baldwin of Flanders is a just man, but I do not know who his advisors are, nor where a single ill-judged moment might lead him. I hope he will understand the nature of your service and accept your offer to help the people now under his rule. I believe that the truth and sincerity you embody will persuade him.

I am sending you this letter with a merchant friend who will hand it to one of his Venetian colleagues. You do not need to reply; it will be enough for me if he lets us know that you are well.

May the love of God—and my own—cover and protect you.

Baldwin IX, the First Latin Emperor of Constantinople. *Miniature by the Maitre de Fauvel, 1337.*

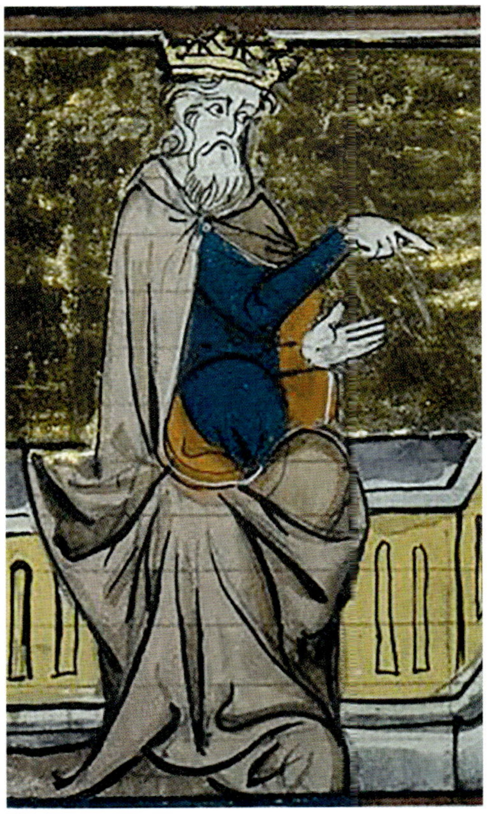

This letter gave me great strength and dispelled the doubts I had about my meeting with Baldwin. The Latin Emperor, who was crowned according to the Byzantine rite, was an honorable man and felt deep embarrassment over the outrages committed by his fellow countrymen.

He received me with the prejudice that the Latins held against us, yet he was trying to grasp the situation. I spoke to him about the sanitary needs of the great city, the system we had in place, and the level of medicine that existed in Byzantium. Unfortunately, he understood nothing. These people were warriors, guided by a lofty code of honor, but held primitive social and economic views. The only things they valued were the power of arms, military exploits, and authority—and they took it for granted that the impoverished people they supposedly "protected" should serve and feed them. The weak, the poor, the sick had no place in their society. In France and other Western countries, there were no hospitals equivalent to our *xe-*

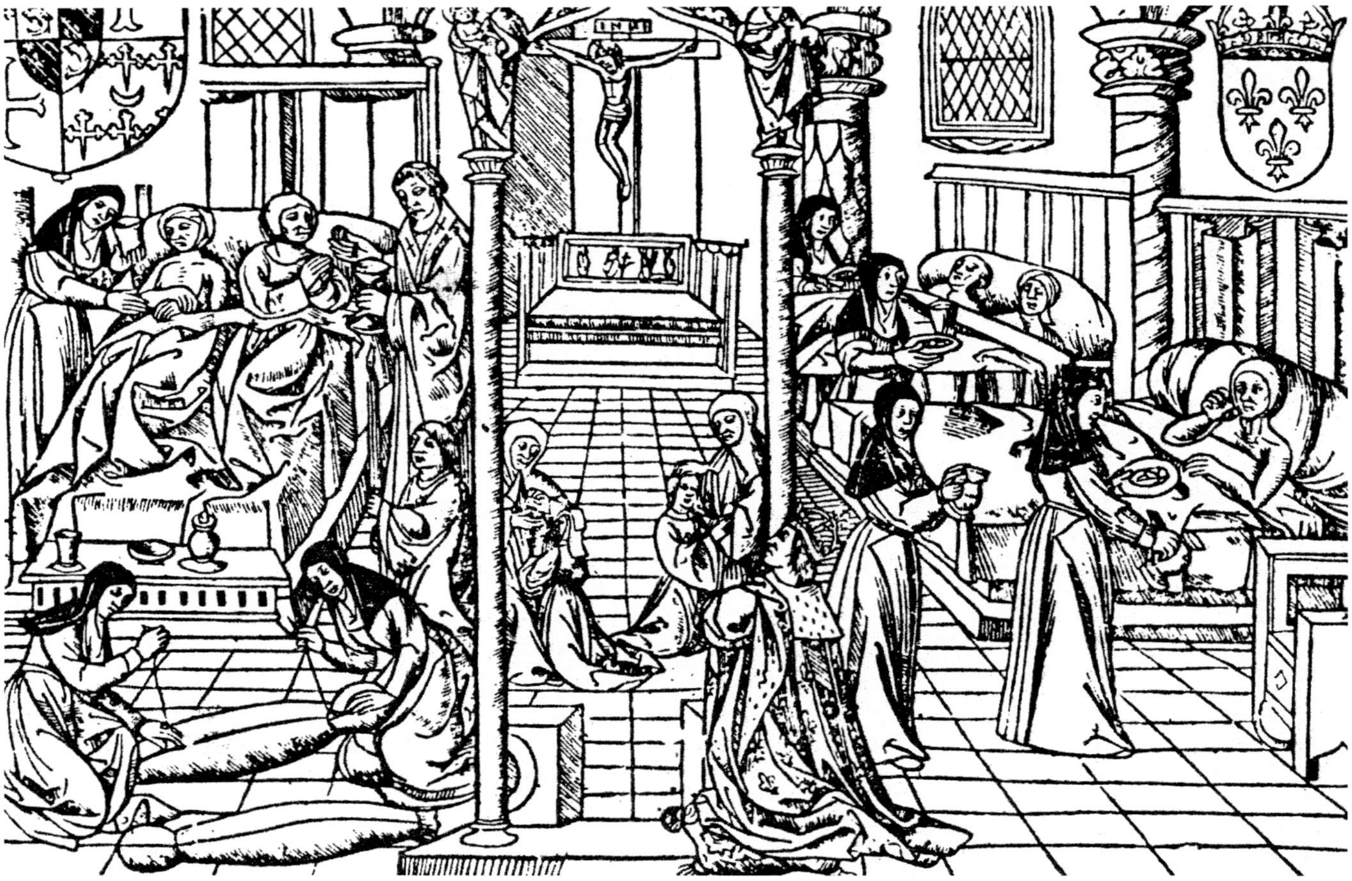

The Hôtel-Dieu Hospital in Bourges, France, in the year 1500. Patients, three centuries after the Komnenoi, are still lying two to a bed.

Header from a letter of gratitude by the Archbishop of Bourges, Photo: Hulton Archive/ Getty Images.

nones (hospitals); there were only asylums, where those who had no share under the sun would go and receive the barest care. Doctors were private practitioners and treated patients at home, while surgery was performed by barbers in public squares before curious onlookers, as if it were a public spectacle. Baldwin had good intentions, but he could not overcome the mentality of his society. The "Latin Empire of Constantinople" was a military state with a weak central administration and semi-independent vassal states and fiefs, following the system they had in their own countries. The care of the sick had been entrusted to two orders of knight-monks, the Hospitallers and the Templars. Of the numerous *xenones* (hospitals) of the City, only two were preserved—those of the Mangana and of Sampson, both near the historical center. These were taken over by the Templars and Hospitallers, who downgraded them to the level of their own hospitals—something closer to asylums.

The remaining *xenones* were stripped of all their property and dissolved. With deep sorrow, I saw the Xenon of the Pantocrator—the pride of our hospitals—abandoned. The Church of the Pantocrator was transformed into a Latin church. The monks were expelled, and the monastery was occupied by Catholic monks of the Order of Saint Anthony. However, the hospital ceased to function as a medical institution and became part of the monastery complex. Some time later, I visited the Xenon of the Mangana, where I had completed my studies. The sight was heartbreaking. Crowds of sick people, nonexistent medical care, rudimentary nursing, total disorganization... The Queen of Cities had been irreparably wounded. As I wandered through the deserted streets, I was gripped by sorrow at the sight of burned and ruined buildings, shattered monuments and statues, the frightened and silent inhabitants—those who had not fled or been killed—and the filth that revealed neglect and abandonment. What relation did this city have to the one I first beheld thirty-five years ago, when I arrived by ship at the harbor of Theodosius, or when I wandered through its streets, teeming with multitudes, marveling at its palaces and churches? Nothing held me anymore in the "Queen of Cities." At the first opportunity, I crossed the Bosphorus by boat to the opposite shore, in search of my family and of Laskaris, who had repeatedly invited me to the new state he had founded in Asia Minor. As the ship pulled away, I saw the dome of Hagia Sophia gleaming, reflecting the setting sun. I remembered the impression Hagia Sophia had made on me the first time I saw it—when the rising sun had triumphantly entered the church, illuminating everything, lifting the dome as if it were suspended above the earth, causing the earthly to dance in harmony with the heavenly. I wept, for I knew I would never see the Queen City again.

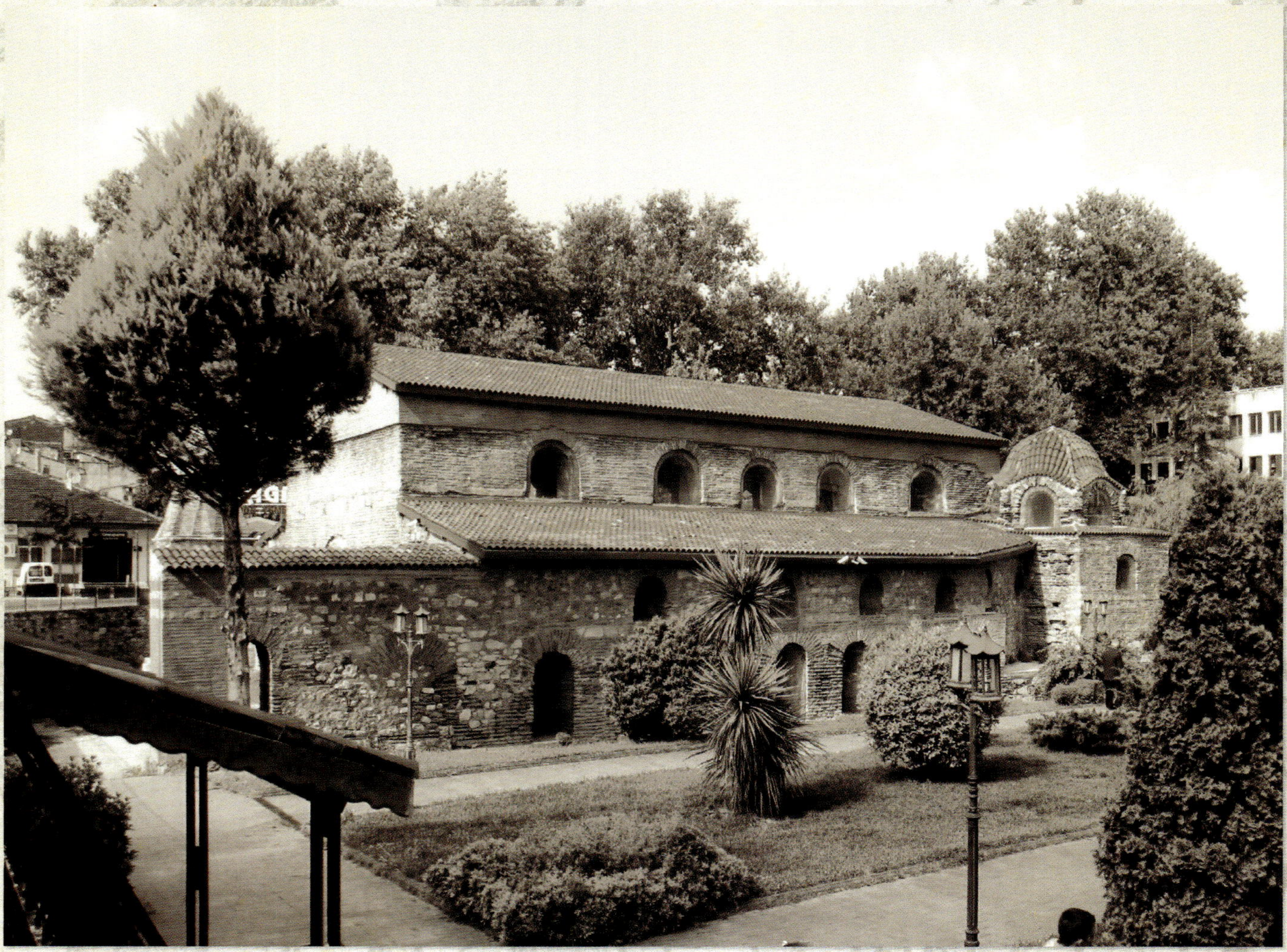

The Church of Hagia Sophia in Nicaea.

Photo: Elelicht, 2012

THE EMPIRE OF NICAEA

After the fall of the City, the condition of the inhabitants of the conquered Empire was very dire. We still called ourselves Romans, because we wanted to preserve the legacy and prestige of the Universal Empire handed down to us by Constantine the Great and continued by Justinian the Great. But now, after 900 years, the circumstances were completely different. The ideal of the Ecumenical Empire had long since ceased to exist. The various peoples who inhabited its lands had developed the consciousness of distinct nations, had their own languages and religions, and wanted their own states and governments. Most of the inhabitants of the Eastern Empire—more often called Romania—spoke the Greek language and felt themselves heirs of Greek civilization and the Orthodox Christian faith. All of our neighbors, Europeans and Slavs alike, now referred to us as Greeks (*Graikoi*), not Romans. So when the City was conquered and all was lost, the one element that held the promise of resurrection was our Greek identity. Hope was not lost; on the contrary, efforts immediately began to expel the Crusaders and return to our former glory—with the Queen of Cities as our center once more.

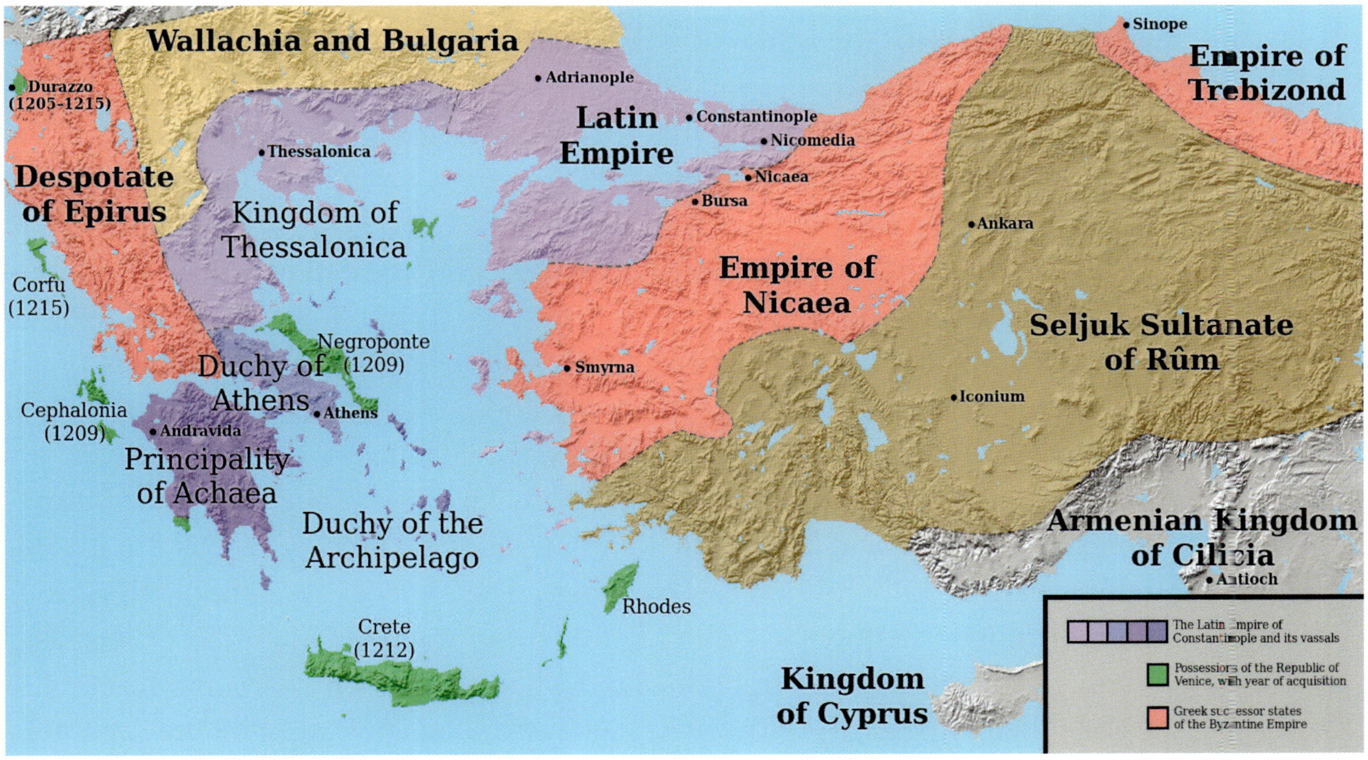

The Latin Empire and the Greek Successor States in 1204.

Alongside the Latin Crusader states that were established, three Greek–Roman states emerged with the hope of reviving the Empire: the Empire of Nicaea, founded by Theodore Laskaris; the Empire of Trebizond, founded by the brothers Alexios and David Komnenos; and the Despotate of Epirus, founded by Michael Doukas Angelos. The Empire of Trebizond included a narrow strip of land between the Black Sea coast of Asia Minor and the Pontic Alps, and was tightly encircled by the Seljuk Sultanate. The Despotate of Epirus stretched west of the Pindus mountain range, from Dyrrachium to Naupactus, with its capital in Arta, and was in constant warfare with the Frankish states. The Empire of Nicaea, closest in proximity to the dream of Constantinople, held the northern and western regions of Asia Minor. All three states viewed their existence as provisional, with the primary aim of recapturing Constantinople and reviving the Empire, of which they believed themselves to be the rightful heirs. Unfortunately, they failed to coordinate a common effort and instead fell into rivalry and hostilities, each seeking to expand its territory within the lands of the former Empire they all claimed.

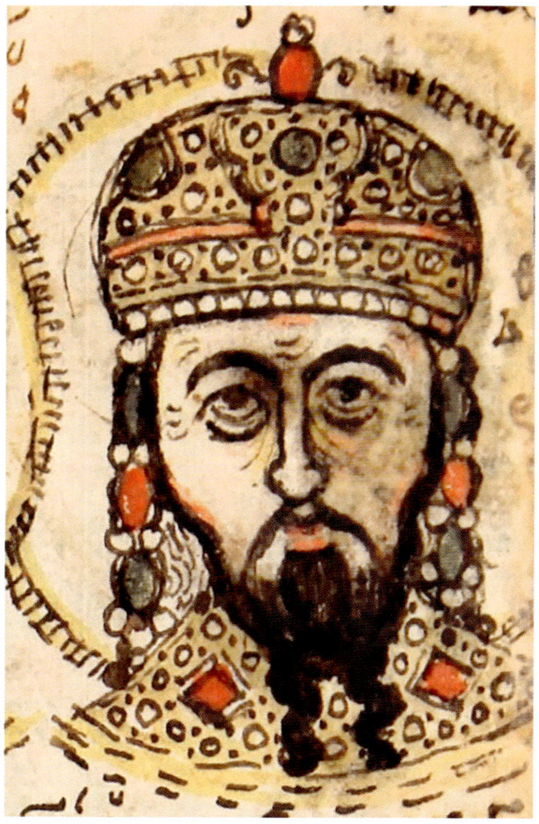

Theodore I Laskaris.

Miniature, Zonaras, 15th century. d'Este Library, Modena.

I followed Theodore Laskaris to the State of Nicaea, where I worked alongside him and many distinguished individuals who had also joined his cause. Under his inspired leadership, and later that of his successor John Vatatzes, a significant social and cultural renaissance took place in Nicaea—worthy of comparison with the achievements of the Komnenoi. My visit and conversation with the Latin Emperor Baldwin, who had taken up residence in the Boukoleon Palace, convinced me that there was no room for mutual understanding. In matters of health and public welfare, the Latins' organization was far inferior to ours. Baldwin had good intentions, but he was neither particularly capable nor well-educated. He desired peaceful coexistence among the peoples, yet he lacked the ability to manage such a task. In contrast, his brother Henry was exceptionally clever, but his sole concern was the conquest of the Roman lands they had divided among themselves and the enforcement of Latin rule. He was the most dangerous enemy we faced.

I arrived in Nicaea a few months after the fall of the City. The Laskaris brothers, Constantine and Theodore, had not yet settled in Nicaea, as the inhabitants were initially cautious toward them. Their past experiences with various opportunistic aristocrats—who would stir up the people with lofty promises only to bring calamities upon the land—had made them wary and hesitant to place their trust easily. However, they were soon convinced by the capability and integrity of the two brothers and accepted them as their leaders. Although Constantine, being the elder, had been proclaimed Emperor of the Romans, the true leadership figure was Theodore, who would go on to become the founder of the Empire of Nicaea.

Nicaea was the best possible choice for the capital of a state that aspired to reclaim Constantinople. Not only was it geographically close—just 100 miles away—but it also held profound symbolic significance for Orthodoxy and the people. It was there that the First Ecumenical Council took place in 325, during which the Creed was formulated, and also the Seventh Council in 787, where the veneration of holy icons was restored. When I arrived in Nicaea, my family had already settled into a beautiful house near the city's northern gate, known as the Gate of Constantinople. The connections my brother and the Vlemmides family had through trade played an important role in securing it. The house, where Antigone awaited me, resembled the one we had first settled in upon arriving in the City from Patras. I felt immense relief and a sense of security, especially as more and more prominent citizens and intellectuals were flocking to the city, making it increasingly difficult to find a good home.

Together with Antigone, we studied the history of the city and walked through it, just as I had done in Constantinople when I first arrived there as a young man—full of wonder, yet filled with dreams. Now, I felt the same sense of beginning a new life, but this time with the benefit of education and a companion by my side. Nicaea is an ancient Greek city, built in the fertile plain of Bithynia, on the eastern shore of Lake Ascania. Its first name was Olbia. The name it bears today was given to it 301 years before the birth of the Savior by

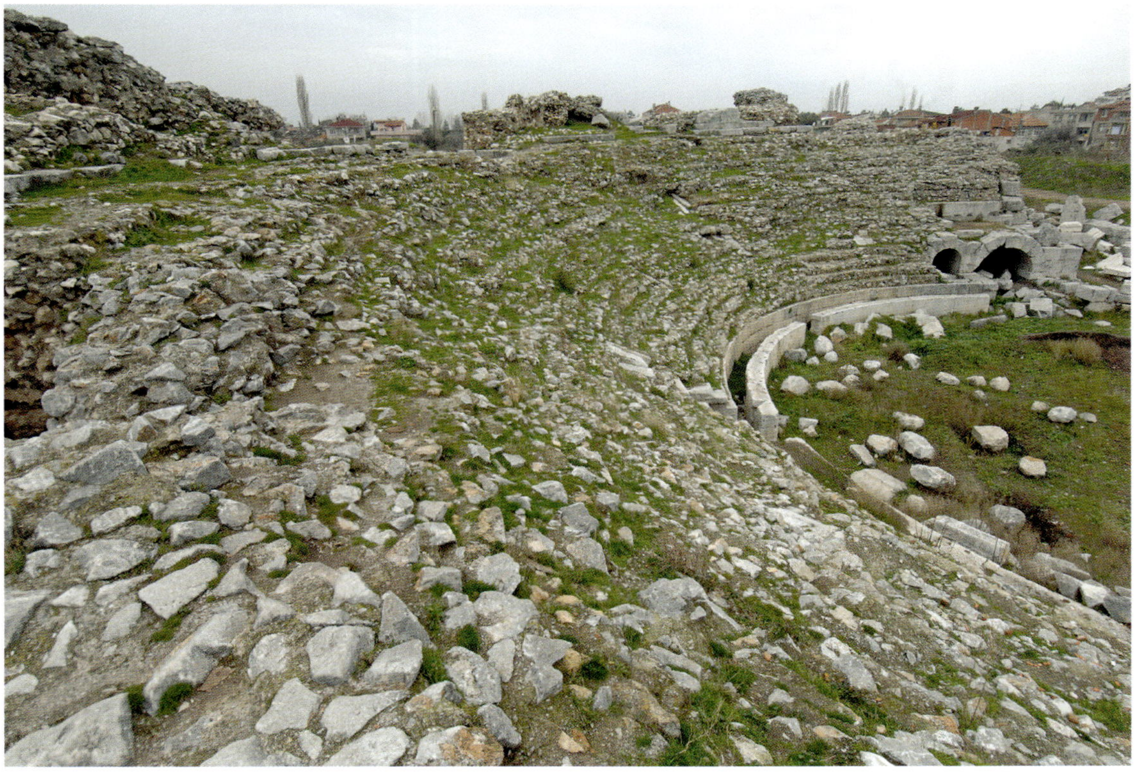

The ancient theatre of Nicaea.

Renovated by Pliny the Younger. Photo: Dosseman, 2019.

the Macedonian King Lysimachus, in honor of his wife. The city is laid out according to the "Hippodamian" system, which first appeared in Ionia in the 5th century BC—its streets run parallel and intersect at right angles, creating orderly city blocks. It has two wide central avenues that cross each other perpendicularly, so that from their intersection one can see all four of the city's gates. Originally, its perimeter was square, but after a major earthquake, the walls were extended into a polygonal shape to better adapt to the terrain, without disrupting the city's urban rhythm.

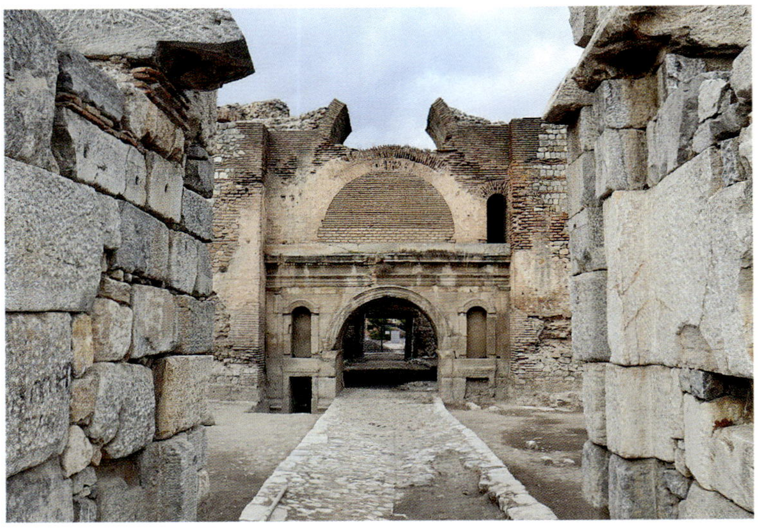

The gate of Constantinople in Nicaea.

Photo : C. Radato, 2019

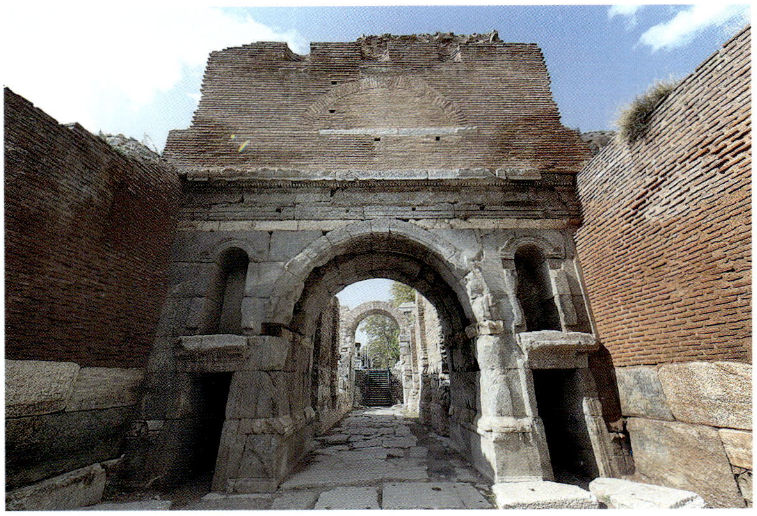

The White Gate in Nicaea.

Photo: Dosseman, 2019

Its walls, of course, cannot be compared to those of Constantinople, yet they are strong and tall, with rounded towers placed at close intervals. The city has four main gates: the Gate of Constantinople to the north, the Gate of Prusa to the south, the White Gate to the east, and the Lake Gate to the west. The orientation of the streets is such that buildings receive sunlight in the winter and remain cool in the summer, while the roads are constructed with appropriate slopes to allow for proper drainage of rainwater.

The city's water supply had been secured since ancient times through a significant aqueduct, which was rebuilt by Emperor Justinian the Great, along with many public buildings and shops. Before the founding of Constantinople, the city had served as an imperial seat and held great prestige. It was for this reason that the First Ecumenical Council was convened there in 325, in the complex of the imperial residence known as the "Basileia," under the leadership of Constantine the Great. There, the heresy of Arius was condemned, and the first articles of the Nicene Creed were composed. It is very pleasant to walk through the city, for its beautiful layout, with perfect city blocks, makes it nearly impossible to get lost. Nicaea is a major commercial center, still supplying the capital with agricultural goods, while also trading with Armenia, Mesopotamia, and the coastal cities of the Aegean. Due to this commercial activity, a large inn has been built for merchants and other travelers passing through, and there is also a noteworthy Jewish community. Shops of every kind line the streets, offering agricultural produce and all manner of goods. The bustle in the streets is delightful, and Antigone was thrilled that she could easily purchase whatever was needed for the household without long journeys. We once again felt the sense of freedom and safety—something we had lost in Constantinople in recent years due to the lawlessness and corruption of the last emperors, and especially during the siege by the Franks.

At the very center of the city, at the intersection of its two main roads, stands the metropolitan church, also dedicated to the Holy Wisdom of God—Hagia Sophia. During the time of Iconoclasm, many distinguished members of Constantinopolitan society, persecuted and exiled, had taken refuge in the nearby monasteries and hermitages on Mount Olympus of Bithynia. These places became strongholds of resistance against the iconoclasts. It was for this reason that, in 787, the Seventh Ecumenical Council—destined to be the last, since the later schism with the Western Church divided Christendom—was convened in Nicaea's Hagia Sophia. That council condemned Iconoclasm and restored Orthodox faith concerning the veneration of holy icons. Within the city, one also finds the famed Monastery of Hyacinth, where, in the 9th century, Saint Constantine the Jew, who had converted from Judaism to Christianity, lived as an ascetic and reposed in the Lord. Besides the great church of Hagia Sophia, many smaller churches adorned the city. Antigone and I sought out and visited them all, along with other landmarks—the ancient theatre and the formidable city walls. We would go to Hagia Sophia for the Sunday liturgy. The services were solemn and magnificent, especially later on when the Patriarch himself was present—part of a greater effort to recreate, in spirit and dignity, the lost glory of the Queen of Cities.

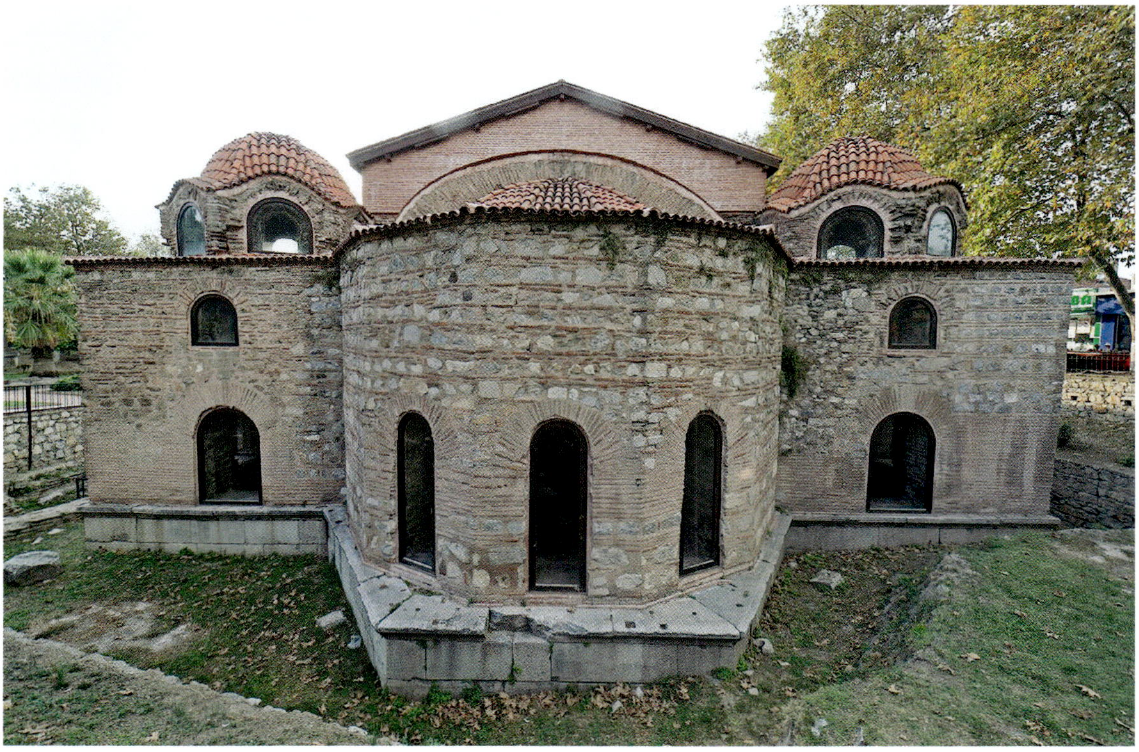

The Church of Hagia Sophia, site of the Seventh Ecumenical Council, Nicaea.

Photo: Dosseman, 2018.

The first concern of the new Emperor was to strengthen the city walls, for the defense of the capital was essential to the survival of the state. The walls were raised in height, a second outer fortification was constructed, and a moat with movable bridges was built in front of the main gates. My friend, the historian Niketas Choniates—who had also taken refuge in Nicaea—described these works with a fair measure of exaggeration, likening them to "sheer mountains or abrupt cliffs, as solid as those built by Semiramis in Babylon and praised by Hesiod." Yet behind this justifiable grandeur lies the deep insecurity that gripped our people after the fall of the God-protected and once-impregnable Queen of Cities—a wound to the soul that could not easily be healed.

Theodoros Laskaris was faced with insurmountable problems, yet he demonstrated remarkable political and military abilities and managed extraordinarily well. The tragic misrule of the Roman Empire by the Angelos dynasty had already, even before the fall of the City, given rise to separatist tendencies across the provinces. The gulf between the provinces and the capital had grown vast, and the provincial population—oppressed by the harsh taxation imposed by the emperors to fund their ambitions and rivalries—had grown resentful. They justifiably believed that the "city folk" exploited and looked down upon them. As a result, autonomous Greek principalities had sprung up in several regions. In Asia Minor in particular, there were three: one around Philadelphia under Theodore Mangafas, another near Sampson under Savvas Asidenos, and a third around Laodicea under Manuel Mavrozomes. There was no recognized leader around whom all Greeks could rally. The two surviving emperors—Alexios III and Alexios V (Mourtzouflos)—had fled in disgrace to old Greece and were regarded with contempt. Those Constantinopolitans who managed to escape fled to the still-free provinces, since the Franks had not yet conquered all the regions assigned to them. It was a sorrowful sight to see these refugees, humiliated, seeking shelter wherever they could lay their heads, only to face the (understandable) hostility of the impoverished rural populations who had suffered greatly under their rule.

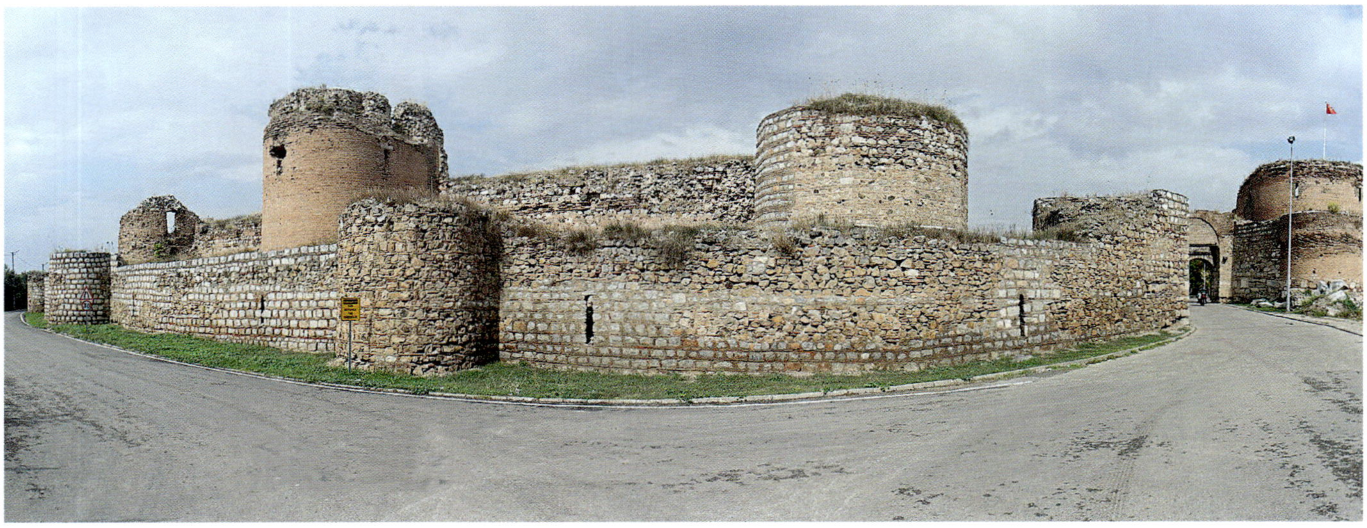

The walls of Nicaea.

Photo: Dosseman 2019.

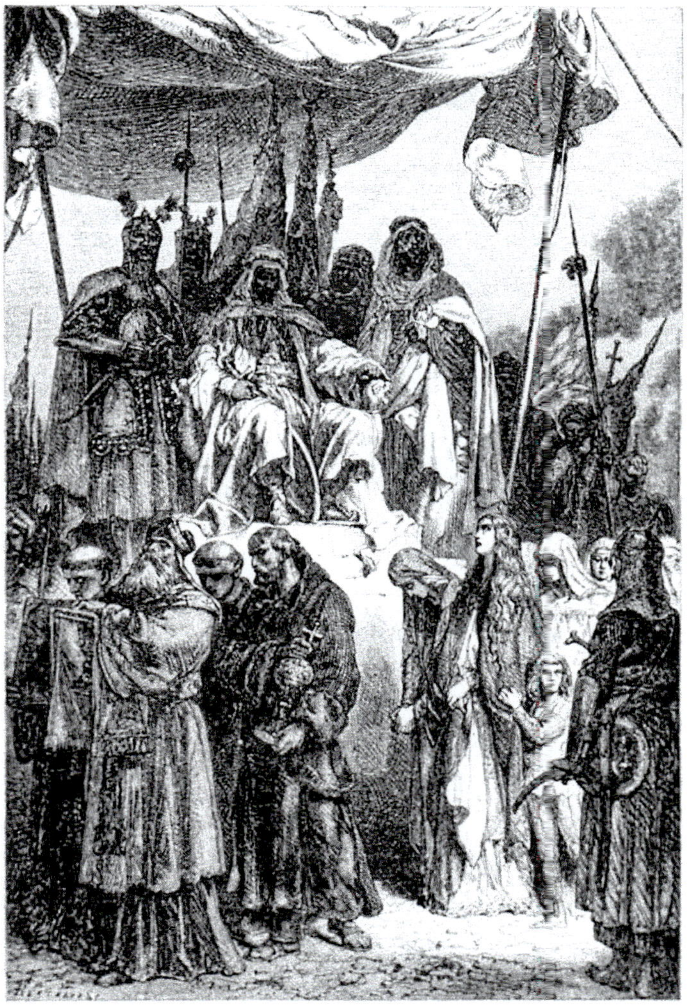

The expulsion of the Christians of the Holy City by Saladin.

Lithograph after a work by Alphonse de Neuville, in F. Guizot, London, 1883. (A similar fate befell the Orthodox Christians of Constantinople).

In Nicaea, the results of Theodoros' prudent governance became evident rather quickly. At first, circumstances were extremely difficult. The fledgling state was caught between the Seljuks and the Crusaders, both of whom not only refused to recognize its existence, but considered the region their own and sought to extend their dominion over it. Indeed, in the winter of 1204–1205, Henry of Flanders, the brother of the Latin Emperor, crossed into Asia Minor with the intention of seizing the lands that had been allocated to them—namely, the whole of Asia Minor. Theodoros hastily assembled an improvised army, composed mostly of mercenaries, yet he had no time to properly organize or inspire a capable fighting force. He was defeated in two engagements with the Crusaders, and the newly established state suddenly faced the threat of complete annihilation.

Indeed, in the second battle against Henry, Theodoros' brave brother Konstantinos was killed. The unfortunate and noble Konstantinos had been proclaimed Emperor of the Romans by the desperate people and nobles shortly before the fall of the City, but was never crowned, and for this reason he is not counted among the official lists of Emperors. After these defeats, a renewed wave of fear and uncertainty overtook us. Fortunately, at the very time Henry was threatening to destroy our fledgling state, his brother Baldwin recklessly engaged in battle near Adrianople with the far superior forces of Tsar Kaloyan of the Bulgarians. The Cru-

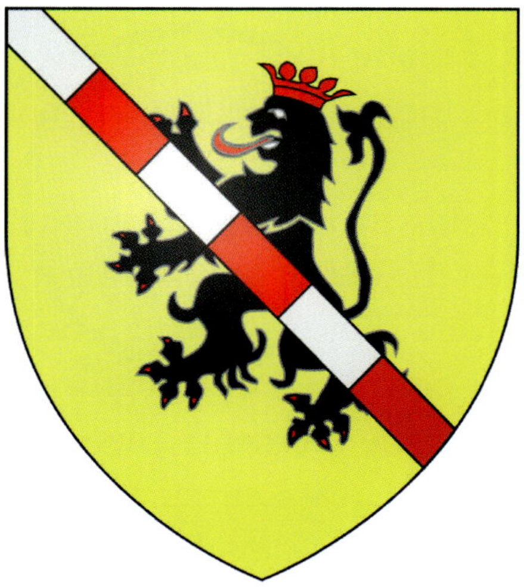

The coat of arms of Henry of Flanders.

In Claes Heinenzoon, Armorial de Gelre (collection), 1396. Royal Library of Belgium, Brussels.

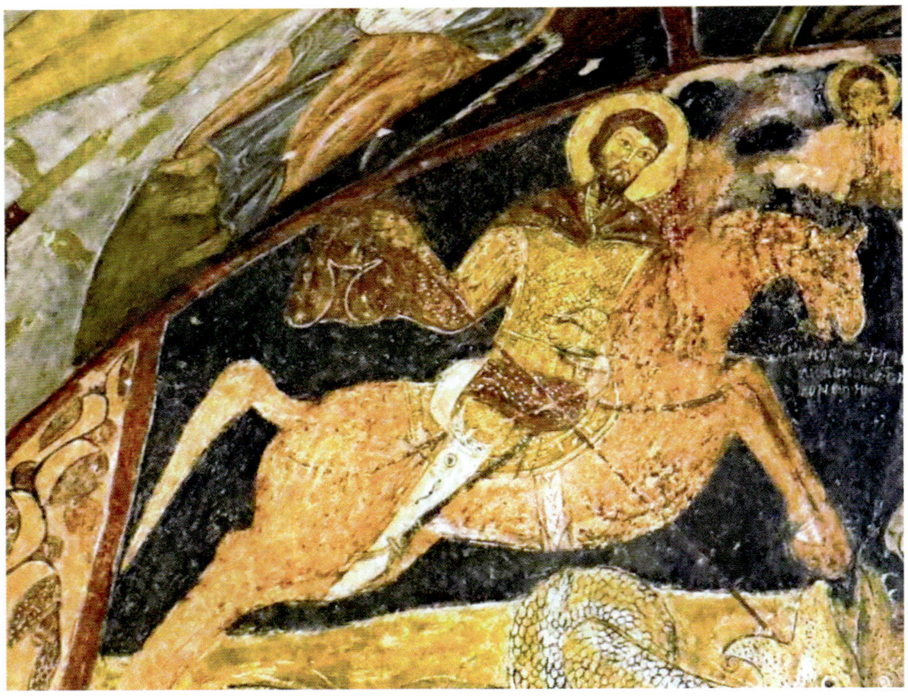

Theodore I Laskaris.

Fresco, 13th century, Cave Church of Saint John, Cappadocia

saders were defeated, and Baldwin vanished—most likely killed, as his body was never identified. Henry hurried back across to Thrace to face the Bulgarian threat, which was by then the greater danger, and thus left Theodoros in peace—for the moment.

We all breathed a deep sigh of relief at this turn of events, for we had begun to fear a second fall of a Greek city—this time, Nicaea. This reprieve proved invaluable for Theodoros, who was a worthy and capable leader, and he seized the opportunity to its fullest extent. He immediately set about organizing both the army and the administration of the state. He secured the recognition and submission of the local Greek rulers, who were compelled to accept his leadership. He assumed the title of Emperor of the Romans, as the heir of his brother, and summoned the exiled Patriarch John Kamateros—who had fled to Adrianople—to come to Nicaea, settle there, and crown him. The Patriarch, however, was elderly and ailing and could not make the journey. He died a few months later, in 1206. Theodoros then launched a series of military campaigns necessary to stabilize his realm. Regrettably, the first battle he had to fight was not against the Latins or the Turks, but against fellow Greeks—the rulers of the Empire of Trebizond—who had extended their domain across nearly the entire southern coast of the Black Sea and were threatening to reach Nicomedia. Losing access to the Euxine (Black) Sea was not an option. The Komnenoi of Trebizond were defeated and retreated as far as Sinope, while the Nicaean state expanded its control into Paphlagonia and the western shores of the Black Sea. Fortunately, following this defeat, the Empire of Trebizond effectively abandoned its claim to Constantinople, and there was no further conflict between the two Greek states.

In Constantinople, after the loss of the reckless Baldwin, his capable brother Henry was crowned as the new Latin Emperor. Yet the defeat by the Bulgarians had been severe, and he needed time to recover. Thus, he signed a two-year truce with Theodore, which marked the first official act of recognizing Theodore as the head of a sovereign state. Seizing the moment, Theodore moved swiftly to legitimize his imperial title. During Great Lent of 1208, he convened a synod of Eastern hierarchs in Nicaea to elect a new Ecumenical

Patriarch. Michael Autoreianos, a most distinguished and learned clergyman, was chosen. Unfortunately, the rulers of Trebizond and Epirus did not acknowledge him as Ecumenical Patriarch, but he was nonetheless accepted by the clergy and faithful throughout the conquered Roman lands. On Easter Sunday of that same year, Theodore was crowned Emperor of the Romans by the Ecumenical Patriarch, in a ceremony conducted with all the solemnity and grandeur of Constantinople. We all gathered in the local Church of Hagia Sophia, dreaming ourselves into the Great Hagia Sophia of the Queen City. His coronation address, the *Silention*, was written by Niketas Choniates, who stood beside me, deeply moved and anxious throughout the ceremony. In that speech, the new Emperor emphasized the divine origin of his authority and proclaimed his foremost mission to be the recovery of the lost homelands—lost through our own failings—and above all, the reconquest of Constantinople itself. "Let us reclaim the homelands from which we were cast out by sin; these are our first abodes, our Paradise, the City of the Lord of Powers, the joy of all the earth, the embattled and renowned City." Thus, Laskaris inaugurated the Great Idea of restoring the lost lands—a vision that would haunt and inspire the Greek nation from that day forth.

The new Emperor achieved significant victories in the years that followed. In 1209, he defeated a Crusader army attempting to seize Bithynia. But the following year, a fresh and grave threat cast its shadow over our lives. The unrepentant Alexios III—the very man who had ruined the Empire and disgracefully abandoned it without a fight—had the audacity and shamelessness to now claim the throne he had once forsaken. He fled to the court of Sultan Kaykhusraw of Iconium and begged for his help to seize the throne of Nicaea. The Sultan, eager for opportunity, saw in this a chance to replace the capable Theodore with a proven incompetent who would serve as easy prey, aligning perfectly with his future ambitions. The confrontation unfolded at the river Meander. The situation was dire, for the Turkish army was powerful, while our own was newly formed and inexperienced. With boldness, the valiant Laskaris challenged the Sultan to single combat. The duel, fought before both armies, was fierce and prolonged, as the soldiers watched in breathless antic-

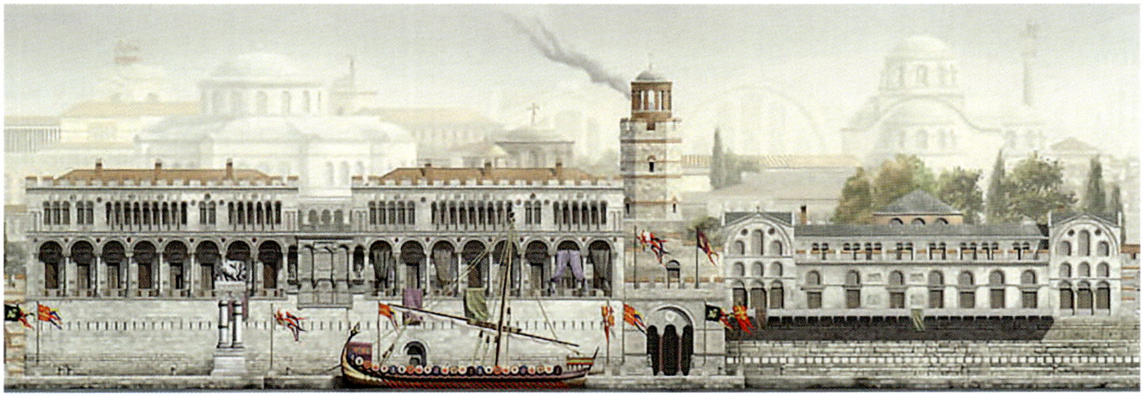

"The Queen City: The Eternal Dream of Hellenism".

Reconstruction by Antoine Helbert, 1876.

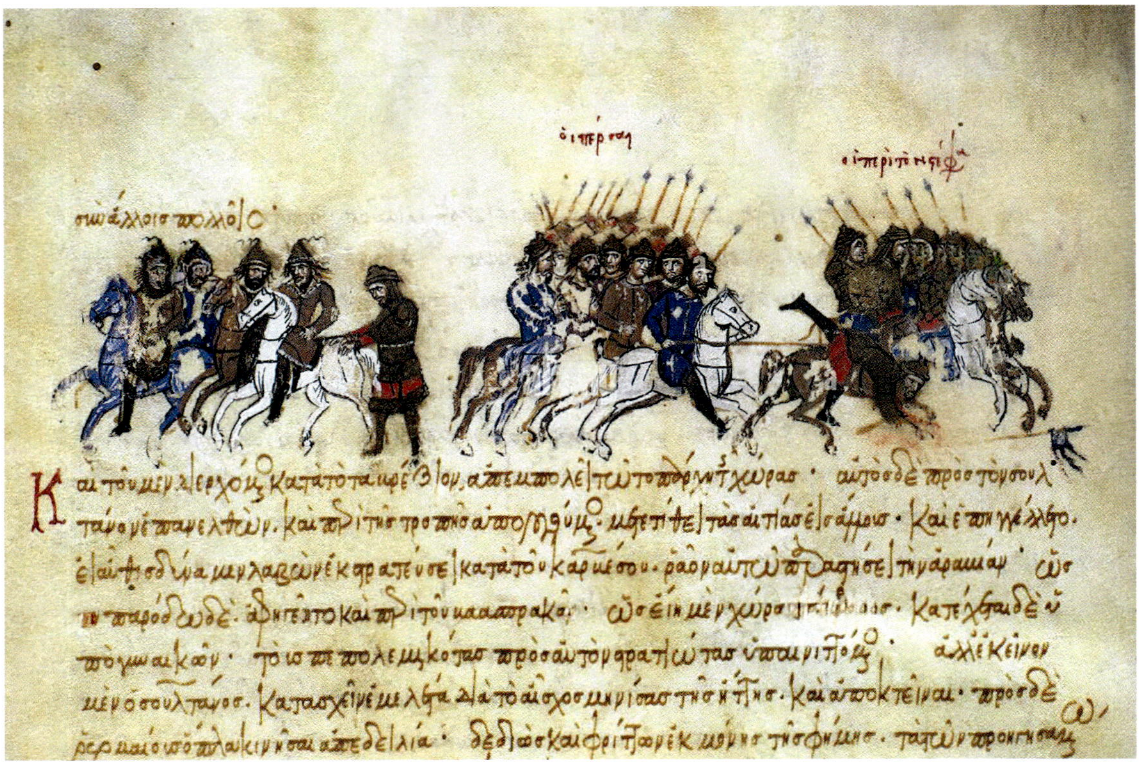

Battle between Byzantines and Turks (referred to as "Persians"). *Skylitzes, 12th century, National Library of Spain, Madrid.*

ipation. At last, the Emperor of the Romans delivered a masterful blow, striking down the Sultan of the Seljuks and sending him lifeless to the ground. The surge of joy among our troops was indescribable—they burst forth with cheers and cries, launching an attack that routed the now demoralized Turkish forces. The pitiful Alexios was taken captive. The state of Nicaea expanded at the expense of the Seljuks, but more importantly, it was now recognized as a viable and formidable power. The victory at the Meander—personally won by the brave Theodore—revived the morale of the entire Greek nation. In Nicaea, the people rejoiced, exalting their king. In the squares and in the streets, a jubilant crowd celebrated the first decisive victory after years of humiliation.

At long last, the Nation was granted a capable leader who restored its dignity and pride. Michael Choniates described the triumph as retribution against the Seljuks for the defeat at Myriokephalon, suffered nearly a century earlier by Manuel Komnenos. In 1214, peace was finally agreed upon with the Latins, and a large portion of Western Asia Minor—including the lands stretching from the Aegean to Attaleia—was formally recognized as the domain of the Empire of Nicaea. The traitor Alexios III—who was, in fact, Theodore's father-in-law—deserved execution, yet Theodore, displaying the magnanimity of the great Komnenian emperors who preceded him, instead compelled him to retire to a monastery, where at last he ceased to be a threat to the Empire.

All three Greek states founded after the fall of Constantinople made notable cultural and social contributions, but the Empire of Nicaea surpassed them all. In Nicaea, a new world was emerging—an empire that, while still claiming the mantle of the Ecumenical Empire and the inheritance of Roman grandeur, was in truth— and this we all knew—a predominantly national state. Surrounded by other national entities, it was distinguished by its Greek character, not only in language and cultural heritage, but also in its consciousness and in the very name "Greek," which in earlier centuries had been closely associated with paganism and thus avoided. Now, however, paganism had long disappeared, and the name "Hellene" or "Graikos," as the Slavs and Latins called us, had regained the glory of a people who first attained the highest achievements of the human spirit and enlightened the world. The Emperor of Nicaea now stood as the only hope for the restoration of humiliated Hellenism. From the outset, Theodore sought to revive the imperial majesty in Nicaea, thereby establishing his realm as the true heir to the Roman Empire. We were all swept up in the excitement, reliving the thrill of the old glory of the Ecumenical State. We watched in awe as the soldiers raised the Emperor upon a shield—an ancient custom that recalled the days of old triumphs. The new "God-crowned King" pursued a prudent economic policy to ensure the state's survival and the prosperity of its people. Yet, for the sake of prestige and continuity with tradition, he preserved the opulence of the imperial court and maintained the bestowal of courtly titles and honors, such as "Despot," "Sebastocrator," "Protosebastos," "Caesar," and others.

Laskaris was given the epithet "New Constantine," and all hopes were set upon him for the recovery of the Queen City. Nicaea was now regarded as the new center of Orthodoxy, the "New Zion," toward which the greater part of the Orthodox world turned its gaze. Here, "in exile," had settled both the legitimate Emperor of the Romans and the Ecumenical Patriarch. Theodore's foremost concern was to ensure the just treatment of his subjects. He devoted considerable resources to social welfare and the well-being of the people, to

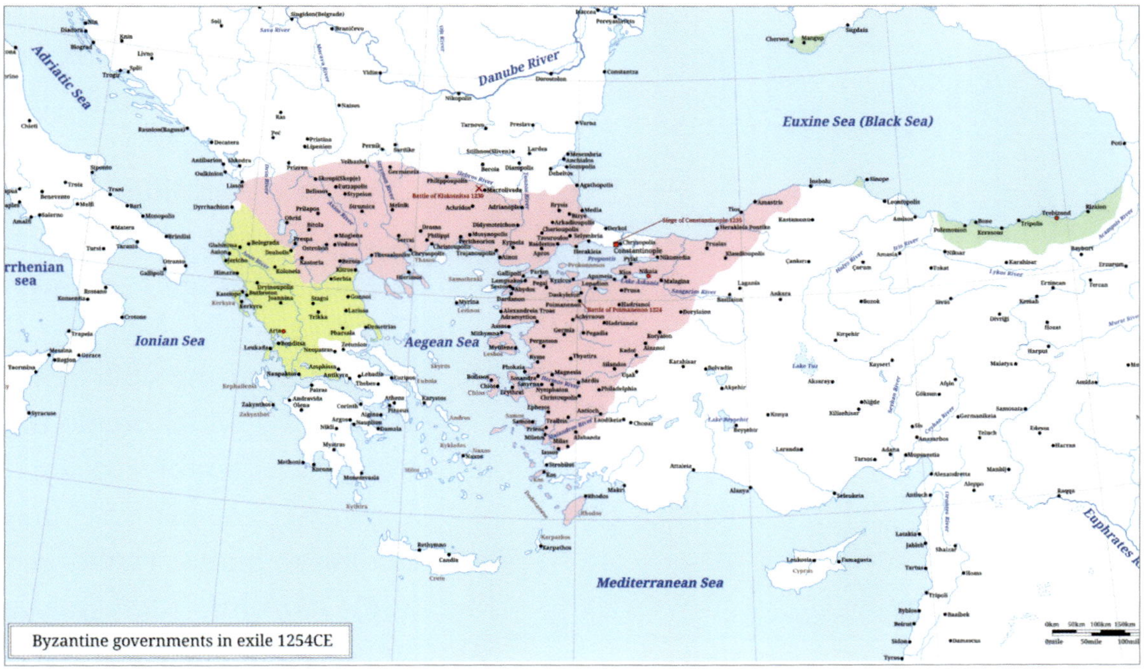

The Empire of Nicaea in 1250.

Historical maps of the Byzantine Empire.

such an extent that he came into conflict with the aristocrats—the *dynatoi*—who, unrepentant, sought to perpetuate the traditions of the Angeloi and preserve their extensive privileges. Nicaea had now become a magnet for many of Constantinople's distinguished citizens—political figures, intellectuals, and others flocking from various parts of the Hellenic world.

King Theodore, as a continuator of the imperial tradition—and later his successor John as well—devoted themselves to the constant care and reconstruction of the cities. They erected new and imposing public buildings, renovated and embellished existing ones, and founded institutions of social welfare such as hospitals (*xenones*), orphanages, and homes for the elderly. They built or restored numerous churches and monasteries: the Monastery of the Sosandri in Magnesia, that of the Lembiotissa near Smyrna, the Nea Moni of Chios with its magnificent mosaics, the Monastery of the Ruffinianoi in the outskirts of Constantinople, and many others—all received great attention and support from the emperors of Nicaea. They themselves undertook the construction of public roads (*basilikai hodoi*), and of course, reinforced and repaired the defensive walls in the principal cities of the Empire. They also established libraries and supported education, which flourished remarkably during their reign.

I had the honor of being appointed chief physician at the distinguished Xenon of Saint Mavra in Nicaea, and I was granted the title of Actuarios, as was customary in the Imperial hospital of the Mangana. Naturally, it was far inferior to the Xenon of the Pantocrator, where I had served in the Queen City, yet I was still vigorous and full of zeal for my work. We all felt that we had to give our very best to build a state out of ruins—it was the only way to survive. I therefore adapted the typikon of Saint Mavra as closely as possible to that of the Pantocrator, placing great emphasis on cleanliness, order, and the courteous conduct of the staff.

The city of Nicaea.

Miniature, Hartmann Schedel, The Nürnberg Chronicle, ed. Anton Koberger, 1493.

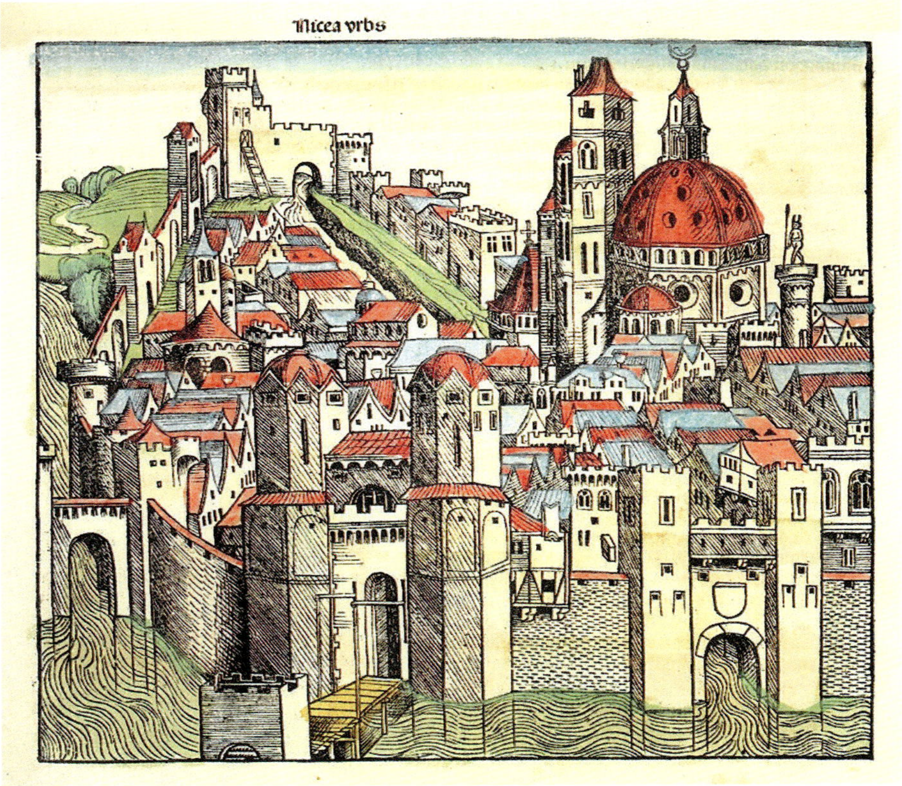

I also hired additional physicians among those who had taken refuge here from Constantinople. Many had already been my colleagues in the City, which made my work considerably easier. I likewise engaged nurses and auxiliary staff. I worked from morning until night, undertaking major surgeries

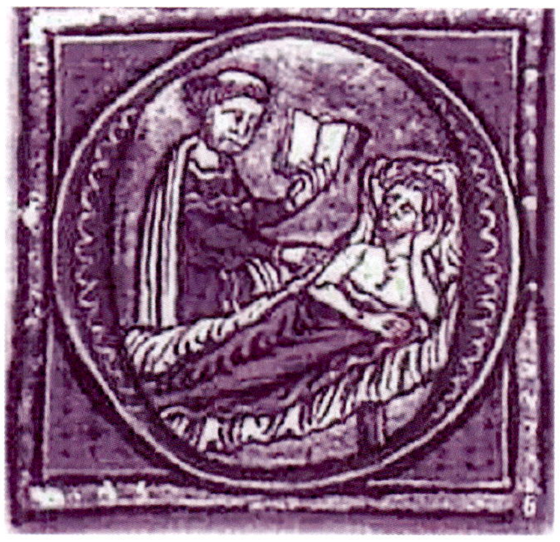

The physician "at the patient's bedside."

Miniature, 13th century, National Library of Medicine, Bethesda, Maryland, USA

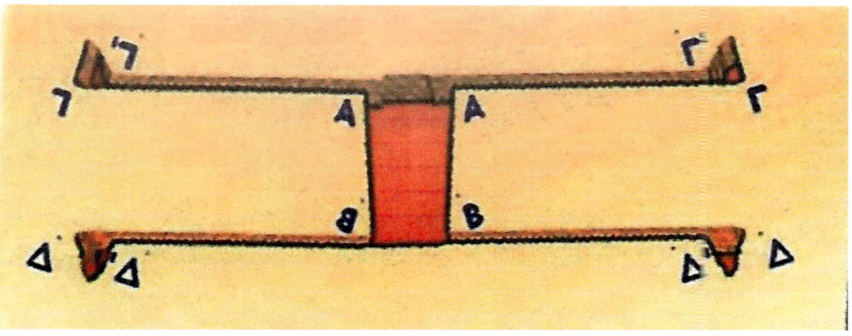

Reconstructive skin flaps, described by Antyllus, physician of the 2nd century AD.

for cases considered incurable. I sought to inspire diligence and compassion toward the sick by setting a personal example and treating everyone with courtesy and fairness. My invaluable collaborator and assistant was—and still is—Antigone, who continues to show her enduring devotion to medicine and to the care of the suffering.

She now works again as a volunteer and has become the very soul of the *xenon* through her tireless service and gracious manner. King Theodore, who esteemed me and was well aware of my work, granted every form of support I requested, so that our hospital became renowned throughout the Empire for the excellence of its services.

Alongside my professional work, Antigone and I began to cultivate a modest social life. We formed a warm friendship with the distinguished historian Niketas Choniates; our residences were close to each other, which made our acquaintance all the easier. The Akominatos family had long been settled in Chonae of Asia Minor, from which they derived their surname, "Choniates." My contemporary Niketas had an elder brother, Michael, twelve years his senior. When the brothers were, respectively, twenty-one and nine years old—in 1159—their father sent them to Constantinople to pursue their studies. Niketas was always under the protection of his remarkable brother. Both displayed great diligence, acquired profound learning, and rose to high offices within the Empire.

The plant cassia, used in the preparation of antidotes against poison (*theriaca*).

Source: Fytorio-amadryas.gr

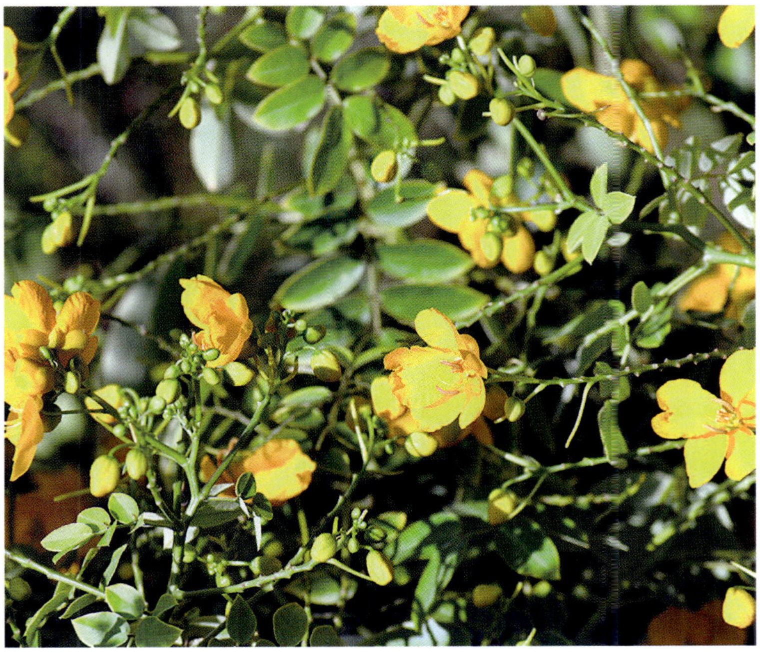

The elder brother, Michael, turned toward the ecclesiastical vocation. He was a noble and gentle soul, who knew Homer and the classical authors by heart, and was held in high esteem by the intellectual and ecclesiastical circles of the capital. At the age of forty-two, in 1182, he was consecrated Metropolitan of Athens and moved there. The Athens of his day bore no resemblance to the ancient, storied metropolis—it was but a village in a wretched state, both architecturally and economically, as well as culturally. The people lived in deep poverty and ignorance, bereft of any spiritual or intellectual light, struggling merely to survive. The cathedral church was the Panagia Atheniotissa—namely, the Parthenon—which had been converted into a Christian church. Around it stood a defensive tower and several small buildings. Michael, who as Metropolitan also bore administrative duties, found upon his arrival a central governance that had fallen into complete paralysis. The scandals of mismanagement and the abuses of public funds were countless. With passionate zeal he set himself to the task of bringing order and improving the economic and spiritual condition of his people. Yet where was he to begin? He wrote many letters—admonitions as well as laments—over the degradation of the once-glorious city of Athens. His classical education made him feel all the more keenly the misery of the former "famed city." But the calamity reached its height in 1204, when the crusading conquerors under Boniface of Montferrat arrived in Athens. There was no choice to be made—the city's defenses were nonexistent, and any resistance would have led only to massacre and ruin. He therefore surrendered the city peacefully, yet even so the rapacious invaders set about the systematic plundering of the already exhausted city. Disheartened, Michael withdrew to the island of Kea, where he secluded himself in the Monastery of Saint John.

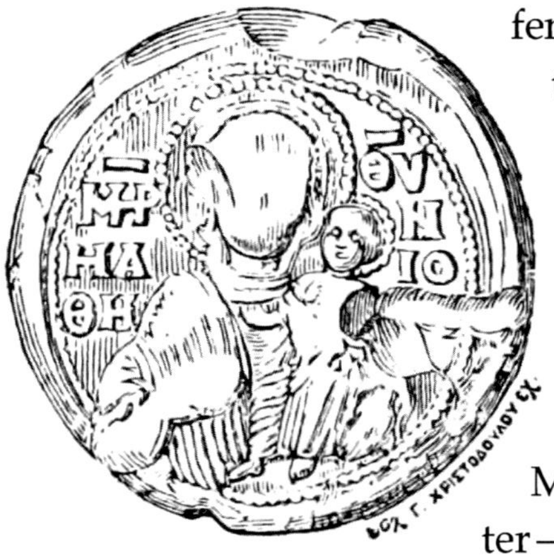

Niketas, who admired and loved his brother deeply, had, by virtue of his great learning and ability, risen to the rank of Megas Logothetes—that is, Grand Logothete or prime minister—under Isaac Angelos. He too sought refuge in Nicaea, where he assumed high administrative office, and his experience proved of great assistance to Emperor Theodore. His most important work, however, is the *History* he composed, encompassing the events in Constantinople and throughout the Empire from the beginning of the reign of John Komnenos in 1118 up to

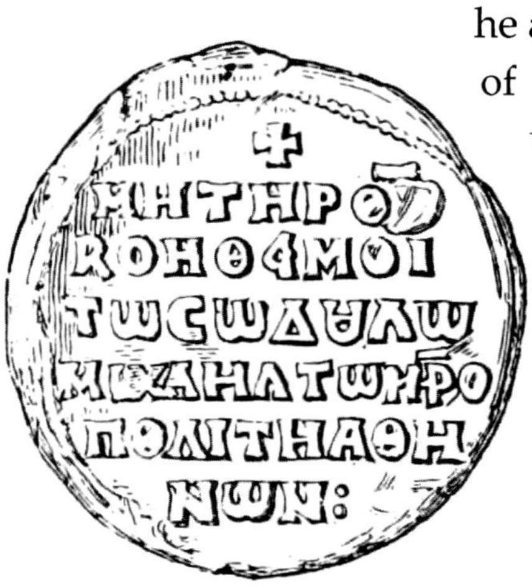

Seal of Michael Akominatos Choniates, 13th century.

Copy after a drawing by Gustave Schlumberger, Sigillographie de l'Empire byzantin, 1884.

the year 1207, wherein he also recounts the early years of Theodore Laskaris's rule in Nicaea. His description of the sack of the City by the crusaders—written with deep anguish—will preserve for all time the measure of savagery and brutality to which humanity may descend, a warning that speaks to all nations and all ages.

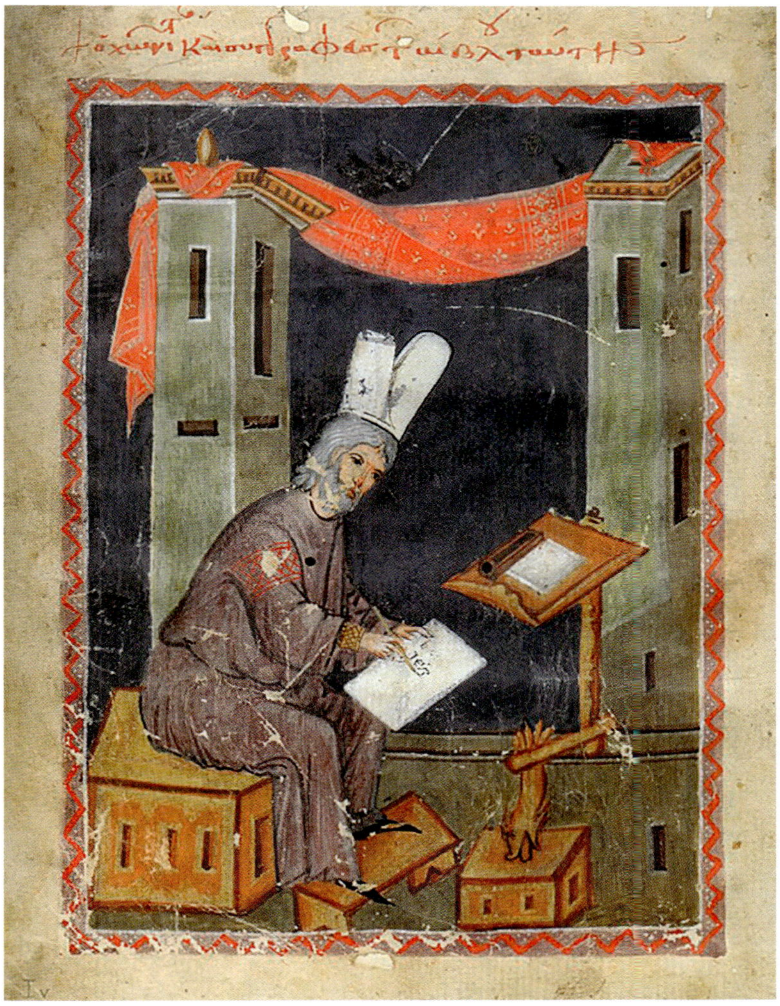

Niketas Akominatos Choniates.
Miniature, History of Niketas Choniates, 14th century, Austrian National Library, Vienna.

I had already known Niketas Choniates from our days in the City, and I had come to admire the integrity of his character. Now in Nicaea, we often exchanged visits; besides our many engaging conversations, he would read to us passages from his *History*—a true delight and a wellspring of knowledge. He loved and revered his brother deeply, writing to him repeatedly and begging him to come join him, even sending an official invitation from the Emperor himself. But Michael, worn down by hardship and illness, declined. Thus we lost the chance to meet and collaborate with a great man, who moreover was reputed to be a saint. Niketas was unable to complete his history of the Empire of Nicaea; he died in 1215, and his brother Michael followed him five years later. Both were devoted to the Hellenic spirit, and their works remain a significant contribution to Greek letters.

The relatively peaceful life in the city, together with the prosperity achieved by Theodore and his successor, John Vatatzes, allowed for the cultivation of social life and personal relationships in Nicaea. Our home had become a gathering place for distinguished individuals—statesmen, physicians, intellectuals, and clergy. Antigone showed remarkable skill in managing the household and keeping it ever prepared to receive guests. With the help of the young women who assisted us, our kitchen was always ready with *kerasmata* and *agapes*—treats and tokens of affection—to welcome our visitors. These gatherings were among the most delightful spiritual pleasures we enjoyed in Nicaea; they took place frequently and lasted late into the night. In this way, we came to know many remarkable people, a few of whom I will now recall.

Apart from Choniates, another eminent scholar with whom we shared a close friendship was Nikolaos Mesarites, a writer and theologian. He too came

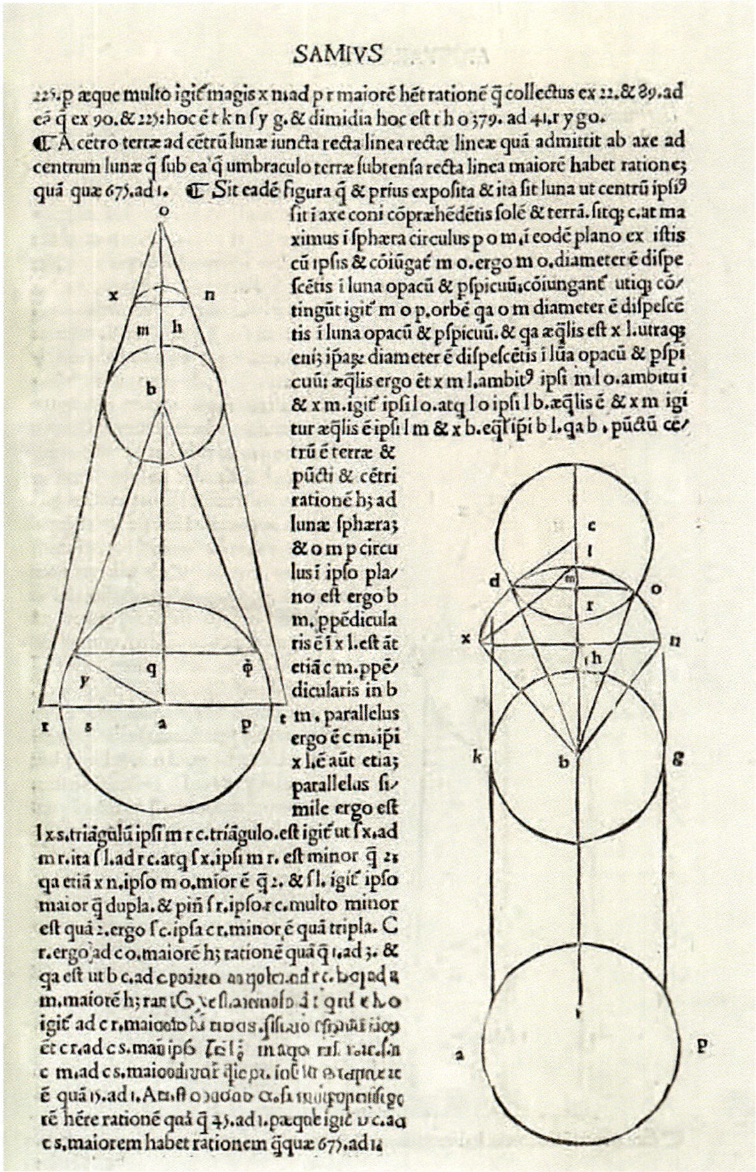

On the Sizes and Distances of the Sun and the Earth.

Nikephoros Vlemmydes, Logica (de Astrolaeo Aristarchi), *Venice, 1498.*

from an aristocratic family—his father, in fact, had served as president of the Senate. In Nicaea he was consecrated Metropolitan of Ephesus and Exarch of Asia. Mesarites, together with Niketas Choniates, undertook negotiations with the papal representatives concerning relations between the two Churches. Understanding with the Pope—who stood as the spiritual superpower of Western Europe—was a necessary condition for the international recognition and survival of the State. The matter was extremely delicate and complex, which is why it was entrusted to the two finest scholars of the age, and they handled it with great skill. Sadly, Mesarites too passed away prematurely in 1216, at the age of fifty-three.

Demetrios Karykes is some twenty years my junior. He distinguished himself by his vast erudition and, in 1214, was granted the title of *Hypatos ton Philosophon*—that is, superintendent of higher education in the Empire. He is a man of great intellect, and later, in 1222, John Vatatzes, who succeeded Theodore, appointed him *Megas Logariastes*, or minister of finance, in recognition of his integrity. In 1234, Karykes took part in the discussions held in Nicaea with the envoys of Pope Gregory IX as part of the ongoing efforts toward rapprochement between the two Churches. The negotiations with the Pope proved exceedingly difficult, for his representatives, conscious of their advantageous position, made excessive demands; regrettably, the talks remained fruitless, especially on doctrinal matters.

A pupil of Karykes was a man of great learning, though of a disagreeable and arrogant temperament—Nikephoros Vlemmydes. With him we had no personal relations, for he was a difficult and unsociable man. His father, however, was a friend of mine—a physician with whom I had collaborated in Constantinople. He was a distant cousin of Manuel Vlemmydes and of Antigone, though they were not closely acquainted. After the fall of 1204, the physician Vlemmydes fled with his family to the Empire of Nicaea, when his son Nikephoros was but seven years old; however, they did not remain near us in

Nicaea. They settled in Ephesus, where he practiced medicine in a prominent xenon as *primicerius*. The young Nikephoros studied rhetoric, philosophy, and mathematics in Ephesus, and later medicine in Smyrna, where he also worked briefly as a physician. He was a gifted and extraordinarily intelligent youth, yet of a difficult disposition. His father often lamented that his son was contentious and constantly quarreled with his colleagues. Nevertheless, he possessed a brilliant mind and an abundance of intellectual interests. Medicine did not satisfy his ambitions nor his insatiable thirst for knowledge. Thus, after a few years, he went on to study Arithmetic, Geometry, Astronomy, and Physics. In 1223, he received the office of Logothete of the Ecumenical Patriarchate and moved to Nicaea. His own teacher, Demetrios Karykes, opposed his appointment on account of his difficult character—a fact that infuriated him. His father asked me to keep an eye on him and to assist him if needed, but Nikephoros was not a man inclined to form friendships. At the age of thirty-eight, he took monastic vows and lived in various monasteries. Wherever he went, he was surrounded by many students who honored him greatly for his vast learning. All these scholars—and many others besides—fostered a remarkable intellectual movement in Nicaea, which was rapidly becoming the foremost spiritual and cultural center of Hellenism.

As is well known, Theodore Laskaris was married to Anna Angelina, the daughter of Alexios III, with whom he had two daughters. The elder, Irene, was wed to John Doukas Vatatzes. In 1222, Theodore died at the age of forty-eight. Although he had a young son and two brothers, he designated his son-in-law, John Vatatzes, as his successor, recognizing in him an exceptional character and great military and political ability. This choice proved most wise and demonstrated that King Theodore cared above all for the welfare of the state rather than for family ties or friendships. Since 1214, he had secured peace and international recognition for his realm, and had devoted himself to its organization and fortification with remarkable success. When he died, he left his successor a nearly exemplary state. Vatatzes proved himself worthy—indeed, perhaps even greater—than his illustrious predecessor. I had a warm and personal friendship with King Theodore, whom I esteemed without limit. His people loved him dearly and mourned deeply his untimely death.

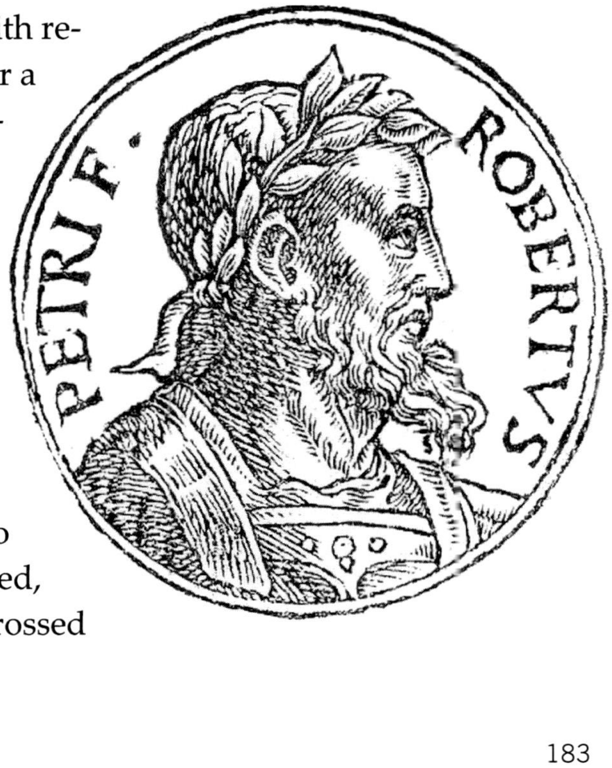

Robert of Courtenay.

Latin Emperor. Guillaume Rouillé, Promptuarii Iconum Insigniorum, Lyon, 1533.

Theodore's two younger brothers, Isaac and Alexios, disputed John's legitimacy as successor. They did not hesitate even to seek assistance from the Latin Emperor, Robert of Courtenay, in order to seize the throne for themselves. Robert readily agreed, and in the early months of 1223 the Frankish army crossed into Asia Minor. The fruitful years of peace had come to an end. The tragic story of the traitor Alexios IV, who had brought the crusaders to Constantinople, seemed in danger of repeating itself. But Vatatzes was no Alexios Angelos, nor were these Latins the same as those of 1204. In the battle fought at Poimanenon, our army—the creation of Theodore Laskaris—utterly defeated the former crusaders.

Kyr John liberated and annexed all the territories the Latins still held in Asia Minor, except for Nicomedia and a narrow strip of coastline facing the Queen City. But he did not stop there. With the Propontic fleet stationed at Lampsacus, he ferried his troops across the Hellespont and captured several cities in Thrace, confining the Latins within the walls of Constantinople itself. At the same time, our Aegean fleet seized all the nearby islands—Lesbos, Chios, Ikaria, Samos, and even Kos.

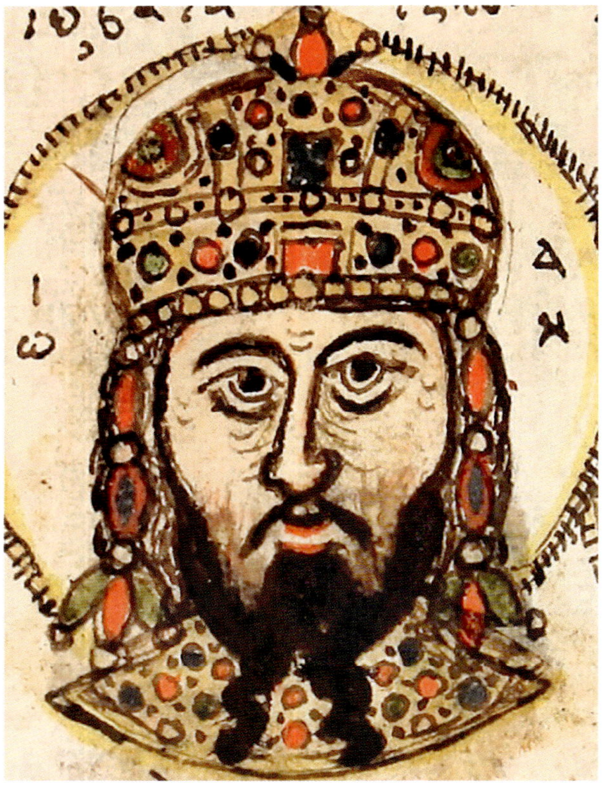

John Doukas Vatatzes.

Miniature, Zonaras, 15th century, d'Este Library, Modena.

The enemies encircling the Empire were many and powerful, and the reorganization—or rather, the reconstitution—of the army and navy was the first and indispensable condition for the state's survival. Naval strength was the great problem. The emperors of Nicaea made immense efforts to create a national fleet, establishing naval bases at Smyrna in the Aegean and at Lampsacus on the Propontis. The primary role of the fleet was at first defensive: to protect the coasts of the realm and to harass and pressure the Latins in the Propontis. The fleet first begun by Theodore Laskaris was greatly improved and strengthened under John Vatatzes. Yet the skills and experience of seamanship are not easily regained—the maritime tradition had long been lost. Italian officers with naval experience were necessarily hired. Despite all these efforts, however, our naval forces never recovered their former prowess or spirit. The Venetian fleet proved far more capable, and in an expedition undertaken in 1235, when we attempted to blockade Constantinople, our navy was defeated by a Venetian squadron considerably smaller in size. Where are those old days when our ships armed with liquid fire struck fear and terror into the hearts of the barbarians!

The defeat by the Venetians was repeated later, both in the Sea of Marmara and in Crete. Nevertheless, the creation of a national fleet—even one inferior to that of sea power Venice—was a brilliant achievement, instilling confidence and pride in the Romans. It should be noted that of the other two Greek states, the Despotate of Epirus possessed no fleet at all, while the Empire of Trebizond maintained only a few ships, used mainly for supply and communica-

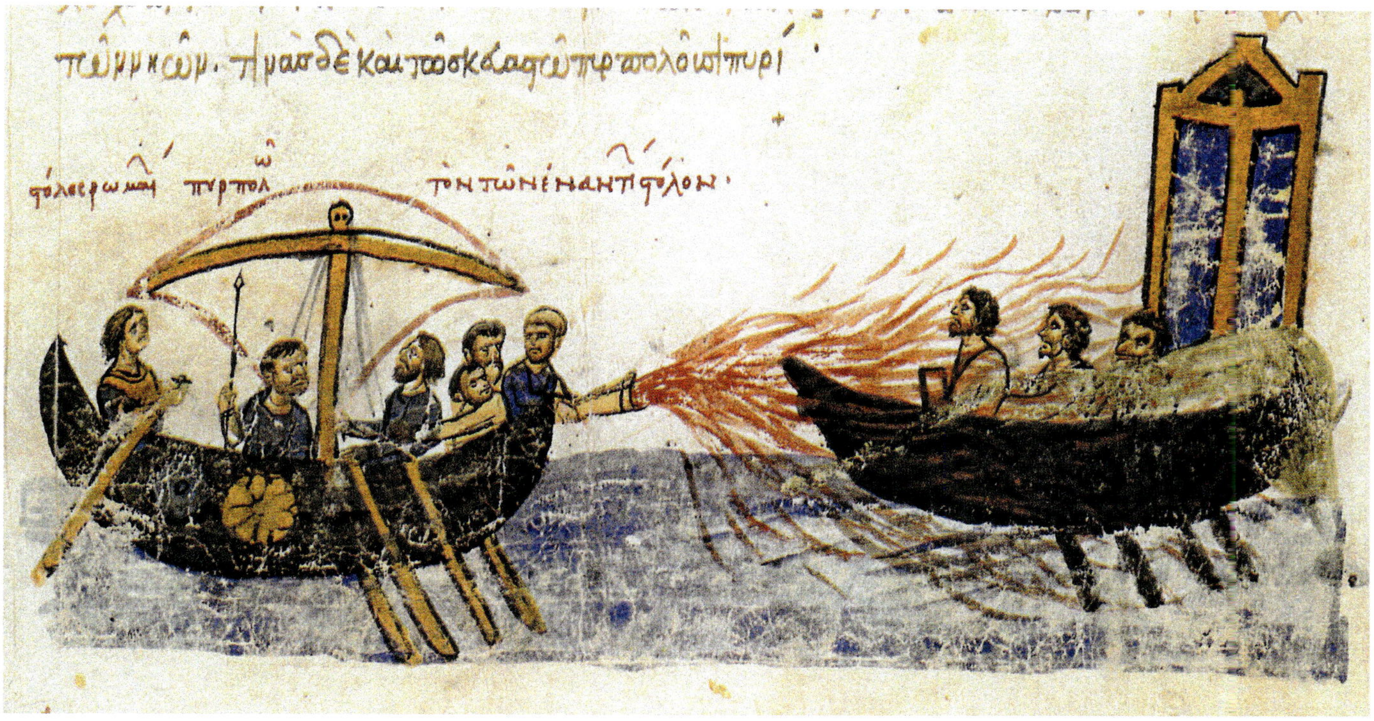

Greek Fire, when Byzantium ruled the seas.

Miniature, Skylitzes, 12th century, National Library of Spain, Madrid.

tion. Naturally, neither the Bulgarians nor the Turks had a navy; thus, apart from the Italians, ours was the only state in the region to command a fleet of real fighting strength.

The creation of a permanent and capable army was a far easier task. The Laskaris rulers understood that a standing army must be formed from native, trained soldiers—not from a motley host of foreign mercenaries driven by profit, who often changed sides when circumstances grew difficult. During this period, Asia Minor experienced a significant increase in population, due both to the migration of Greeks from the occupied territories and to the just and prudent governance of the Laskaris emperors. This demographic growth led to the rise of new urban centers and the expansion of older ones—such as Smyrna, Magnesia, Sardis, Philadelphia, Miletus, and Nymphaion—all now flourishing anew. The chief source of wealth and occupation for the majority of the people was agriculture; hence, a program of careful and intensive cultivation of the land was implemented. The rural population thus became the reservoir from which the soldiers of the new permanent national army would be drawn.

The Laskaris emperors restored the system of military themes and stratiotika ktemata—the military estates. Each theme was now governed by a Doux, who held both civil and judicial authority and was appointed by the Emperor. The Doux (Duke) entrusted local administration to capable military officers rather than to self-serving officials or tax collectors. They also revived the institution of the *akritai*—the native frontier soldiers who defended the borders against raiders, chiefly the Seljuks of Iconium—a venerable institution that had flourished during the Empire's glorious centuries.

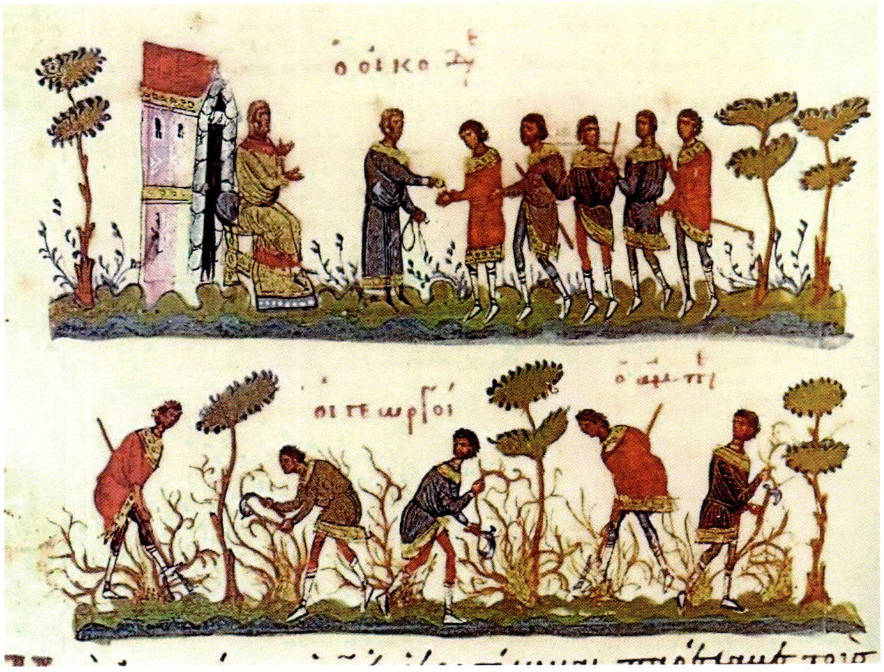

Peasants working in the fields and receiving their wages.

Illustrated Gospel, 11th century, National Library of France, Paris.

However strong the native forces might be, they were not sufficient for the expansionist campaigns necessary for the recapture of Constantinople. Permanent and reliable mercenary troops were also required. Thus, besides the Roman army, which formed the main body of the forces, there existed both the Latin and the Scythian contingents. The Scythian corps consisted of Cuman warriors—brave men and exceptionally skilled archers—who had been converted to Christianity and settled in Asia Minor by John Vatatzes. The Latin corps, on the other hand, was made up of Frankish knights who had come to Byzantium during the Crusades, together with their infantry retainers. Our historians call them cataphract cavalry, for indeed they wore impressive armor that rendered them almost invulnerable and struck fear into their enemies. These men had by now become nearly assimilated to our way of life and were bound, according to their own feudal customs, by an oath of vassalage to the Emperor. They were known as "the king's *lizioi cavallarioi,*" and together with their followers they enjoyed the privileges granted to them by the Emperor—namely, *pronoiai* (land grants) in regions of Asia Minor. They served the Romania faithfully and were under the command of the Contostavlos, a high-ranking officer who was always a Roman—by which we mean a Greek.

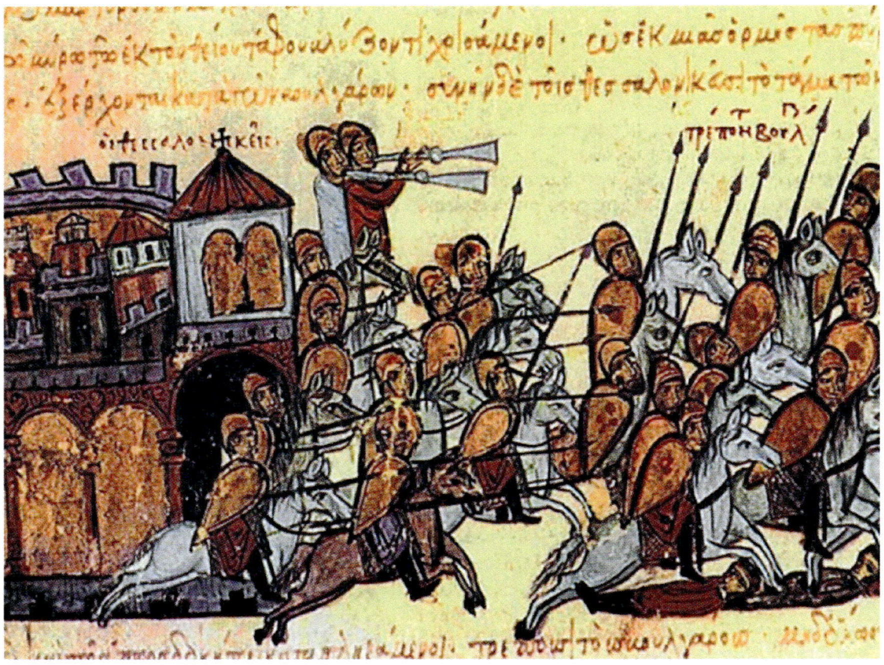

Battle of Greeks against Bulgarians at Thessaloniki, 1040.

Miniature, Skylitzes, 12th century, National Library of Spain, Madrid.

The administrative character of the Nicaean state, though influenced by the feudal system of the West, nevertheless remained centralized, with all authority emanating from the Emperor. He was the supreme commander of both army and navy, appointing the *Megas Domesticos*—the commander-in-chief of the land forces—and the *Megas Doux,* the grand admiral of the fleet. The *Domesticos* in turn appointed the *allagatores* or *stratopedarchai,* who commanded the divisions of the army. The defense of fortresses and citadels was entrusted exclusively to Greek Romans under the command of the *Castrofylax*. Central administration was directed by the *Megas Logothetes,* who fulfilled the duties of prime minister. The *Protovestiarios* oversaw the finances, while the *Megas Logariastes* managed the general fiscal administration. The *Epi ton Deēseōn* acted as the intermediary between the Emperor and the people, conveying petitions and requests. Tax collection was entrusted to the *Pronoiars,* trusted men who reported directly to the Emperor. Unfortunately, even under their supervision, abuses and corruption were not entirely eradicated.

The victorious campaigns in Thrace and Macedonia continued—but now, regrettably, not against the Latins or the Bulgarians, but against our own kinsmen in the rival Despotate of Epirus. Civil strife has been our misfortune since antiquity. The Despots of Epirus, too, coveted the recovery of Constantinople and the restoration of the Roman Empire—but for themselves. Thus the two Greek-Roman states came into conflict instead of cooperation. In 1224, Theodore Komnenos Doukas, Despot of Epirus, captured Thessaloniki, and the following year he was crowned there as Emperor of the Romans, extending his dominion as far as Adrianople. Having allied himself with the Bulgarian ruler John Asen, he hoped, with his assistance, to recover Constantinople from the Latins and to be crowned there as the legitimate Emperor of the Romans. Yet he soon discovered that Asen harbored similar ambitions, having already assumed the title of Tsar (Caesar) of the Bulgarians and the Romans. Overestimating his own strength, Theodore violated his alliance with the Bulgarians and, in 1230, launched an attack against them, hoping thereby to secure the recovery of Constantinople for himself. But Asen was far more cunning. Feigning retreat, he lured the Epirote forces deep into his territory. Near the village of Klokotnitsa the great battle took place, ending in the complete destruction of the Epirote army and the capture of Theodore himself. After this victory, the Bulgarians occupied nearly all of Thrace, Macedonia, and Albania, while Thessaloniki became their vassal. The ambitions of the Despots of Epirus toward Constantinople were extinguished once and for all, and thereafter they remained confined within their own domains.

The hour of Nicaea had come. Lord John, in turn, allied himself with the Bulgarians against the Latins of Constantinople; yet the Italians, with their fleet, and the Franks of Achaea, with their army, prevented them from advancing. Last year, in 1241, Tsar John Asen died, and the Bulgarian state fell into disorder and near dissolution. The Empire of Nicaea has now become the strongest power in the region, controlling much of Macedonia and Thrace as well as the eastern part of Asia Minor. It has been blessed, during my lifetime, with two remarkable rulers: Theodore Laskaris, until 1222, and John Doukas Vatatzes, who has reigned ever since. May he live long—for the good of the Empire and of our people.

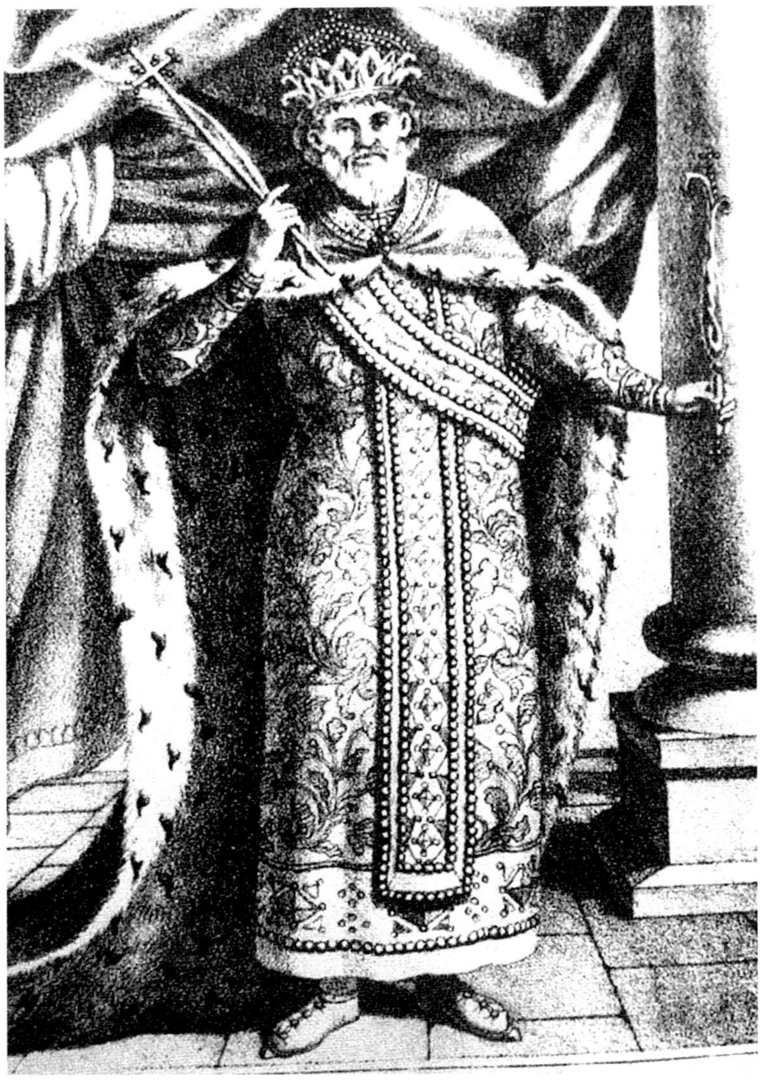

John II Asen, Tsar of the Bulgarians (1218–1241).

Now, in the year of salvation 1242, as I write these lines—or rather, as I dictate them to my student Nicolaos Melissenos, who stands by me like a son—I am ninety-two years old. Thankfully, my health, apart from the frailty of age, remains good, and above all my mental faculties are still intact. I began writing this account in the early years of my residence in Constantinople, in 1168. My desire was to set down on paper my thoughts, as well as my observations and impressions, of the wondrous world of the Queen City and of the world-changing events that so utterly altered the balance between East and West.

Before concluding my account, I would like to set forth my thoughts on the religious and metaphysical dimension of medicine, as it is experienced in our society today.

Religious experience and a profound metaphysical understanding of life and the world are fundamental characteristics of our Byzantine society, and they run from end to end throughout our thousand-year Empire over the whole span of its life. Christianity, as it was received and shaped by the Greek-speaking populations—nurtured in the soil of Hellenic philosophy and religion—became the constitutive element of the new society. It marked a transformation of the ideals of the former pagan world toward the observance of Christ's commandments, the foremost of which is love and compassion toward one's fellow human being, one's *neighbor*. This found its first social expression in organized philanthropy, which began within the activity of the Church but eventually became state policy, realized through the creation of various charitable institutions—some of which developed into the precursors of hospitals. Within these institutions medicine was practiced collectively, systematized, and advanced. Medical services were offered to all citizens, either for a modest fee or free of charge. The level of medical and hospital care is now quite high; yet medicine, of course, cannot cure every illness. Thus people turn to physicians and hospitals, but at the same time they also seek the transcendent help of God, the Theotokos, and the saints. In the private sphere, however, many renowned physicians who visit patients in their homes demand exorbitant fees. Consequently, among certain parts of the population—particularly in remote regions with limited access to hospitals—there has arisen a measure of distrust and resentment toward physicians, as has been the case in nearly all societies.

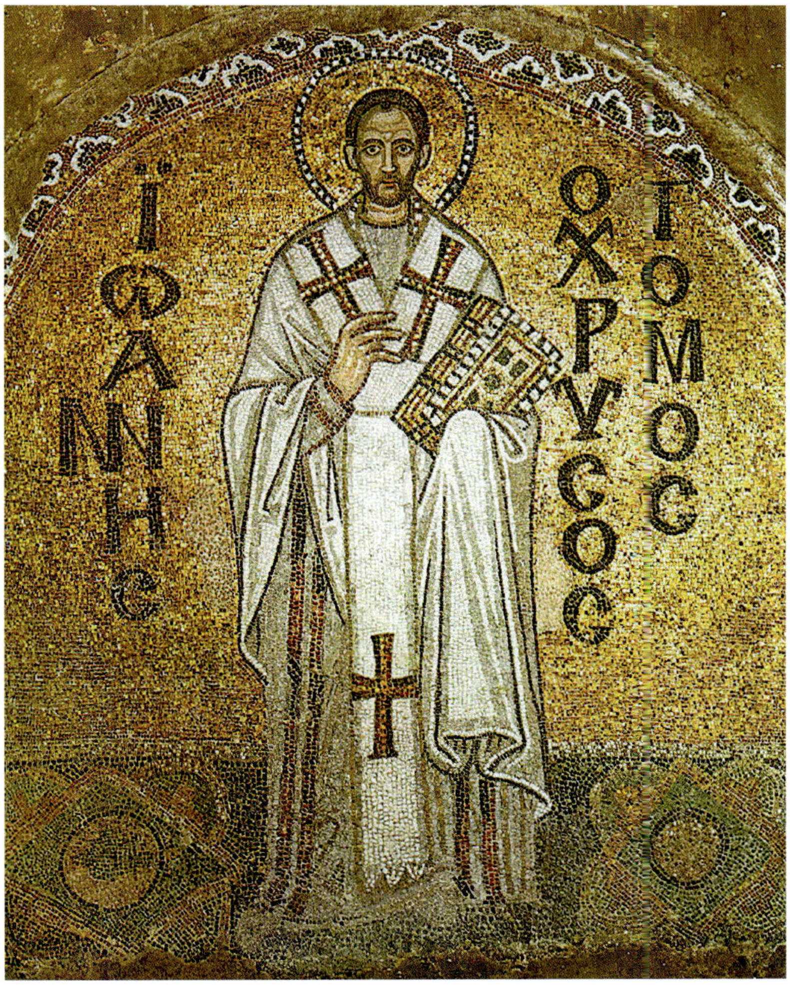

Saint John Chrysostom.

Mosaic, 12th century, Hagia Sophia.

It is only natural that in a multiethnic and multicultural society different mentalities, conceptions, and interpretations of the divine and the transcendent should emerge. From the earliest Christian centuries, heresies appeared—that is, divergent interpretations of doctrine—while the old religions survived in the form of magic, sorcery, and various methods of folk healing. Even today, although our medicine has made considerable progress, there remains—just as throughout Europe—a veil of ignorance, superstition, and obscurantism that often shrouds the "official" practice of medicine. I speak not, of course, of deep religious faith, according to which all illness is healed through the grace of God, but of the exorcisms, amulets, and charms still commonly used, both among the nobility and the common people alike. Since ancient times there have circulated among the populace didactic medical poems and household medical manuals filled with magical practices, references to mysterious and esoteric drugs of Eastern origin, and invocations of spirits. These popular and empirical collections of medical advice—of which I have spoken earlier—are known as *Iatrosophia*.

All these arbitrary remedies were rejected and vigorously opposed by the enlightened Fathers of the Church, who neither denied nor disparaged the contributions of official medicine—indeed, many among them had themselves studied the art of healing. Among the ancient Fathers we may name Ba-

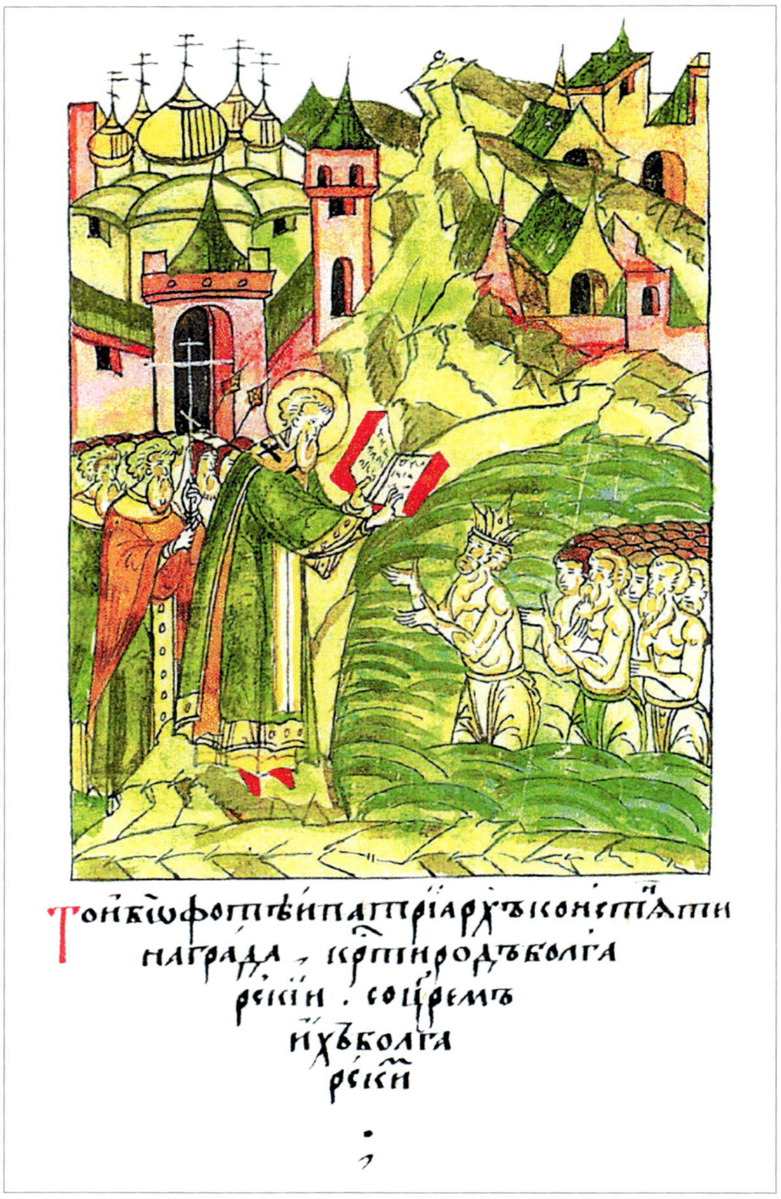

Patriarch Photios baptizing the Bulgarians and their king.

Miniature, 16th century.

sil the Great, founder of the first comprehensive charitable and medical institution in the world and himself a practicing physician; Eustathios of Antioch; Gregory the Theologian; Gregory of Nyssa; John Chrysostom; Epiphanius of Cyprus; Meletios the Iatrosophist or Monk; John of Damascus; and, in later centuries, Photios the Great, John Prodrianos, and many others. Our contemporary (in the twelfth century) Archbishop Theophylaktos of Ohrid even calls medicine a "philanthropic science" and describes the physician as an "artist," recognizing the therapeutic value and significance of medical practice without diminishing the necessity of religious faith and hope. Indeed, these great ecclesiastical figures concur with scientific medicine in the treatment of illness, while at the same time urging prayer, faith, and the invocation of the saints. Their aim is directed toward the spiritual dimension of sickness, following the understanding that when the body suffers, the soul suffers as well—thus inaugurating a kind of holistic approach to illness and its healing.

The miraculous interventions of the saints are widely accepted and believed throughout the world. We physicians ourselves—while practicing our art with consistency and diligence—also believe in the possibility of miraculous healing. The *synaxaria* of the saints recount many such wonders, though at times with a measure of embellishment. Yet it is noteworthy that these healing saints are real historical persons, who lived only a few generations before us and earned the reverence of the people through their virtuous lives. Most of them were themselves physicians who had practiced medicine successfully and without accepting money or other compensation—such as Saint Panteleimon and the Holy Unmercenaries, Kosmas and Damian, or Cyrus and John. It is also characteristic that many saints are regarded as "specialists" in particular illnesses—those of children, of women, of the eyes, and so forth—according to the experiences they had during their earthly lives. Women, for example, commonly turn to female saints for help with gynecological ailments, such as Saint Elizabeth or Saint Theodora.

It must be noted here that our Byzantine society holds a position toward women that is at once paradoxical and pioneering. On the one hand, women are generally excluded from public life and often undervalued; on the other

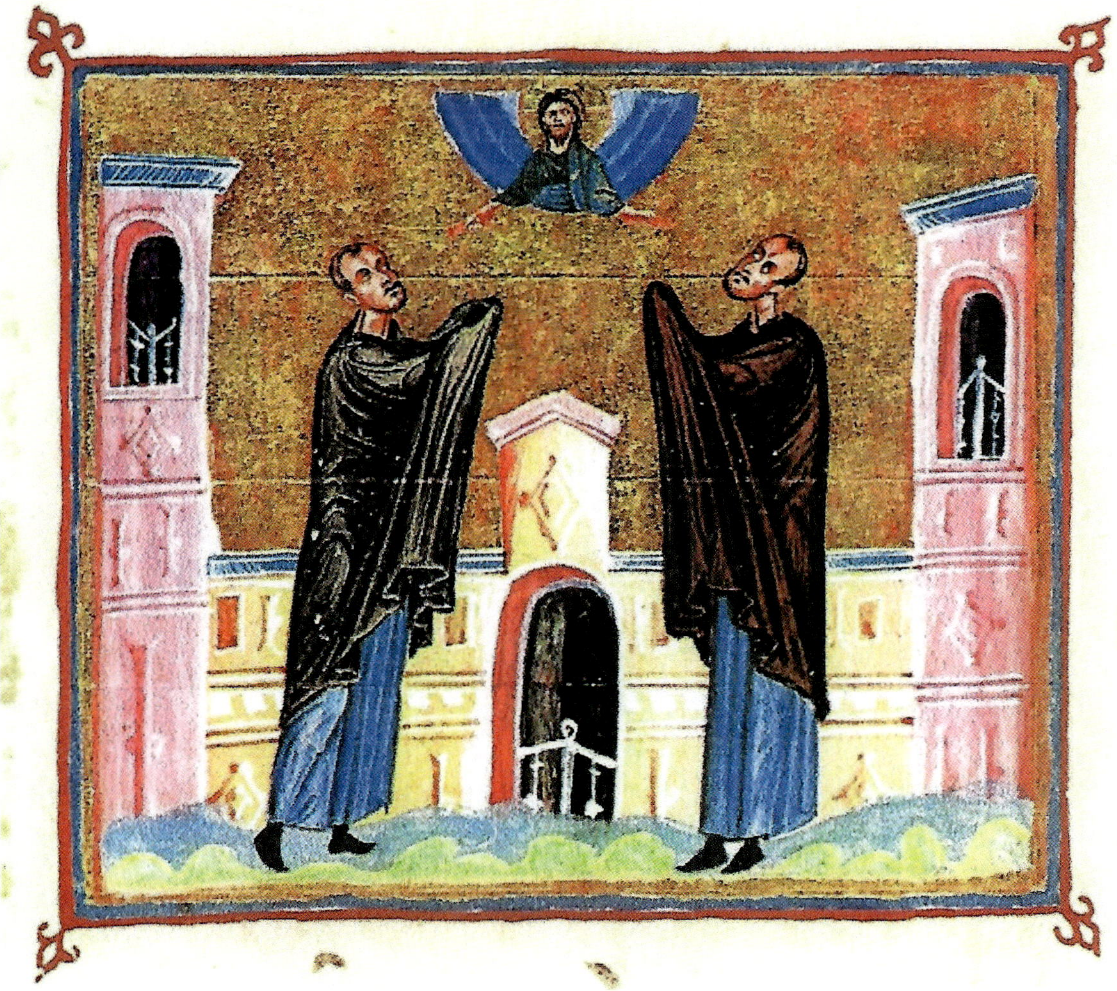

The Holy Unmercenaries receiving the grace to heal.

Miniature, 11th century, Library of Dionysiou Monastery, Mount Athos.

hand, it is this same society that reveres above all the Mother of Christ, honors the women saints, accepts without protest that women may assume imperial authority alone (as did Irene and Theodora), and recognizes the equal participation of *iatrainai* and *iatromeai*—women physicians and midwife-physicians—in the hospitals, with the same legal rights and obligations as their male counterparts. It is characteristic, for example, that in the fourth century there appeared the woman-physician Metrodora Kleopatra, the first woman known to have written a medical treatise on gynecology, entitled *On the Female Afflictions of the Womb*.

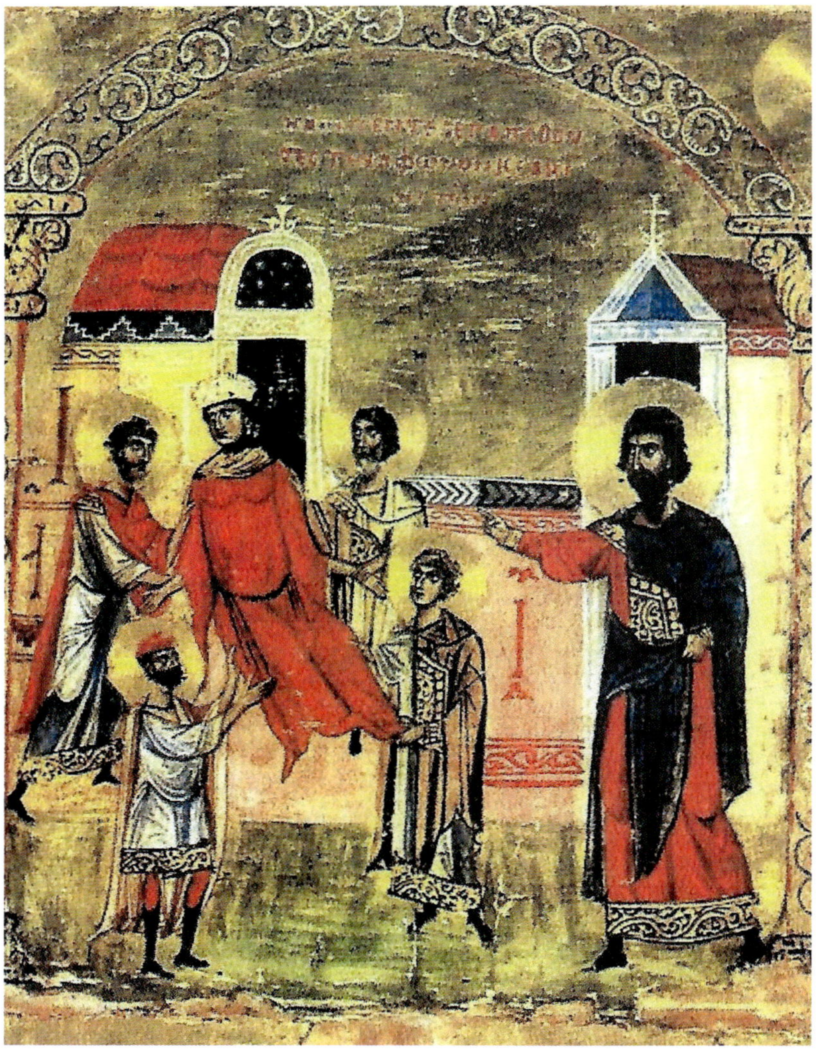

The Five Holy Physicians healing a woman who was mute and unable to move.

Icon, 12th century, Monastery of Sinai.

Neurological and psychiatric disorders possess a particular character that readily invites an appeal to the metaphysical dimension. The most important psychiatric institution of the Empire was the *Katagōgion of Saint Anastasia* in the Queen City, though monasteries also play a certain role—especially in caring for the incurably insane, whose madness has, regrettably, long been associated with curse or sin. For mental illnesses—especially mania and melancholia—various treatments have been proposed by the great physicians of earlier centuries, such as Aetios of Amida and Paul of Aegina, and by more recent ones like John Actuarios: therapies involving baths, diet, or sedative medicines. As for epilepsy, the so-called "Sacred Disease," ever since the time of Hippocrates and Galen it has been regarded as having an organic cause—specifically, the accumulation of phlegm around the brain, and later, the obstruction of the brain's ventricles. Nevertheless, Alexander of Tralles—being the first to employ what we would now call "placebo therapy"—permitted the use of "magical" remedies, even though he considered them worthless, so long as certain patients felt better through them. Epilepsy, of course, is still regarded by the common people of Byzantium as a demonic illness. It is important to emphasize that the notion of the *daimonion* constitutes a distinct conceptual framework, encompassing a wide range of mental disorders in an age when our knowledge of the brain remains minimal; consequently, such ailments are considered exceedingly difficult to cure. Now, following the teaching of John Actuarios, most of us physicians view the brain as the source of movement and emotion, as well as the seat of the soul. It is natural in every age that a considerable gap should exist between scientific understanding and popular belief. Today, we physicians focus chiefly on prevention and advocate a healthy life, with a diet low in fats; nor do we reject anointing with therapeutic oil—practices that the Church itself likewise recommends.

The metaphysical dimension is real and deeply significant in our Byzantine society, and it is only natural that it has influenced our medical understanding. Yet one must not focus solely on the popular beliefs born of excessive religiosity, widespread though they may be. The human being is a psychosomatic unity: when one part suffers, the whole suffers, and healing must be directed toward the whole. The metaphysical element is indispensable for the complete spiritual and bodily healing of the patient within a holistic understanding of illness and its treatment. Physicians—being themselves faithful Christians—acknowledge the miraculous power of faith and prayer, yet they insist first and foremost on the application of all available scientific means for the treatment of disease.

Here, however, I must bring my narrative to an end. My age no longer permits me to continue. I trust that my student, Nikolaos Melissenos—who carries on my medical work in the Xenon of Saint Mavra—will continue these notes until the recapture of the Queen City, which I foresee coming very soon. I believe that our great king, John III Vatatzes—whom the people, out of affection, call Kalogiannis and most often simply "Kyr John," for they feel him to be their own, truly a father to them—will be the one to liberate the Queen City from the Latins and to restore the glorious Roman Empire. He deserves this both as a soldier and as a statesman. A worthy successor of the worthy King Theodore, he has won the boundless love of his people, who have already proclaimed him a saint.

Now I shall withdraw into my memories and revisit the events of my life. I began in Patras as the son of a cloth merchant, and I followed my dream: to study and to become a physician, so that I might offer to others the fruits of science and the love my parents and teachers instilled in me. Divine providence allowed me to behold the Queen of Cities, to study there, and to serve as a physician in the greatest hospital of the inhabited world. It also granted me a worthy companion, who stood by me in all the hardships of my vocation. I lived through the glory and flourishing of the Komnenoi dynasty, the corruption and decline of the Angeloi, the utter humiliation of the sack and plunder of the City by the crusaders, and finally the rebirth of the Hellenic-Roman nation in the Empire of Nicaea. I came to know and to work with remarkable people—the very flower of Hellenic education—who had gathered first in Constantinople and later in Nicaea. I witnessed both the splendid grandeur and the miserable baseness that coexist in our state and among our people, as well as among all the nations around us. I learned that there are no "good" or "bad" peoples; human beings are the same in every era. Our nature inclines us toward rivalry, the struggle for dominance, violence, and hatred. I learned that only knowledge and science can free our minds from prejudice, obsession, and delusion. These—together with faith in the ideals of Christianity—can lead us beyond our nature, toward tolerance and, more than that, toward the love of the other as a lifelong discipline. Only then can our world become better—or at least bearable.

Here ends the narrative of Nikephoros Messenes. What follows is the account of his student, Nikolaos Melissenos, who—at his teacher's request—completed the chronicle with a description of the world-shaping events leading up to the recovery of Constantinople by the Roman-Greeks.

The Reconquest of Constantinople

My name is Nikolaos Melissenos, and I serve as Actuarios, physician at the Xenon of Saint Mavra in Nicaea. I am the student and successor of Nikephoros Messenes, who honored me with his trust, taught me the secrets of the Medical Art, and entrusted his writings to me. My teacher was an exceptional man, deeply reflective—one who taught us not only Medicine and Surgery, but also the art of approaching the sick person in such a way that the treatment we administer may achieve the best possible result.

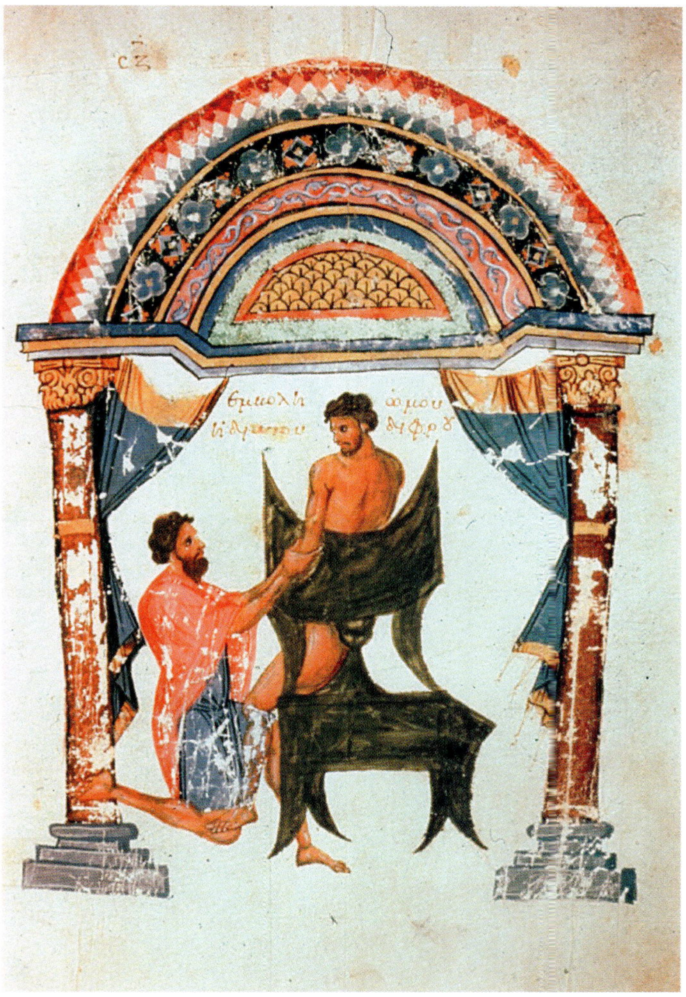

Reduction of a dislocated shoulder.

Miniature, Niketas, Surgical Collection (Apollonios of Kition, On Joints). 10th century, Laurentian Library, Florence.

Messenes first taught us to love our work and our science as something set apart—because it does not aim at our own benefit, but at the relief of those who suffer and are afflicted. He taught us to be faithful to our vocation by continually studying the writings of physicians, both ancient and contemporary, and by observing our elders attentively so that we might profit from their knowledge and experience. He would not tolerate ignorance, indifference, or carelessness. Such things, he would say, may cost a patient his life; therefore they are not mere oversights or mistakes, but grave sins. He also taught us to approach the sick not from above, but as equals, as persons simply finding themselves in an unhappy condition in which we ourselves may well be tomorrow. We must draw near to them with genuine concern, with compassion and love; we must be discreet and refrain from offending or humiliating them through our questions

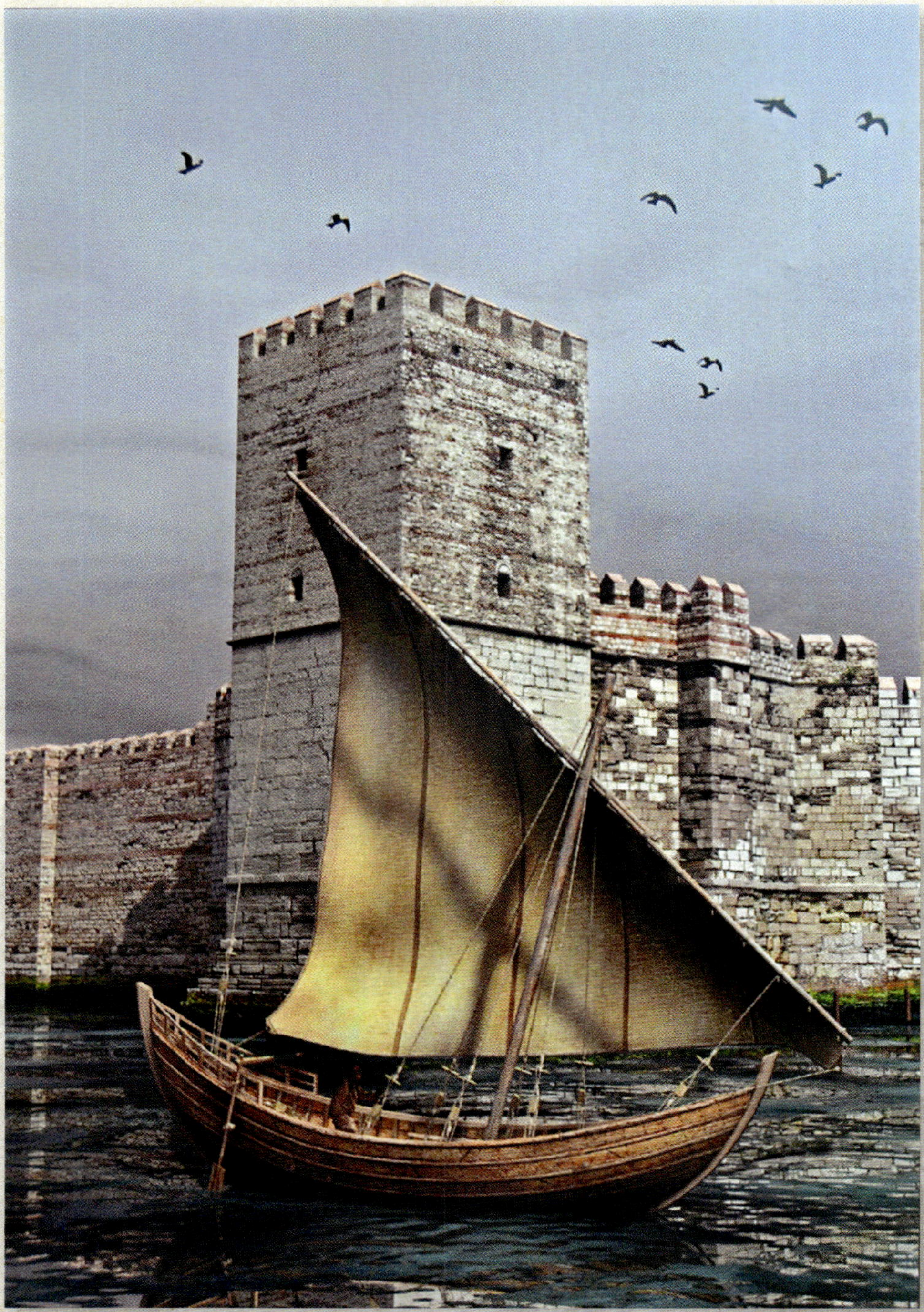

The Marble Tower at the Harbor of Theodosius.

Reconstruction: Byzantium 1200

or our manner of examination. The best way to "unlock" the patient and diagnose his ailment, he would say, is to win his trust through sincere interest and respect—something the patient perceives at once with the sensitive emotional "antennae" that suffering sharpens within him.

Having studied Mathematics and Philosophy alongside Medicine—and having served for many years as chief physician (*primicerius*) in the famed Xenon of the Pantocrator—he had acquired deep experience and vast knowledge, which he generously shared with all of us. In Nicaea, after the fall, he played a vital role in organizing the realm's medical services and structured the Xenon of Saint Mavra, which he had taken under his care, according to the model of the Pantocrator's hospital. Kings Theodore I and John III esteemed him greatly, offering him every assistance and support in his work. Now he has entered his rest, and I have continued his work in the xenon as best I could, honored to have received his love and his trust. He asked me to record the events that would unfold in our region up to the reconquest of the Queen City by the Greek-Roman armies and the restoration of the Eastern Roman Empire—an outcome he considered certain, and even imminent, though he knew he would not live to see it. This I shall attempt to do, as faithfully as I can. For much of what follows I consulted the venerable Lady Antigone, his wife, who assisted me with many details, especially concerning the activities of women in Byzantium. Lady Antigone followed my teacher Nikephoros into eternity one year after his repose, in 1244.

My teacher's prediction—that John Vatatzes would take the City back from the crusaders—was, alas, not fulfilled. *Kyr Giannis*, as the people lovingly called him, reigned for thirty-two years, from 1222 until 1254, when he died at the age of sixty-one. His reign marked the most glorious and prosperous years of the Empire of Nicaea. In 1242, just as he had secured dominance over Thessaloniki, a new and deadly danger appeared from the East. The Mongols—whose irresistible hordes had swept aside every kingdom and tribe of Asia—defeated our neighbors, the Seljuks, and reduced them to tributary status. At the same time, another of their armies shattered the already weakened Bulgarian state. Faced with this common threat, John entered into alliance with the Seljuks, yet God preserved him, and he was spared the need to face the Mongols in battle. The Mongols, because of internal troubles, suddenly withdrew from the region just as swiftly as they had arrived, contenting themselves with a simple tribute from the states of Asia Minor. The conditions were now greatly in our favor. The Bulgarians, the Seljuks, and the Latins were all weakened, while our own army remained unscathed. In 1246 John landed in Macedonia and, in a remarkably short span of time, annexed to his realm nearly the whole of Macedonia and Thrace. The Despots of Epirus were compelled to recognize the ruler of Nicaea as Emperor of the Romans and the legitimate heir to the throne of Constantinople.

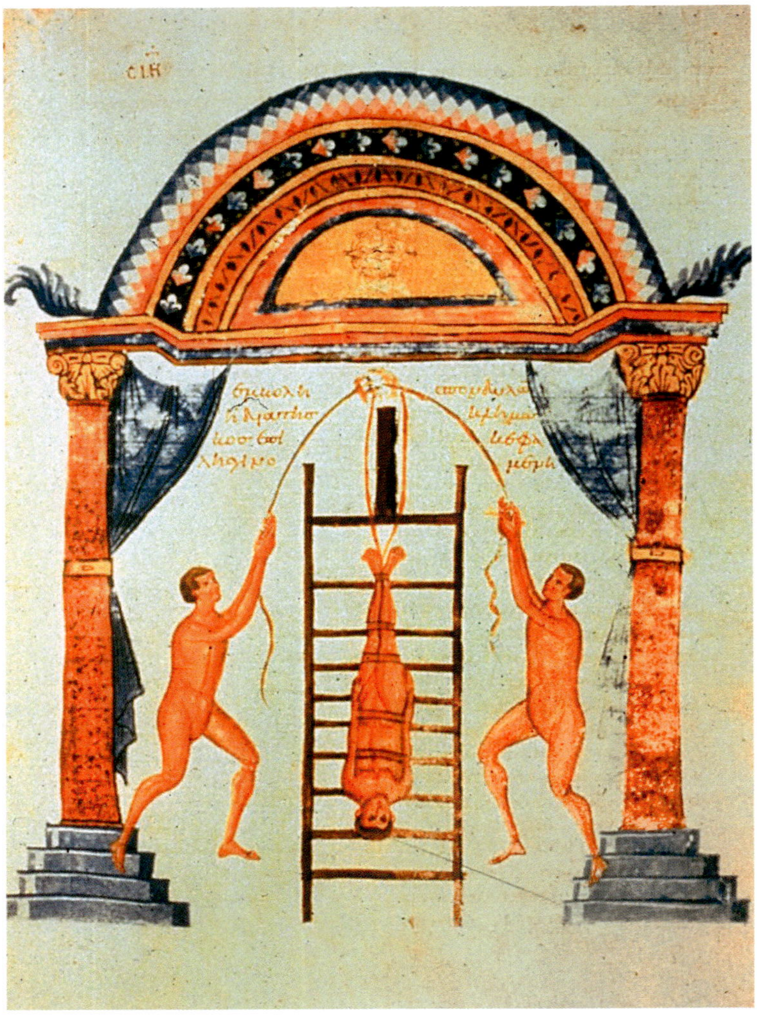

Joint traction (the "falling ladder" technique).

Miniature, Niketas, Surgical Collection *(Apollonius of Citium, On Joints). 10th century, Laurentian Library, Florence.*

His life with Irene, the daughter of Theodore I Laskaris, was harmonious, and in 1222 they welcomed their only son and heir to the throne, Theodore, who was given the surname Laskaris Vatatzes in honor of his grandfather—the founder of the Empire—and to secure his rightful claim to succession. Tragically, the noble Irene was severely injured in a fall from her horse while hunting, suffering a grave fracture of the pelvis. She was unable thereafter to bear more children. This disability burdened her deeply, and some years later she withdrew to a monastery as the nun Eugenia, where she died in 1239 at only thirty-nine years of age. Irene–Eugenia was a modest and prudent woman, deeply faithful to God and the Church. She greatly supported her husband in his social and charitable endeavors. On one occasion, while traveling past the Strofades islands near Zakynthos, she prayed fervently to the Theotokos for the healing of her sister, who suffered from a serious illness. The Mother of God granted her request, and in gratitude the Empress built there a monastery-fortress, *Panton Chara* ("Joy of All"), which remains greatly revered by the people.

John, seeking to stabilize his realm—especially since the Pope was fiercely hostile toward the "Greeks" and even threatened a new crusade against them—formed an alliance with Frederick II Hohenstaufen, Emperor of the Germans, who was an avowed opponent of the Papacy and rejected the imposition of ecclesiastical authority upon his state. In 1245 John even married Frederick's daughter, Constance, who was renamed Anna. The German monarch, having descended from Norman Sicily, was familiar with Greek culture and knew the Greek language. He corresponded with John in Greek; in one of his letters he even stressed that Constantinople had been wrongfully taken from its rightful owners—the Greek Romans—and that it was equally wrong for them to be regarded as schismatics, since the true author of the schism was the Pope himself. Pope Innocent IV responded by excommunicating Frederick and denouncing the entire race of the "Greeks."

The success of the alliance, however, was that the Germans forbade the passage through their lands to the troops the Pope was preparing to send in aid of the Latins in Constantinople. Yet the Pope remained the greatest spiritual—and indirectly military—power in Europe, and thus relations with him needed to be restored. For that reason John convened two councils at Nymphaion with the papal representatives, but both ended in failure despite the participation of the Empire's most distinguished scholars. Vatatzes' stance in the face of the Pope's arrogant and offensive pressures was dignified and unwavering: "Who does not know that the rightful lot of succession from the Great Constantine has come to our people, and that we are his true heirs and successors?" He further assured the Pope that: "We shall never cease fighting and warring against those who hold Constantinople." In other words, he declared plainly that we are the true successors of Constantine, and that we would never abandon the ardent and rightful claim to the Queen of Cities. John did everything within reason to reconcile with the Pope, but he would not, under any circumstances, surrender the inherent rights of our people.

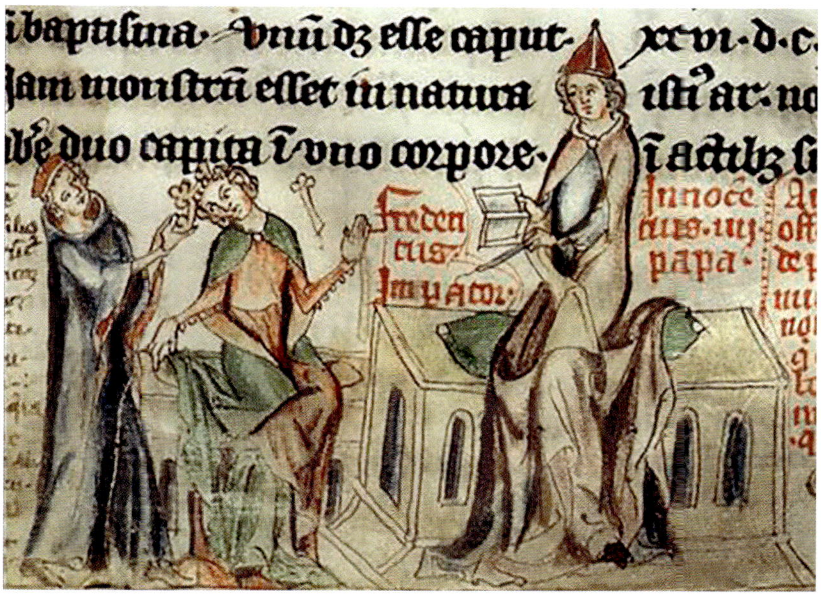

The pope excommunicates Frederick II because of his relations with the Greeks.

Miniature, 14th century, Bodleian Library, Oxford.

Yet the most important achievement of Vatatzes was the thorough reorganization of the realm on every level. He showed particular concern for the prosperity of the lower and middle classes. He pursued a successful program of economic recovery, supporting the farmers and commerce, both of which experienced remarkable growth. He fought abuses and the wastefulness of state officials with exceptional strictness and succeeded in reducing taxation. By his own example of frugality, he encouraged his collaborators and the people to do the same. He even rebuked his only son, Theodore, when he saw him dressed with undue luxury. To show how far one might advance through prudent and consistent stewardship, he himself engaged in agricultural work on his estates whenever public affairs allowed. Indeed, from the earnings he made by selling the eggs produced on his land, he commissioned a crown of pearls, which he offered to the Empress. This crown became known as the *ōaton*."

It is said that in every righteous endeavor, fortune also lends her hand. The Mongol invasion wrought great destruction in both Bulgaria and the Seljuks of Ikonion, yet left the Empire of Nicaea untouched. As a result, exports—especially of foodstuffs—increased, bringing new wealth into the land. The economic situation and the people's prosperity rose to levels unmatched in earlier times. None among the elders remembered such good years, nor had they ever heard their forebears recount them. The people felt secure from barbar-

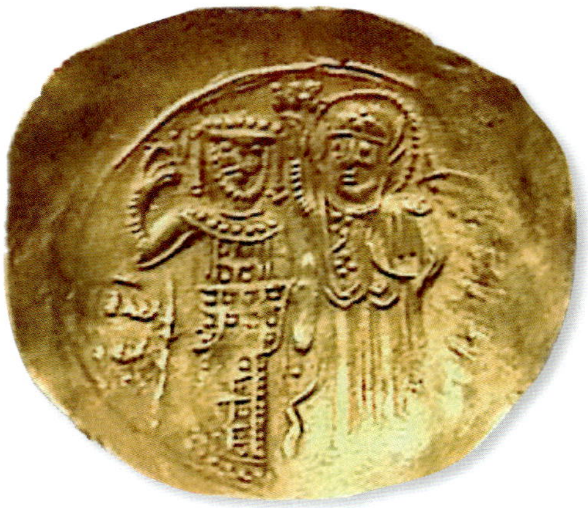

Hyperpyron of John Vatatzes.

13th century, Metropolitan Museum of Art, New York.

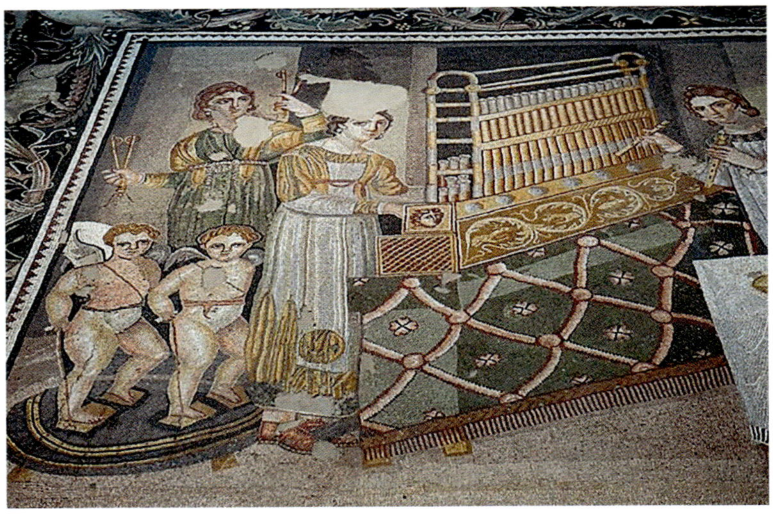

"The arts flourished in Nicaea." Musicians.

Mosaic from a Byzantine villa at Maryamin, 4th–6th century, Hama Archaeological Museum, Syria.

ian raids, they cultivated the earth and saw the fruit of their labor rewarded rather than lost to foreign incursions or corrupt tax collectors. Our army won victories, and the usurping Latins were confined to Constantinople. The day of the Empire's restoration no longer seemed far away.

The Emperor showed particular concern for education and the sciences. Letters and the arts flourished magnificently. Monasteries, churches, hospitals, and other charitable institutions were founded, with the substantial support of Queen Irene. He also established libraries and schools, such as the "Chorus of the Wise" near Ephesus, directed by Nikephoros Vlemmydes, who composed numerous treatises on logic, physics, and geography. Many men of letters gathered in Nicaea, as they had earlier under Theodore I. Besides Vlemmydes, the reign of John saw the activity in Nicaea of the eminent historian George Akropolites, the Grand Primicerius Constantine Tornikios, and other distinguished figures of learning and of the Church. As the successor of Messenes and actuarius of the Xenon of St. Mavra, I had the opportunity to meet and associate closely with several of these notable men—above all with Akropolites, with whom I formed a sincere friendship.

John's second marriage to Constance was formal and motivated purely by political considerations, and the couple had no children. The Emperor, however, fell in love with a beautiful attendant of the Empress—the famous "Marchesina," as she was called by her detractors, who believed she exercised a malign influence over the sovereign. Indeed, the Marchesina behaved with arrogance in the palace and had provoked the resentment of the courtiers and the people. The Emperor perceived the public's reaction and corrected his conduct. Yet although the people disliked the "foreigner," they cherished their worthy Emperor, whom they truly regarded as a father. His moral failing did not weigh against him in the least; the people judged him by his essential virtues—his simplicity, his effectiveness, and his genuine love for his subjects. In particular, the restraint he imposed on the arbitrariness of the aristocrats—who had long oppressed and exploited the people—gave ordinary folk a sense of justice, security, and dignity. These things, together with the safety of the borders, the easing of taxation, and the flourishing economy, bestowed upon "Kalogiannis" the radiance and reputation of a ruler granted by God. The state of Nicaea became a model for the surrounding realms. The people proclaimed John Vatatzes a saint, and many accounts were written of his life and deeds—some true, others somewhat embellished. He may well have been the worthiest Emperor of the Romans, though he was not granted the blessing of being crowned and ruling his empire from the Queen of Cities, Constantinople. Kyr John Doukas Vatatzes, already burdened by ill health, died in 1256 at the age of sixty-one. The people mourned him sincerely, as a father and protector.

He was succeeded by his son, Theodore II Laskaris Vatatzes, at the age of thirty-two. In many respects, the young emperor proved worthy of his great father. He was more of a scholar by nature and had received an excellent education from two distinguished teachers, Akropolites and Vlemmydes. Thus he, too, gave strong support to learning and founded many schools and libraries. He was an ardent admirer of Greek culture and used the name "Hellenes" to describe his subjects. He called them "Romans" in reference to their political and imperial identity, and "Hellenes" to distinguish them from the surrounding "neighbors"—the Bulgarians, the Seljuks, and the Latin Italians and Franks who encircled the Empire. Characteristic are his words when confronting the arrogance of Westerners, especially the envoys of the Pope with whom he was obliged to negotiate: "Of all tongues, the

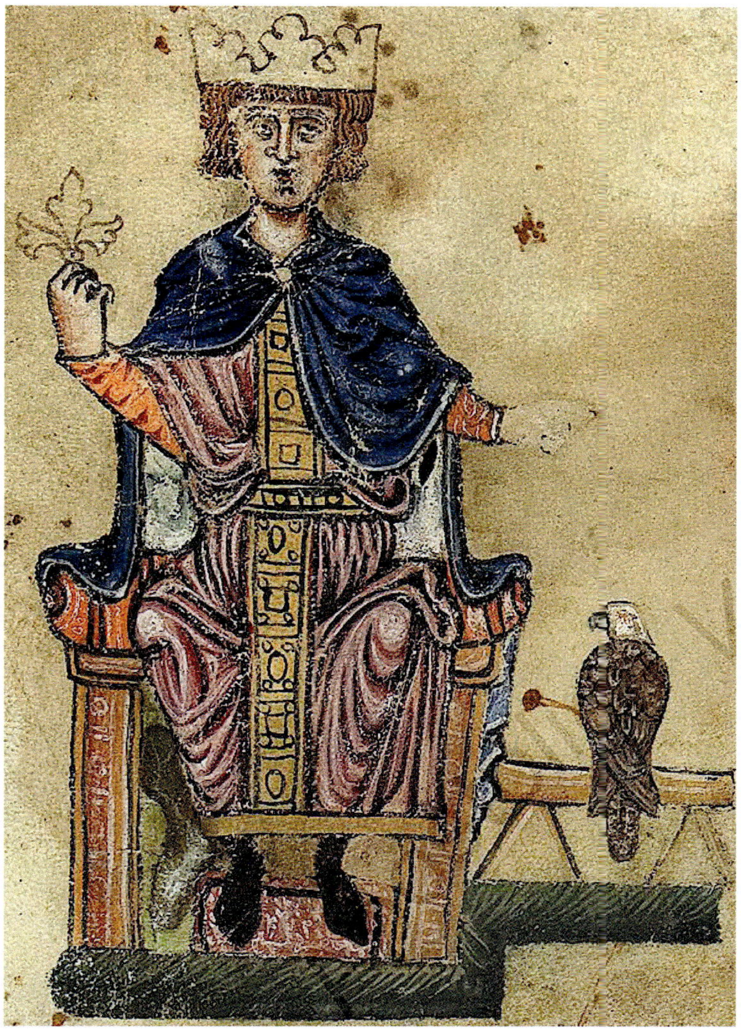

Frederick II Hohenstaufen.

Miniature, 13th century. By the same hand. The art of falconry. Vatican Library, Rome.

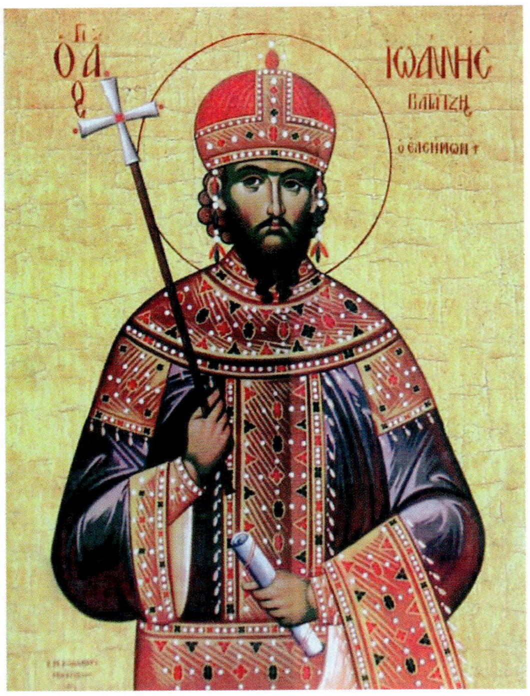

John Vatatzes as a saint.
Contemporary icon.

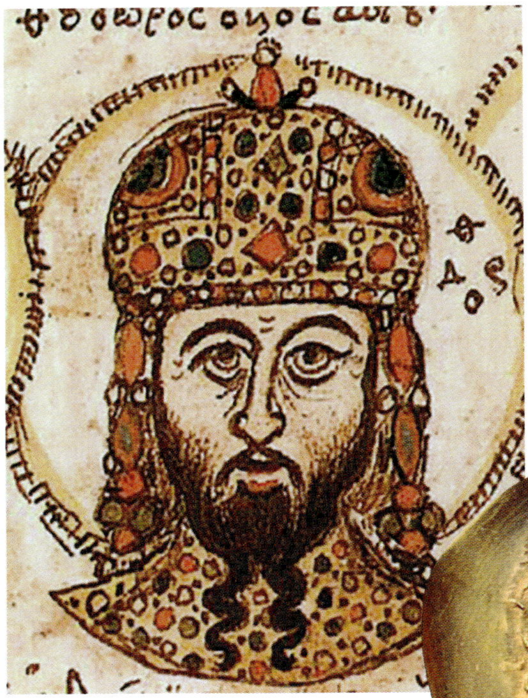

Theodore II Laskaris.
Miniature, Zonaras, 15th c., d'Este Library, Modena, Italy.

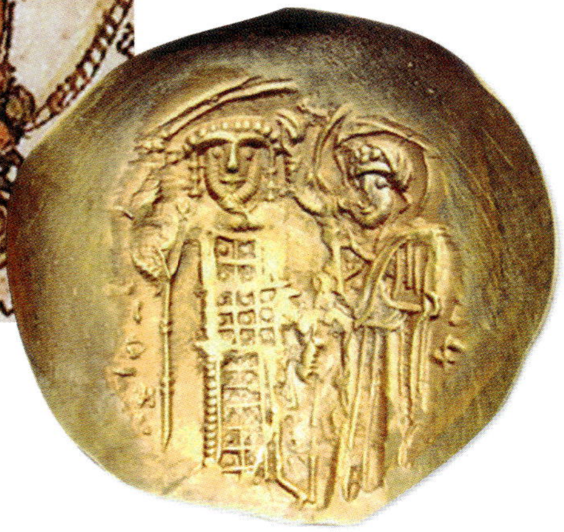

Hyperpyron of Theodore II Laskaris, depicting him with the Theotokos.
13th century.

Greek race stands above," and again, "Every philosophy and every form of knowledge is a discovery of the Greeks… And you, O Italian, for what do you boast?"

Kyr Theodore had married Helen, the daughter of John Asen of Bulgaria, with whom he had one son—the heir John—and five daughters. Unfortunately, his health was poor; he suffered from severe epilepsy, which, however, did not prevent him from being an excellent Emperor—both in military affairs, where he successfully repelled Bulgarian designs, and in political matters, though his negotiations with the papal representatives concerning church union bore no fruit because of the excessive demands of the Latins. He was deeply devout and possessed a profound faith in God. He rebuilt churches and monasteries, among them the renowned Monastery of St. Tryphon in Nicaea. He composed many works—philosophical, theological, and even dramatic, including comedies. His most important work, however, is the Great Supplicatory Canon to the Most Holy Theotokos, a magnificent literary and theological composition destined to endure through the ages, for the Orthodox Church has incorporated it into her hymnography, and it is read especially during the Dormition Fast in August.

Nor do the virtues of kyr Theodore end here. The example of his father, together with the education he had received, inspired in him a sincere love for the people and a deep concern for their welfare. He continued his father's

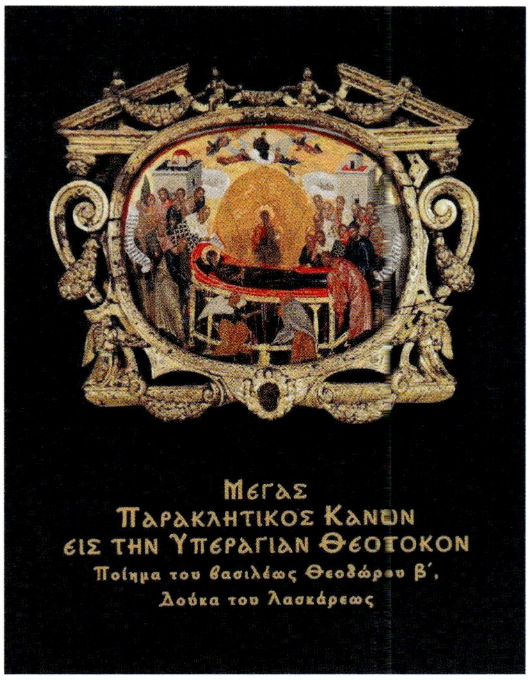

The Great Supplicatory Canon to Theotokos by Theodore II Laskaris

popular program, supporting the townspeople and especially the peasants against the great landowning families of the aristocracy. During his reign, the people found in him a true father and protector. He promoted to high office men from the lower classes, choosing them for their merit rather than their lineage. This, unfortunately, provoked the resentment of the aristocrats, who gathered themselves around a new and powerful figure who had appeared on the political stage—Michael Palaiologos.

The Palaiologoi were a great family that had produced many capable military commanders for the empire. They were connected by marriage to the Komnenoi, the Doukai, and the Angeloi, and wielded considerable influence within the state hierarchy and its administration. Michael, born in 1223, was nearly the same age as Emperor Theodore. From an early age he displayed signs of remarkable military and political ability—along with boundless ambition. John Vatatzes, recognizing his merit despite various accusations brought against him, appointed him Grand Constable, commander of the foreign mercenary troops.

Theodore II retained him in his post, but Michael, representing the interests of the aristocracy, came into conflict with the Emperor's social policies to such an extent that he was suspected of plotting revolt and overthrow. While serving as commander in Bithynia, he was forced to flee to the Sultanate of Iconium and to enter the service of the Seljuks as commander of the Byzantine mercenary forces. My friend George Akropolites notes in his history that Michael was not a traitor and that his character was "philorhomaios"—loyal to the Roman cause—but that he was exceedingly ambitious. In this I agree. When the Mongols com-

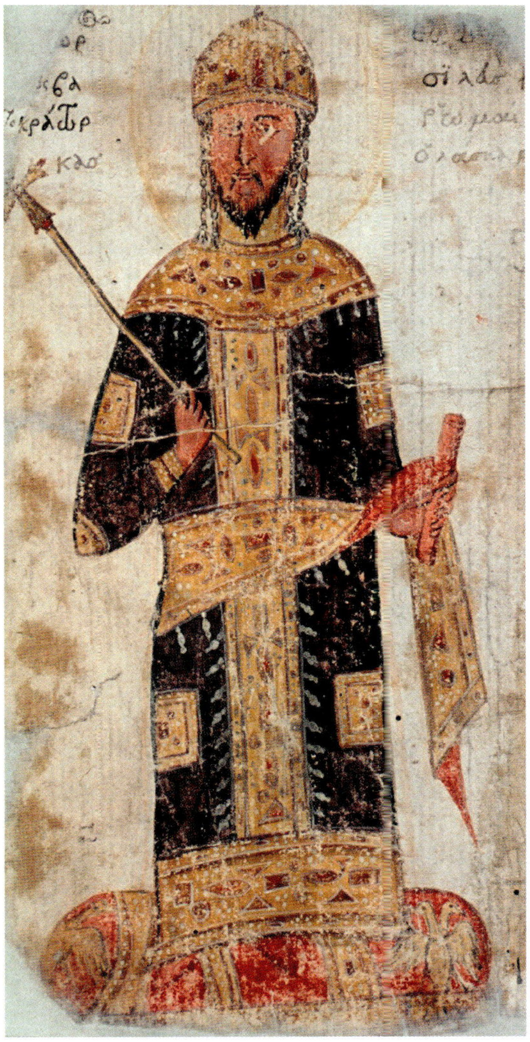

Theodore II Laskaris.

Miniature from George Pachymeres, History, 13th century, Bavarian State Library, Munich.

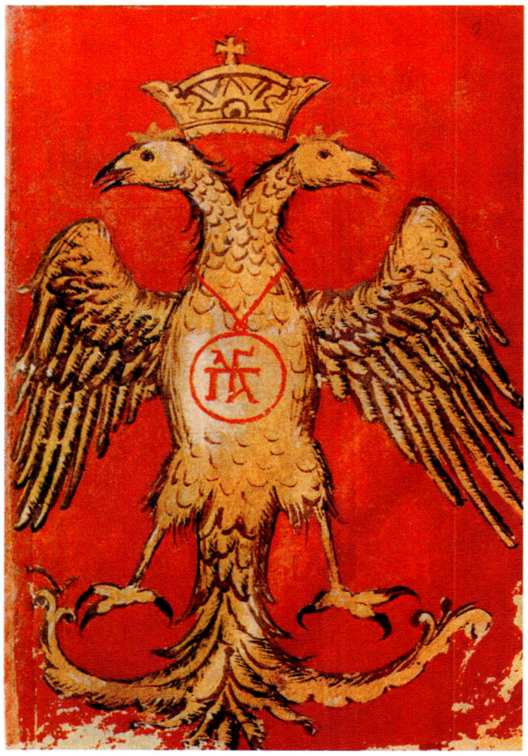

The double-headed eagle of the Palaiologos dynasty.

Miniature, 15th century.

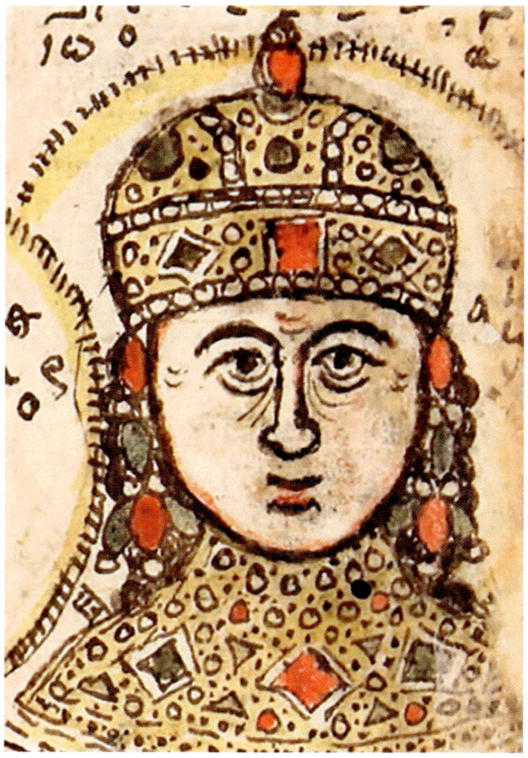

John IV Laskaris Vatatzes.

Miniature, Zonaras, 15th century, d'Este Library, Modena.

pelled the Seljuks to seek aid from the Greeks of Nicaea, Michael returned to Nicaea and restored his relations with the Emperor. The magnanimous Theodore reinstated him once again as Grand Constable.

Unfortunately, kyr Theodore did not live long. He was stricken by a grave illness and died at Nymphaion—then the empire's second capital—in 1258, at only thirty-six years of age. My fellow actuarius at the imperial Xenon of Nymphaion undertook his care, yet he could do nothing. The people mourned the loss of Theodore II Laskaris for two reasons: first, because they were losing a great Emperor and their protector; and second, because the state was entering perilous times, for his heir, John IV Laskaris Vatatzes, was only seven years old.

Theodore entrusted the guardianship and regency of his son to an honorable and capable man, George Mouzalon, upon whom he had bestowed the high office of protovestiarios. Yet Mouzalon did not come from the aristocracy; he was of "humble" origin. This was something the professional aristocrats—who placed their own interests above those of the country, and whose ambitions had already brought such calamity upon the Empire—could not tolerate. They, together with their leader Michael Palaiologos, refused to accept that a "common" man from outside their ranks should hold so exalted an office. Only a week after Theodore's death, during the memorial service held for him at the Monastery of Sosandrai, in the presence of the imperial family, the Latin mercenaries—commanded by Michael—burst into the church and murdered George Mouzalon and his brother in cold blood, showing disrespect both to the young John and to his deceased father. It is unmistakably clear that Michael was behind the assassination. He hastened to assume the guardianship of the young John, ostensibly in order to "protect" him. His qualifications for this role were that he was the most distinguished general of the realm, widely popular with the army, the scion of a great family, and that his wife, Theodora Vatatzaina, belonged to the family of the illustrious John Vatatzes.

The ruthless yet highly capable Michael delayed the coronation of the young John and assumed for himself the title of Despot. The following year he was crowned Co-Emperor alongside John—whom, of course, he completely marginalized.

As the ancients said, "No evil comes without some good." I must acknowledge that the usurper Michael was a highly capable ruler, and he took the helm of the Empire at a difficult moment. Against the state of Nicaea there now formed an alliance of the Despotate of Epirus, the Principality of Achaea under William of Villehardouin, and the Kingdom of Sicily under Manfred Hohenstaufen, the illegitimate son of Frederick II of Germany—well known to us as the father-in-law of Vatatzes. Their army clashed with ours in 1259 at

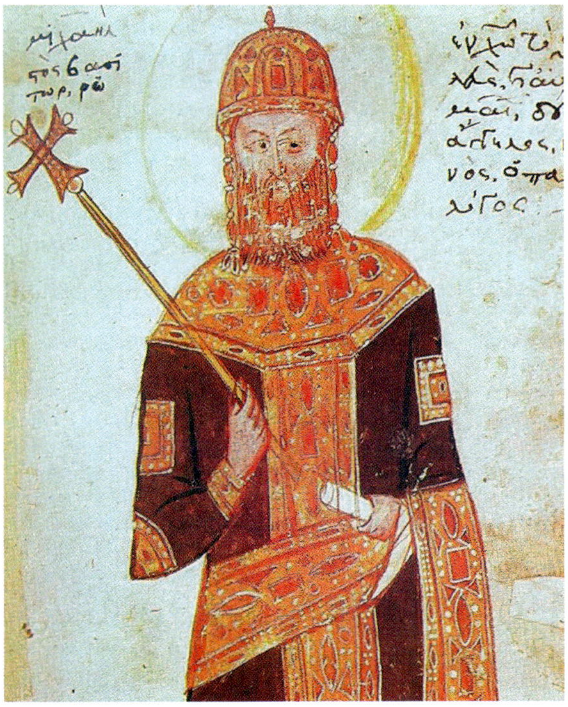

Michael VIII Palaiologos.

Miniature, from George Pachymeres' History, 13th century, Bavarian State Library, Munich.

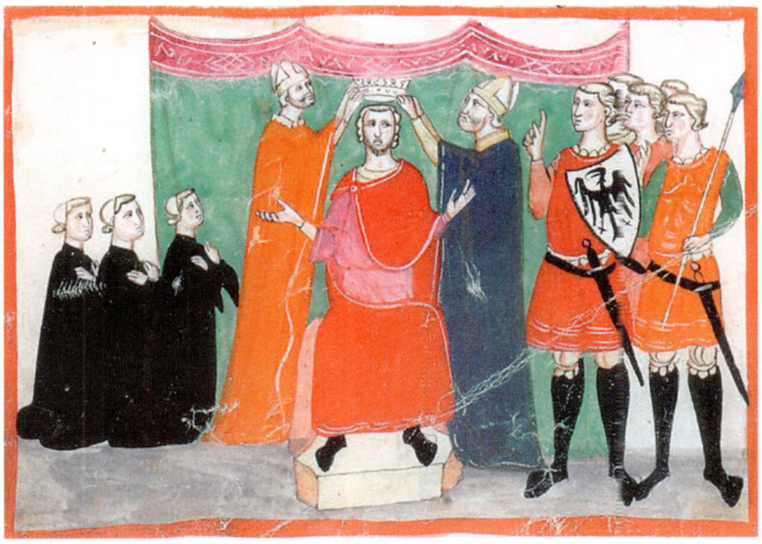

The Coronation of Manfred Hohenstaufen in Sicily, 1258.

Miniature, Giovanni Villani, Chronica, 13th century, Vatican Library, Rome.

Pelagonia, a region north of Kastoria. There the painstaking work of the Laskarid emperors became evident, for they had organized a truly national army; and there, too, shone the great skill of the generals John Palaiologos, brother of Michael, and Alexios Strategopoulos.

Although our army was smaller, it moved with intelligent strategy. By supplying the Despot of Epirus with false information, it succeeded in breaking the alliance and inducing the Epirots to withdraw. It then attacked the Franks of Achaea and the Germans of Sicily and utterly crushed them. The enemy forces were scattered, and Villehardouin was taken captive. The consequences of this battle were considerable, above all for the morale of the army.

The Despotate of Epirus was humbled and ceased once and for all to pose a competitive threat to the state of Nicaea. More important still was the complete defeat of the French and German knights, who—with their heavy, encased armor and their great, high-necked warhorses, "clad in mighty weap-

The Battle of Pelagonia
From the Chronicon of the Morea

What more could I tell you, and how could I unravel it all?
All the horses and fine mounts of the Franks and the Alemanni—
they slaughtered them completely, and the horsemen were cast down.
For even he, the wondrous one, the pride of the soldiers,
the lord of Karytaina, fell together with his fine steed.
...
Then the Sebastocrator, at the very start of the battle,
...
how he set upon the Hungarians, and likewise the Cumans,
and persuaded them to shoot so as to slay the enemy horses
...
Then the multitude of the Romans, with their flights of arrows
cut down the horses, and the horsemen crashed to the earth;
and once they found themselves on foot among the battle-lines,
they knew not what they could do—whether willing or unwilling.
So that they would not die an unjust death in this world,
they all surrendered—even the prince himself.
None escaped, save only the poor folk
those who managed to flee and reached Vlachia,
some escaped on foot and returned to the Morea,
others the Vlachs seized in Vlachia,
others again they killed and stripped them.
So the battle ceased, and they had won victory over the Franks.

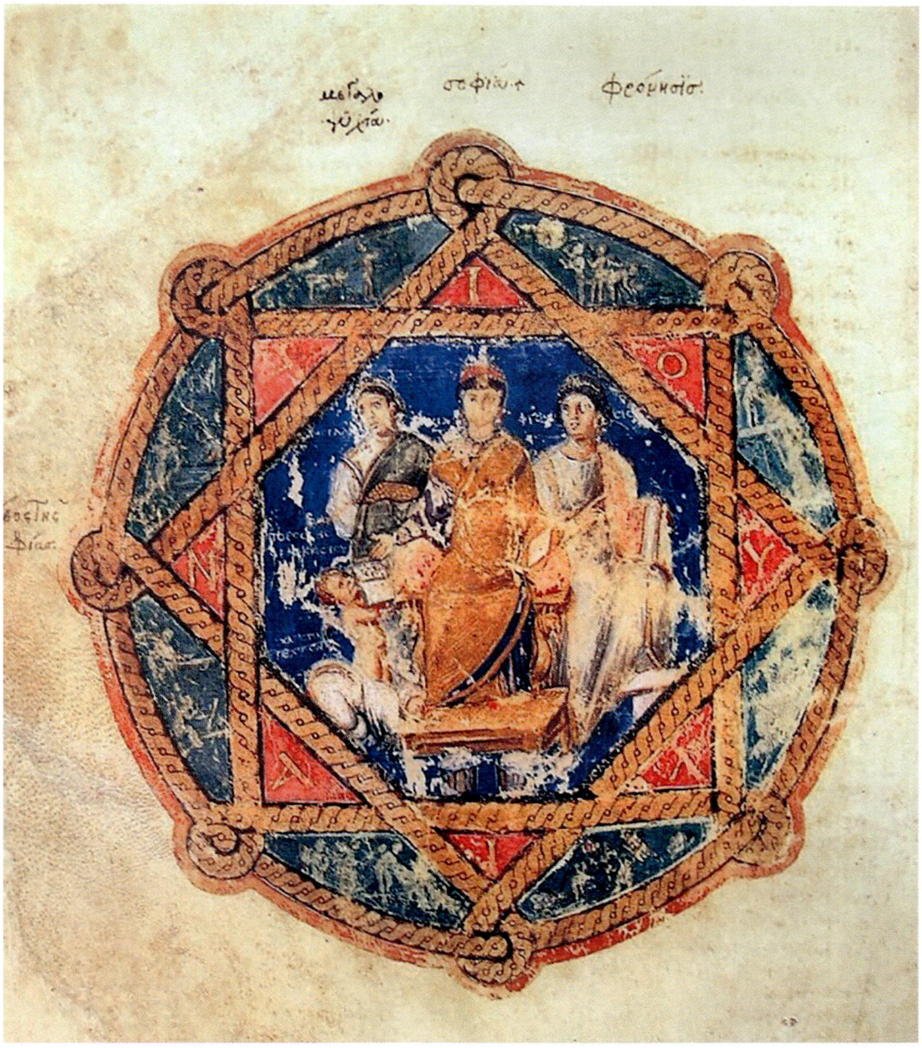

Anicia Juliana, depicted as donor between Magnanimity and Prudence.

Miniature, 6th century, from an illustrated copy of Dioscorides.
Austrian National Library, Vienna.

ons and mounted upon lofty and proud steeds"—had been regarded as an irresistible force. The disciplined Roman infantry and the renowned Cuman archers, who targeted the horses of the Latins, prevailed over the knights' furious charge. Manfred fled in disgrace, while Villehardouin—the ruler of the strongest Frankish principality in the Greek peninsula, the Principality of Achaea—and many Frankish nobles were captured, having hidden themselves in a hayloft. They were held until 1262, when Michael released them in exchange for the fortresses of Monemvasia, Mystras, and Great Mani. The Empire thus expanded into the Peloponnese—an important achievement for Michael.

Fulfilling my teacher's charge, I now recount the events that unfolded until the recovery of Constantinople. Yet, in order for one to understand these events rightly, it is necessary also to highlight certain social and cultural features of our age. And I shall begin with the role of women in our society.

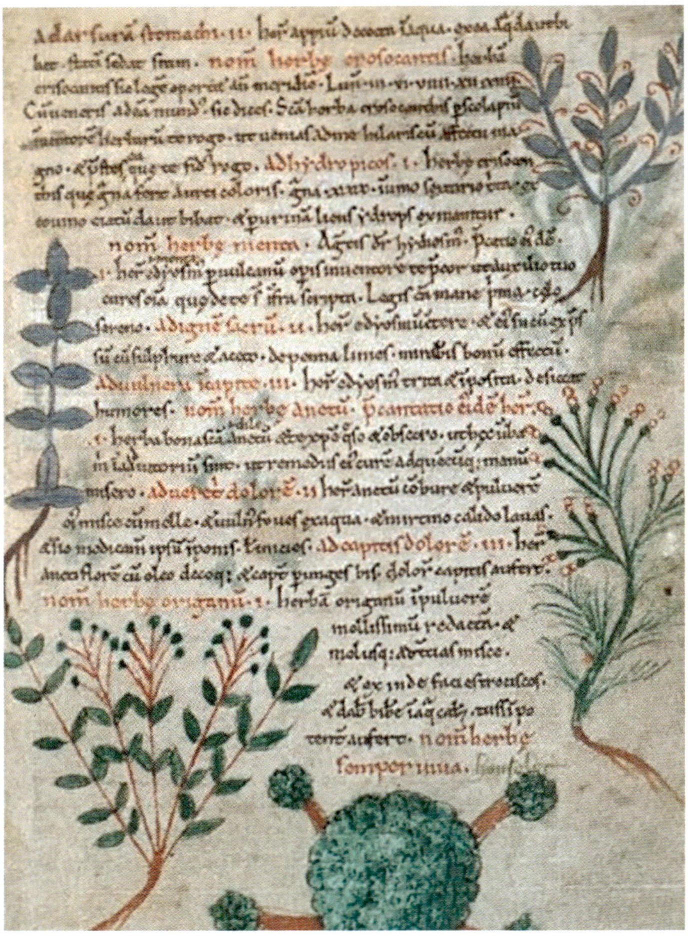

"Origanum". *Miniature, 11th century, from the Herbarium of Pseudo-Apuleius, Bodleian Library, Oxford.*

In the early and middle centuries of our Empire, very few women played a significant part in the political or cultural life of the realm. An exception was the sphere of nursing and social care, where women contributed greatly and indispensably. From the eleventh century onward, however—and especially in our own thirteenth century—women of the aristocratic class, who possessed the means to be educated, not only participated actively in the life of the Empire but often held an almost equal position to the men of their rank. Most women of the Byzantine elite are now literate; they have at least the basic education of our tradition. Among them there have been some exceptionally learned, with theological and philosophical training: Anna Komnene, Eirene the Sebastocratorissa, and later Theodora Komnene Raoulaina, the niece of Michael Palaiologos. These and many others show that the imperial society of our time is not lacking in women of intellect, refinement, and influence.

Society's views regarding the role of women have changed greatly over the past century—and they continue to change in our own days. For instance, in matters of law concerning marriage, divorce, dowry, property, and financial arrangements, the rights of women have increased substantially. As a result, women today—whether married or widowed—participate actively in the economic life of the realm. They are able to manage their own property or dowry independently and to dispose of it as they themselves see fit. Many rent out shops or plots of land; others lend money; still others oversee personal enterprises or even administer state funds. Numerous women, thanks to their advanced education, have acquired political and social independence. Indeed, those belonging to the imperial family—such as Anna Dalassene, Maria of Antioch, and Maria of Alania—played an exceptionally important role in political affairs. Thus, in our land, women—and especially those of the aristocracy—are anything but confined to the interior of their households.

Another interesting phenomenon observed in our own time is an unexpected spiritual and cultural blossoming. Despite the troubled political circumstances and the growing strength of the enemies who encircle us, people—disheartened and humiliated by the shrinking of the Ecumenical Empire—have sought refuge in spiritual and aesthetic pursuits. Thus we are witnessing a remarkable flourishing of classical letters and the arts, a true renaissance of Greek learning and Byzantine artistry, brought about chiefly by the prosperous classes who possess the means for education.

Painting in particular—now expressed chiefly as iconography in the churches, whether through frescoes upon the walls or egg-tempera on wooden panel icons—has reached an enviable level of aesthetic refinement, while still preserving its transcendent and metaphysical character. In matters of painting I am rather well informed, for having myself a certain inclination toward the visual arts, I often took part in the conversations my teacher held with his brother-in-law, Manuel Vlemmydes, the distinguished master of Art and Philosophy. Unfortunately, the art of mosaic has almost been abandoned, since mosaics are very costly and the resources of the state have become exceedingly limited.

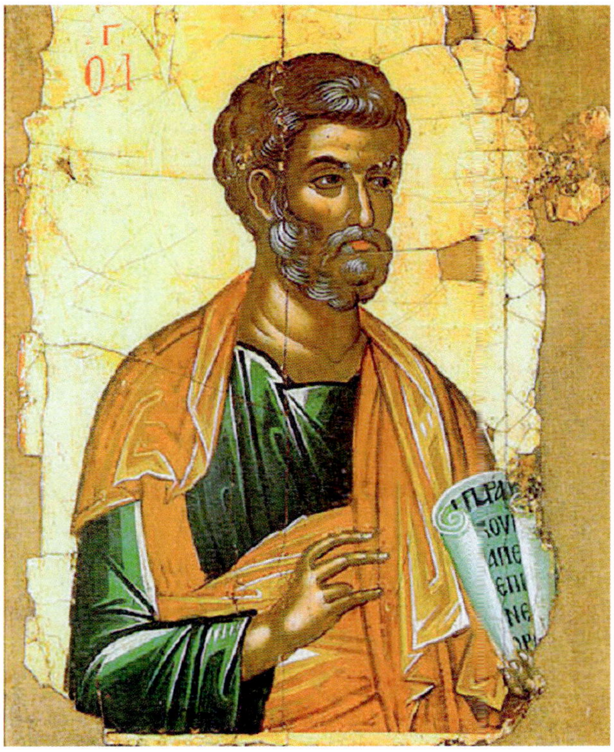

The Apostle Peter.

Theophanes the Cretan, 16th century, Monastery of Stavronikita, Mount Athos.

In Venice—and indeed throughout Italy—a keen interest in art and the sciences has begun to flourish. Through trade, travel, and economic prosperity, the horizons of this gifted people have widened greatly. Not long ago I was visited by a Venetian colleague and friend of mine, Mario Pellini. Pellini, besides being a physician, is also an amateur painter and a man of broad education. He is an ardent admirer of Byzantine art, especially of our mosaics, and he could not conceal his amazement that all these magnificent works are anonymous.

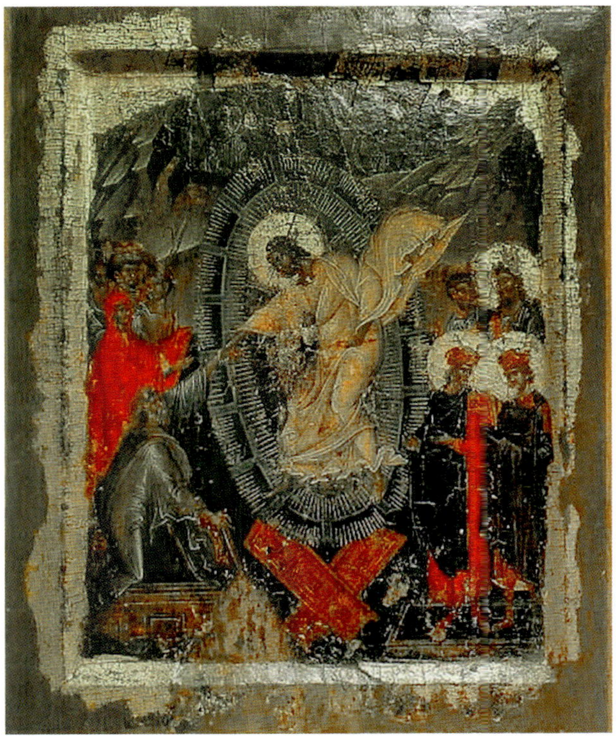

The Descent into Hades.

Michael Astrapas, 14th century, Church of St. Clement, Ohrid, North Macedonia.

"Why did these great artists never sign their works so that we might know who they were?" he asked me.

"The creations of painting," I answered him, drawing on what I had learned from Manuel Vlemmydes, "as well as those of architecture, are not regarded as personal achievements. That is why the names of the builders, the master craftsmen, or the painters have not been preserved. In the mindset we have inherited from antiquity, every work is a collective creation of a whole group. A church, for example, has its "*geometers*"

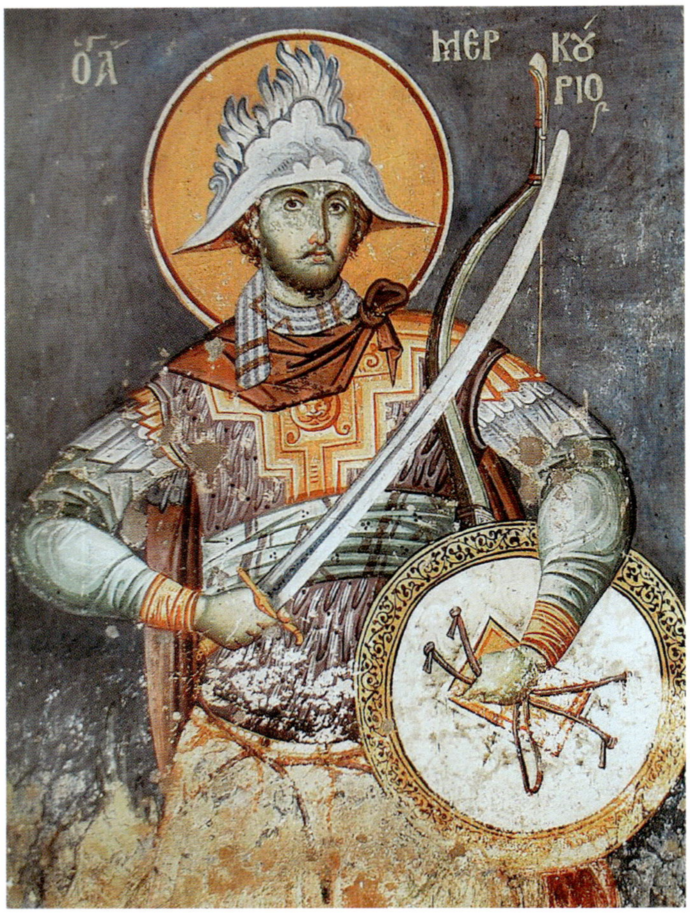

Saint Mercurius.
Fresco by Manuel Panselinos, 13th century, Protaton Church, Mount Athos.

who prepare the designs and the structural study of the building; its *"tektones"* who execute the construction; its chief master-painters who compose the iconographic programs for mosaics or frescoes; the artisans who carry out the careful placing of each tessera or the mixing and laying of pigments; the specialists who select and fit the marble revetments and reliefs; and the workers of every kind who labor under the direction of the *"maistores."* The unifying force behind all this work is the *"poietes"* (*poets-creators*)—the maker in the true sense—the patron who commissions the work and bears its cost.

"So then," Mario asked in amazement, "the meaning of a work of art—and, more generally, of any creation for you—is actually the outcome of the ancient understanding of the works of the polis?"

"Yes," I replied. "I believe what survives is the ancient collective spirit, where the individual is woven into the *common endeavor*, rather than standing out through personal achievements. According to the great Aristotle in his *Metaphysics*, every creation has multiple causes. The most important is the *formal cause*, that is, the prototype the work seeks to portray. If it is an icon, the formal cause is Christ or the particular saint; if it is a church, it is the living Church of Christ itself. Next comes the *efficient cause*—the *poietikon aition*—the patron, the founder who is responsible for the construction and is in a sense the 'maker' of the work. Then follows the *instrumental cause*, the craftsman or artist; the *material cause*, the materials used; and finally the *final cause*, the purpose of the work, the need it fulfills, or even the finished work in its ultimate form. Every individual craftsman is an organic part of the whole, but not someone separate and independent from the rest—as such, he cannot boast of being the exclusive creator. In earlier times, the *"poets"*—that is, the makers—were usually the emperors. In our own age powerful nobles have appeared who are able to commission great works and have their names attached to them."

My companion was deeply impressed by this view. In Italy these days, artists work with the aim of expressing their personal vision and individual style, giving many new shapes to art. Both approaches—though they reflect the cultural differences that have grown between us—are of course legitimate, each with its own strengths and weaknesses. Pellini remained in Nicaea, where I hosted him for nearly a month. I showed him around the Xenon of Saint

Mavra, and he was astonished by the organization and functioning of the hospital—admitting that it far surpassed the medical institutions of his own land.

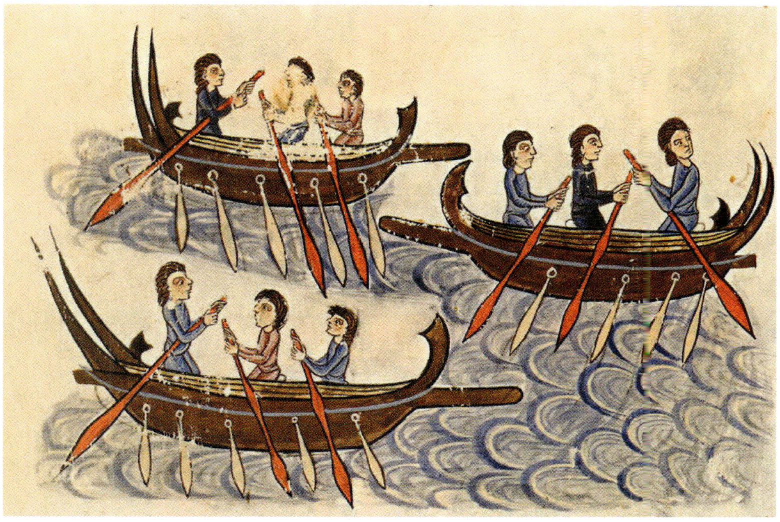

Byzantine Oared Ships.

Miniature from Skylitzes, 12th century, National Library of Spain, Madrid.

Let us return, however, to the events themselves. The greatest and most glorious achievement of Michael was the recovery of Constantinople. This, after all, had been the primary aim of every Emperor of Nicaea. After his great victory at Pelagonia, he attempted in 1260 a campaign against the Queen of Cities, but once again the Venetian fleet thwarted our hopes. Thus he was compelled, the following year, to forge an alliance with Genoa—the great rival of Venice—in order to secure its naval support, granting in return significant commercial privileges. This agreement had the advantage of splitting the Latin world and weakening the overwhelming power of the Venetians, yet in the end it proved unnecessary and extremely harmful to the Empire, for the recapture of the City occurred entirely by chance, without any need for Genoese assistance.

Here is how events unfolded. In July of 1261, Michael sent the Grand Domestic Alexios Strategopoulos with a force of 800 soldiers to the outskirts of Constantinople in Thrace, in order to scout the situation and intimidate the besieged Latins. When they reached the region near Selymbria, the local farmers informed the Domestic that the Frankish army and the Venetian fleet of Constantinople were absent—they had sailed on an expedition to the Black Sea, attempting to seize the city of Dafnousia, which belonged to Nicaea. One farmer even told him that, though he lived within the City's walls, he was able to go out each day to pasture his animals through the Gate of the Life-giving Spring, which, as he said, remained unguarded. Strategopoulos, that very night (25 July), entered the City through that gate, launched a sudden attack on the Latin guards, and after a brief battle seized the land walls. He immediately sent messengers to Nicaea to announce the news. The Latin Emperor Baldwin II, who was in the Boukoleon Palace, and the Latin Patriarch of the City, upon learning that the land walls had fallen to the Greeks, fled with the remaining Catholic inhabitants to the harbor, waiting for the Venetian fleet to return and rescue them. Indeed, the Venetians arrived swiftly by sea and took on board both the nobles and the populace. Meanwhile, the army of Nicaea had reached the walls and occupied the western sector of the City. The Venetians judged that they could not prevent the complete capture of Constantinople, and their fleet withdrew. Thus the recovery of Constantinople took place without bloodshed—without battle and without massacres.

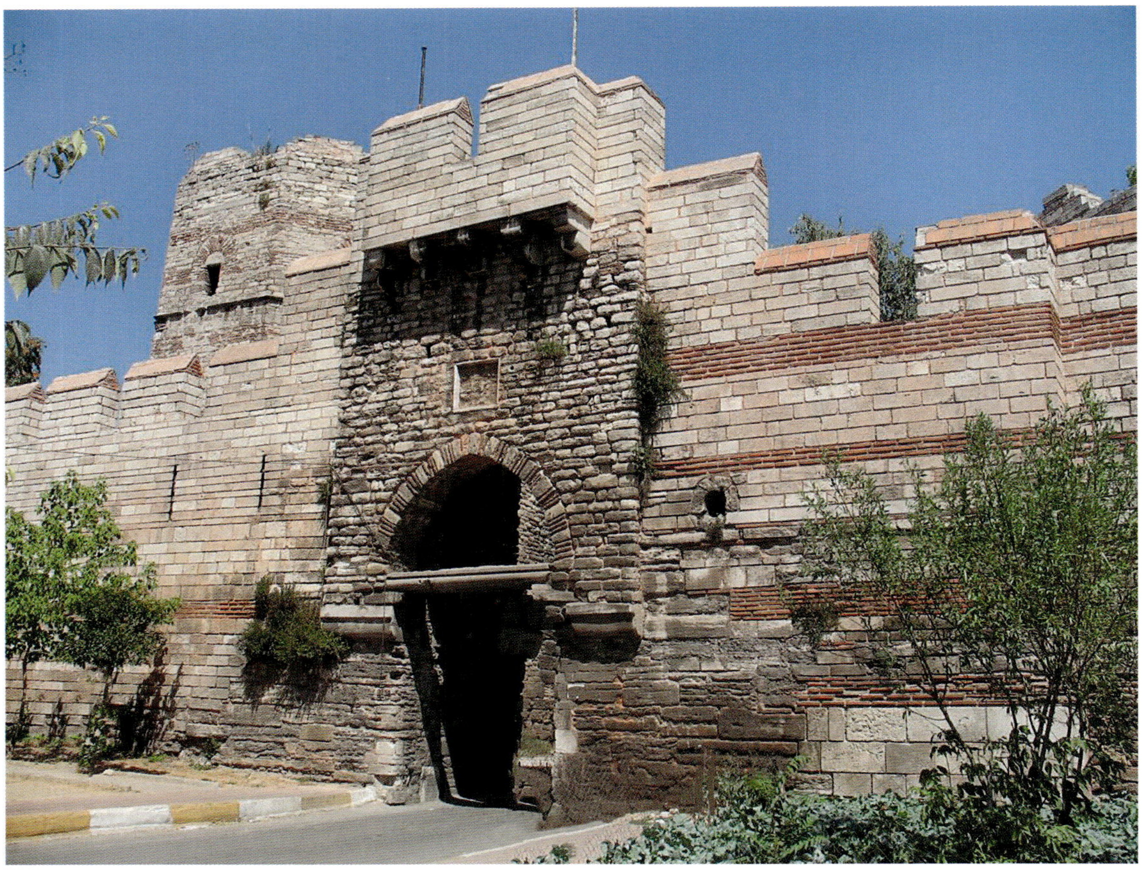

The Gate of Selybria, or Gate of the Life-Giving Spring, Constantinople.
Photo: CrniBombarder, 2006.

On the 15th of August, on the very feast of the Dormition of the Theotokos, Michael arrived from Nicaea in solemn procession before the Golden Gate. There he knelt, and thirteen prayers—composed at his request by Akropolites—were read to offer thanks to God for this unexpected victory. The procession followed the Mese Odos and reached Hagia Sophia in triumphant splendor. Crowds of people followed, glorifying God and their Emperor. There, Michael was crowned with full magnificence as "faithful King and Emperor of the Romans." No one mentioned the rightful emperor, John IV, who had been entirely set aside. What followed was a great migration of people from Nicaea and from every corner of the Greek world, hastening to return to the Queen of Cities. I myself chose to remain in Nicaea—my beloved city—and in the hospice of Saint Mavra, where I continue to offer my services to its people. What befell Nicaea is, indeed, a sorrow and an injustice. This city—this model city—which once sheltered the hopes of Hellenism and its universal mission; the city governed by perhaps the finest emperors Byzantium ever knew, the two Theodores and the great John Vatatzes; the city that became the capital of a just state, that revived the sound institutions which had glorified the Empire in earlier times—fair taxation, the institution of the *akritai* who defended the borders, the organization of a national army and fleet—this very city was quickly abandoned and fell into decline before the irresistible superiority and splendor of Constantinople. The scholars, the thinkers, the merchants, the craftsmen all followed the kings and powerful aristocratic families to the fabled Capital—those very families who, now freed from the restraints once imposed on them by the Laskaris dynasty, reclaimed their old powers under the protection of Palaiologos, with all the unhappy consequences this brought upon the state and the people. Michael at once devoted himself to restoring churches and public buildings, repairing the palaces and the ruined walls. Yet even so, Constantinople could not regain its former glory and brilliance. Large quarters of the city remained uninhabited; many houses stayed destroyed and in ruins; and the old vitality of commerce did not return, for the Italians—now the Genoese—held a monopoly over trade.At Christmas of that same year, 1262, Palaiologos committed a dreadful act—one that revealed the ruthless cast of his character and brought shame upon his entire generation. On the very day when the legitimate emperor, young John, turned eleven years old, he had him blinded so that he could never claim the throne, and confined him to a monastery, where the unfortunate child lived out the rest of his sorrowful life. This deed, carried out in secret, filled the Empire with horror. Patriarch Arsenios Autoreianos, who had likewise undertaken the protection of young John and had compelled Michael to swear that he would do him no harm, excommunicated him when he learned the truth and forbade him to enter Hagia Sophia. But Michael held the army and the foreign mercenaries under his command. He exiled the Patriarch to Proikonnesos on the false charge of plotting against him. A large portion of the people sided with the Patriarch, and thus arose the so-called Arsenite schism—strong for a time, yet ultimately suppressed by the forces loyal to Palaiologos.

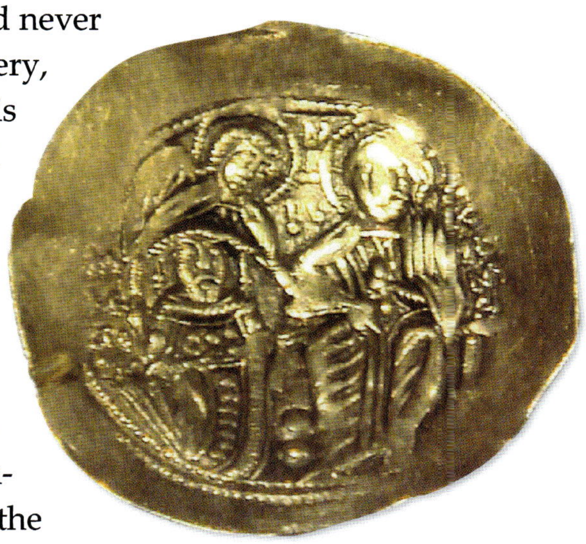

Hyperpyron of Michael VIII Palaiologos. 13th c.,

Metropolitan Museum of Art, New York.

Michael proved to be a successful emperor. He reigned for many years and carried out effective military and diplomatic undertakings. He secured footholds in the Peloponnese through the territories ceded to him by the captive Villehardouin. He won several battles against the enemies who threatened the Empire, which now stretched from northern Epirus to Cilicia. He also sought an understanding with the Pope, for a new and formidable danger had arisen—Charles of Anjou. This powerful ruler of Naples and Sicily had already convened and was planning a great expedition against Constantinople, aiming to restore the Latin Empire and reinstate the deposed Baldwin. With highly skillful diplomatic and military maneuvers, Michael managed to avert the danger. Yet he was forced to grant the Pope the primacy of the Church, signing in 1274 at Lyon in France the union of the Churches. This act of union—despite the removal of the military threat—brought him into direct conflict with the sentiment of the people, who would under no circumstances accept

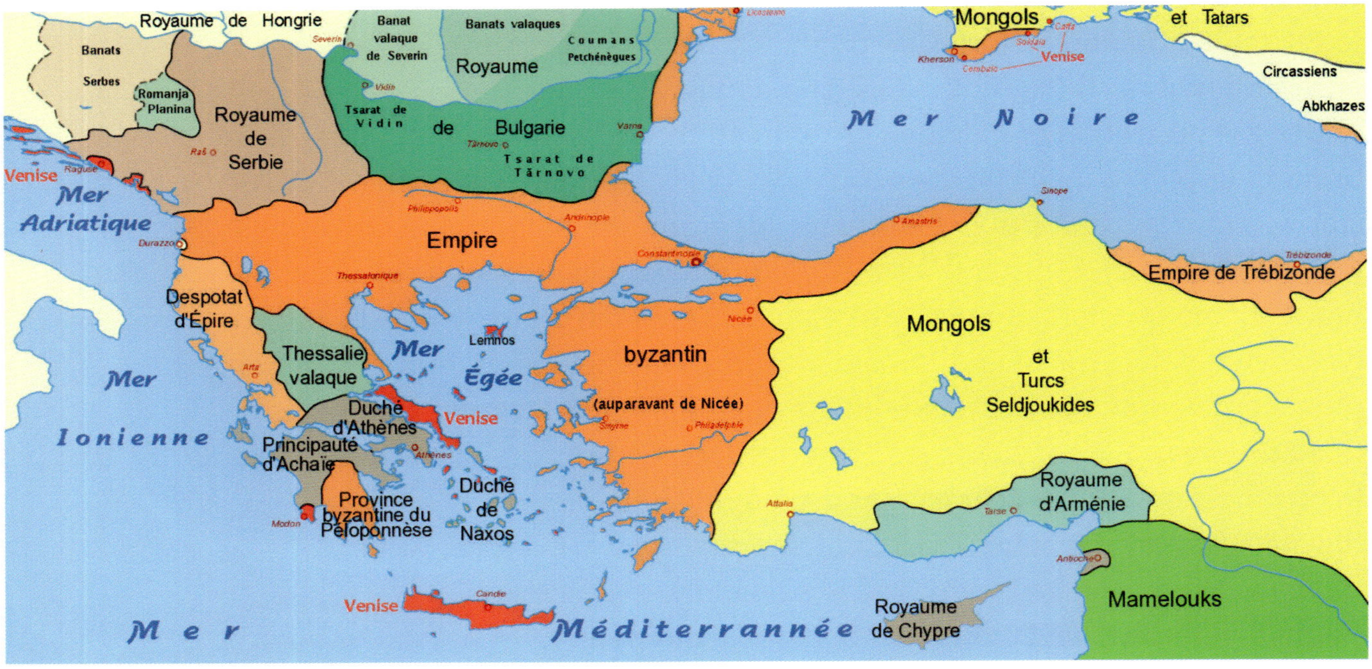

The Empire in 1265.

Map by Neuceu, 2005.

the subjugation of the Orthodox Church to Rome. The populace and the Orthodox clergy regarded him as a schismatic and never accepted the union. In fact, in his attempt to enforce it, he resorted to harsh measures, exiling, torturing, and even blinding distinguished clerics who opposed his policy.

Yet despite these sorrowful circumstances, the cultural work begun by the Laskaris emperors continued in his time, and there was a true renaissance in the realm of learning and the arts—one that endured and even intensified throughout his reign. In fact, the religious unrest stirred by his policies gave rise to much theological and philosophical ferment, and it offered the occasion for certain noble-born women monastics to come to the forefront in steadfast opposition to his actions. Among them were Maria–Martha Palaiologina and her daughter Theodora Balanidiotissa—close relatives of Michael—who supported the Arsenite monks against him with remarkable resolve; and also Theodora Raoulaina together with her mother Eulogia, who stood boldly against his policy of union with the Western Church.

It is no coincidence that all the women who dared to oppose the Emperor were nuns. Life within the monastery has always granted women great prestige, and they were held in deep respect by society. Unfortunately, the old notion still prevails—as it did in antiquity—that the female nature possesses certain inherent disadvantages compared with the male. Yet it is believed that these cease to exist from the moment a woman dedicates herself to the path of God. In the eyes of the citizens of the Empire, nuns are holy virgins, venerable elder-women, whose words carry the same weight as those of men. For this reason, monastic life—especially in our own days—has become for women a path to independence and a space for free expression. As for many men, it is also a road toward higher learning or toward a vocation in the arts and sciences.

Personally, I feel aversion toward Michael; I consider him a usurper and a murderer, and this is one of the reasons I did not follow him to the Queen of Cities. Yet I cannot fail to acknowledge the work he accomplished in every domain. To begin with, he showed real interest in providing higher education, which he entrusted to the Grand Logothete George Akropolites. Akropolites became a loyal supporter of Michael, even participating in the Council of Lyons, and in the history he composed he avoids mentioning the Emperor's disgraceful treatment of the young John IV Laskaris. To this silence contributed both the commanding personality of Michael and the fact that the late Emperor Theodore II had once severely reprimanded Akropolites after a serious diplomatic failure. The circle of scholars who attended Akropolites' lessons was large. At the same time, alongside Constantinople, another great intellectual center arose in Thessaloniki—the second city of the Empire—equal in stature to the capital, while Nicaea, sadly, sank into oblivion.

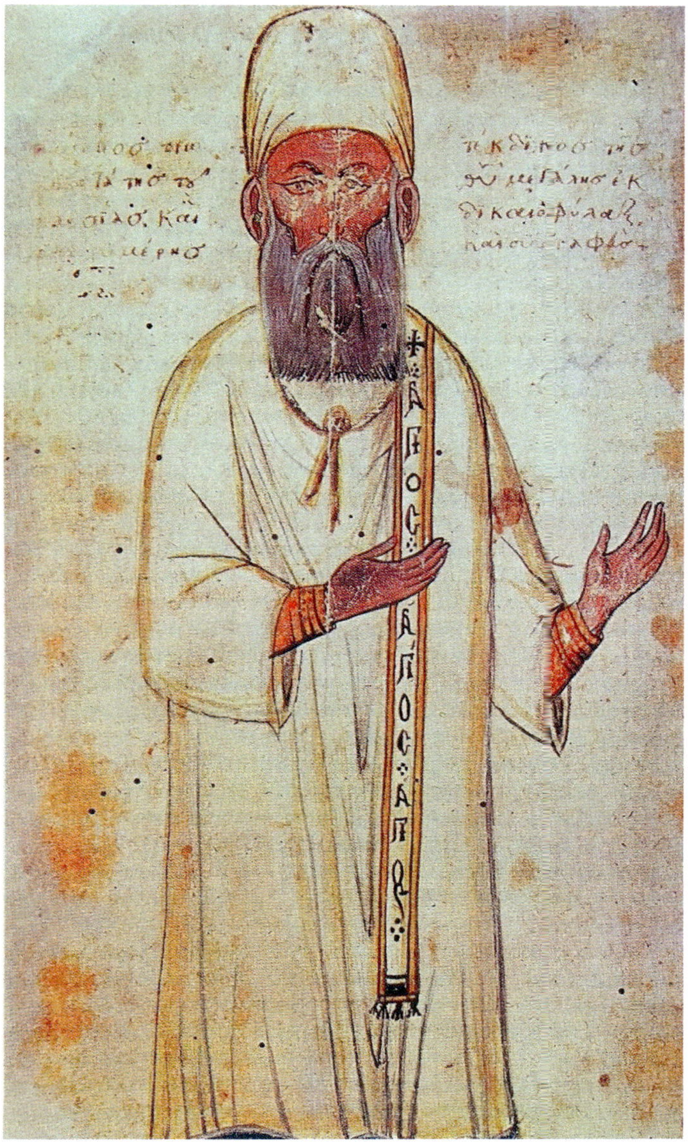

George Pachymeres, scholar and historian, 1242–1310.

Miniature from Pachymeres' History, 14th c., Bavarian State Library, Munich.

What distinguishes the scholars of our time is their well-rounded education. To be a specialist in one narrow field is of little importance. The sciences are not unrelated to one another; they are all parts of philosophy in its fullest sense. In recent years a younger scholar has emerged who shows great promise—George Pachymeres. He has already written works on mathematics and music, and has become familiar with a new system of numeration, the so-called Indian numbers. Until now we have used the Greek system for counting and mathematical operations, employing the letters of the alphabet (α, β, γ ...), where each number is represented by a letter. This system is quite inconvenient compared to the Indian one, which introduces new symbols (1, 2, 3, ...) and, remarkably, includes a number entirely unknown to the Greeks: zero (0). This has made calculation and numerical operations astonishingly easier.

Pachymeres does not yet use the Indian numerals in his official writings, but it is certain that they will soon prevail throughout the world. The Arabs already employ them, and for this reason some people refer to them as Arabic numerals.

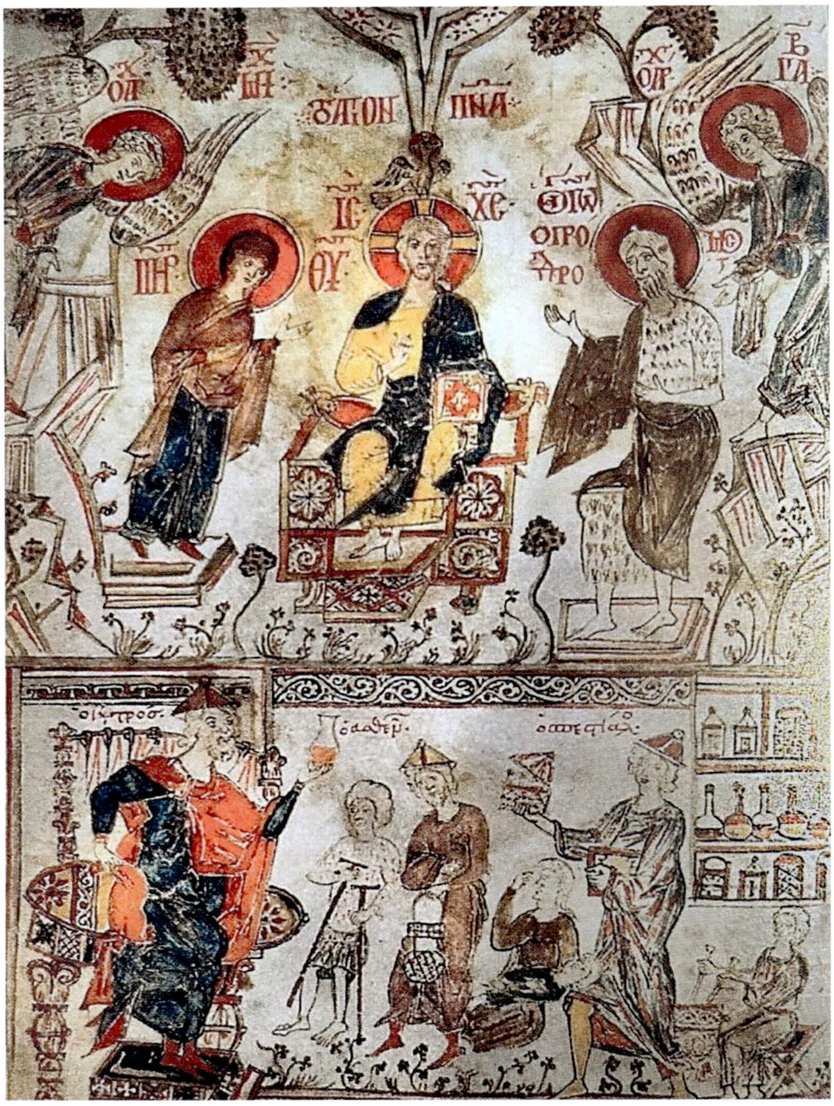

Nikolaos Myrepsos (below) dispensing medicines to patients.

Miniature, 13th c., National Library of France, Paris.

In medicine, the scholars of our own time have made significant advances. The most distinguished physician of our age is Nikolaos Myrepsos. He first worked in Nicaea, where he composed an extremely important pharmacological treatise entitled Dynameron, which the Franks have already translated into Latin and from which they now teach. The book contains more than 2,500 medical prescriptions, arranged according to type and illness. Myrepsos has become renowned for a particular remedy he devised, which he calls Alexandrian Gold—a medicine remarkably effective for colic and vascular crises.

I worked closely with Myrepsos in Nicaea, and his medicines were of great help in my practice. After the reconquest of Constantinople, he followed the majority of physicians who returned there, together with another exceedingly learned colleague of ours, Demetrios Pepagomenos, who now serves as Michael's personal doctor. Pepagomenos has even written an original treatise on gout, based on his own observations. As for me, I avoided offering my services to Michael; it was well known that my loyalty belonged to Emperor John IV, whose end had been so grievous. I have collaborated with many physicians here in Nicaea. Besides the Greeks, there are also many Jewish doctors—Roman citizens, of course. That nation, which in the early years of the Christian Empire had lived under various restrictions, now flourishes especially in commerce, but also in the sciences.

Michael's attention was turned chiefly toward the West, for from there came the greatest danger, since the Seljuks were not yet strong. During his reign the army of the Empire became highly formidable, and the fleet was systematically strengthened. When he first assumed the throne, the entire eastern Mediterranean was ravaged by pirates—Italian and Greek alike—because the state lacked the power to restrain them. At the beginning he collaborated with them; indeed, he even employed some in order to strike effectively at the naval bases of his great adversary, Charles of Anjou. Later, however, once his own fleet had become strong, he turned against the pirates to such an extent that he boasted (with a fair measure of exaggeration) that he had restored Byzantine dominion and peace to the eastern Mediterranean. Unfortunately, however, Michael—unlike the emperors of Nicaea—once again favored the aristocracy. As a result, large estates returned to the hands of the powerful, the small farmers of Asia Minor fell into decline, and the population thinned out, leaving the eastern frontiers vulnerable once more to the invaders from the East.

The conquest of Constantinople by the Latins and the overthrow of the Empire were catastrophic for our nation and our civilization. The losses in human lives, in buildings, in works of art, in manuscripts and books are beyond all reckoning. Hostilities and hatred between the peoples reached their peak. Niketas Choniates, the historian of the fall, wrote characteristically: "Between us and the Latins there yawns a vast chasm. We stand in diametrical opposition. We do not share even a single thought." Now, however—with the forced coexistence of the two peoples and the commercial and political contacts that followed—after a few generations several positive aspects emerged. There had once been deep suspicion and prejudice on both sides. We considered the Westerners uncouth, barbarous usurpers of our inheritance, and they considered us corrupt, devious, and degenerate. They knew no Greek at all, just as we knew no Latin, and this often caused misunderstandings and misinterpretations. Slowly, however, we discovered that not all of them were as barbaric as we had imagined, and they discovered that we were not so corrupt, but rather the true custodians and continuators of ancient wisdom.

In the everyday rhythm of our shared life we discovered that the same human elements exist in all nations; everywhere there are good and bad people, and it is unjust to judge an entire people—favorably or unfavorably—on the basis of extreme examples. The long theological debates regarding the procession of the Holy Spirit and the primacy of the Pope revealed that on both sides there existed philosophical reflection and a love for truth and right thinking, beyond, of course, the political motives involved. Our scholars impressed the Westerners with their profound erudition, yet they in turn were impressed by them. Many among us learned Latin and studied the works of great writers such as Thomas Aquinas. The Westerners, especially the Italian scholars, discovered the authentic sources of Plato and Aristotle and sought to learn Greek. The various intermarriages contracted with many houses of Europe—naturally for political reasons—brought the customs and cultures of our peoples into closer contact. In other words, a kind of cultural osmosis took place which, in the long term, will surely bring positive results, for ignorance and prejudice are always poor counsellors.

The efforts being made toward understanding and union between the Churches encounter, for now, the excessive demands of the Pope and the Latins—who currently stand in a position of strength—and the inflexibility of our own clergy and people, who perhaps rightly fear that such a union would bring about the complete spiritual and political domination of the papal party. I do not know what outcome these discussions will have or whether they will lead anywhere at all. What I do see is that our state—no longer regarded by our neighbors as an ecumenical Roman Empire but rather as a Greek Kingdom—is encircled by powerful enemies who threaten its very existence. The Franks continually menace us with the prospect of a new crusade to restore the Latin rule, and all the efforts of Michael Palaiologos are directed toward averting that danger. Sadly, the eastern frontier is thus neglected, where another enemy lies in wait: the Turks. They may now be weakened by the recent Mongol incursion, yet this people possesses a vigor that troubles me. We do not know how long they will remain quiet, nor when they might set their sights on the Bride of the Bosporus—the city coveted by all, from East and West alike, since the days of the Constantines.

Here I shall bring my story to an end. I feel that I have fulfilled my duty to my teacher, who asked me to continue his work until the recovery of Constantinople—a recovery he believed would come swiftly. Now, nearly twenty years after the triumphant entry of the army of Nicaea into the City, Michael VIII Palaiologos reigns in brilliance—an unashamed usurper of the throne, yet one whose abilities no one can deny. Through his diplomatic and military successes he has established himself as a most capable Emperor of the Romans. Thanks to the groundwork laid by the Laskarids, but also to his own talents, the Roman-Greek Empire has been reborn politically and culturally, reaching a peak that one might think approaches that of the Komnenoi. And yet—alas. The world-shaping events that have unfolded have radically altered the balance of power and the very mentalities of our region. A new world is emerging within our Realm, and throughout Europe as well, and this new Empire is profoundly different from the old. Far removed now from its

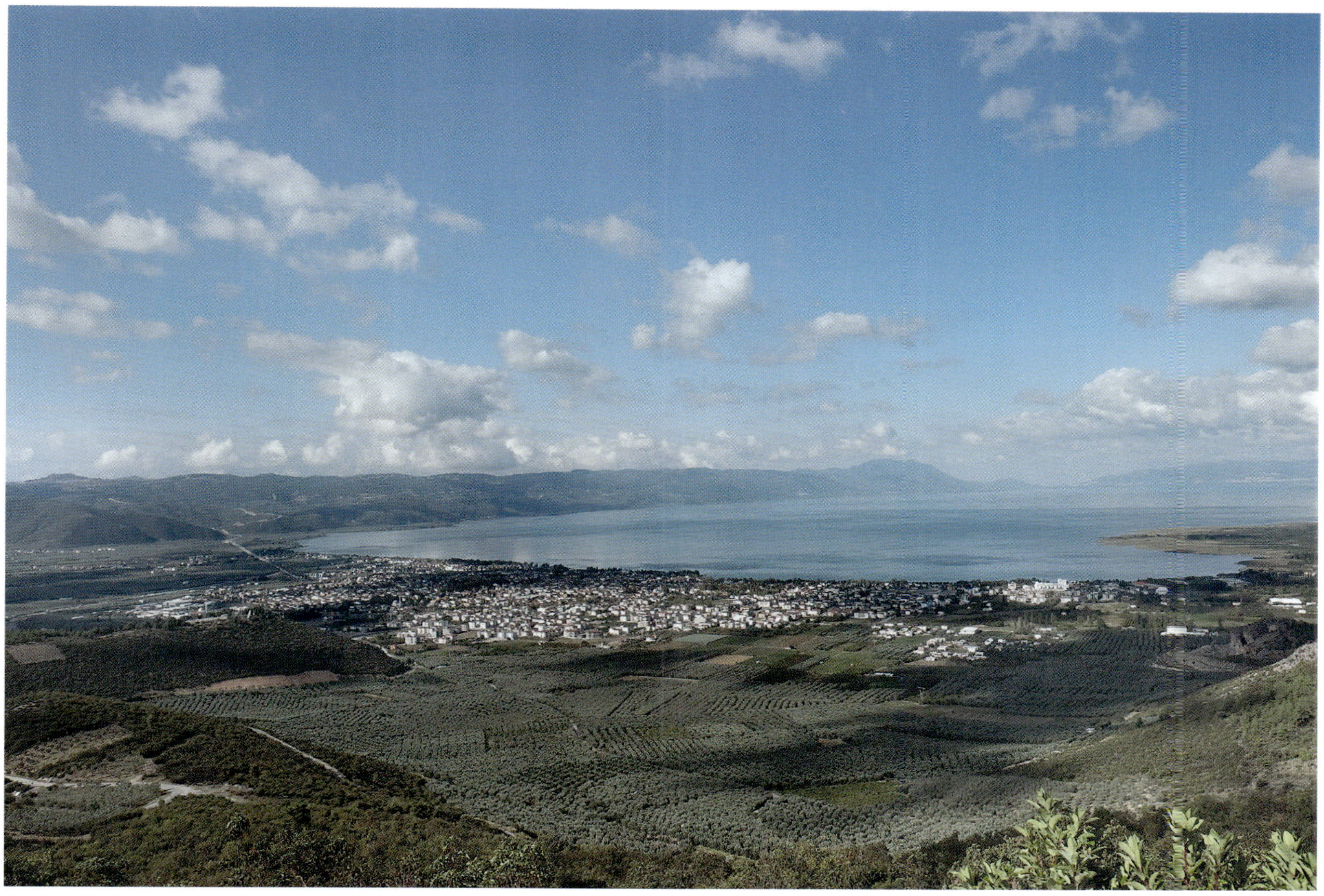

Lake Askania at Nicaea.

ecumenical horizons, it struggles simply to survive amid the swelling threats rising from both East and West.

I have now withdrawn from my medical service at the Xenon, yet I will not abandon Nicaea, where I lived the most creative years of my life. I dwell near the gate that opens toward Lake Ascania, where early each morning I go out to savor its stillness and vastness. I watch the fishing boats returning from their night's labor. And I see that life continues, despite the vain ambitions and greed of men. This land—watered with the blood and the sweat of its people—will forever remain the mother and cradle of Romiosyne (Hellenism).

Select Bibliography

1. Ahrweiler, Hélène: *Byzance et la mer. La marine de guerre la politique et les institutions maritimes de Byzance aux VII–XV siècles*. Thèse pour le doctorat ès lettres. Presses Universitaires de France, Paris 1966.
2. Bakke, Jorgen: *The vanished Gardens of Byzantium. Gardening, Visual Culture and Devotion in the Byzantine Orthodox Tradition*. Edition Bodin & Hedlund, Uppsala 2013.
3. Brunet, Felix: Die Spätantike und die Byzantinische Medicin. *Illustrierte Geschichte der Medizin, Andreas Verlag, Hannover 1992.*
4. Cedars, M.G. Reconstruction of the localized eyebrow defect. *Plastic & Reconstructive. Surgery 1997, 100:685–689.*
5. Concina, Ennio: Η Βυζαντινή πόλη. *Μετάφραση Κατερίνα Δασκαλάκη, Εκδόσεις Εστίας, Αθήνα 2009*
6. Constantelos, D.J.: Byzantine Philanthropy and Social Welfare. *New Brunswick – New Jersey 1968.*
7. Diehl, Charles.: Βυζαντινές Μορφές. *Εκδόσεις Μπεργάδη. Αθήνα 1969.*
8. Diehl Charles: Histoire de l' Empire Byzantin. *Μετάφραση Ε. Καψαμπέλης, Εκδόσεις Εστία, Αθήνα 1951.*
9. Ellis, Harold: The Cambridge illustrated history of Medicine. *Cambridge University Press 2009.*
10. Forum_de_Constantin https://fr.wikipedia.org/wiki/
11. Gautier, C.: "Le typikon du Christ Sauveur Pantocrator". *Institut Français d' Etudes Byzantines, Paris 1974.*
12. Giarenis, Ilias: The Crisis of the Fourth Crusade in Byzantium (1203–1204) and the Emergence of Networks for Anti-Latin Reaction and Political Action. *Academia edu. Giarenis*
13. Heiberg, I.: Paulus Aegineta. *Έκδοση Teubner BG, Lipsiae et Berolini 1924.*
14. Jacoby, David: The Greeks of Constantinople under Latin Rule 1204–1261 . *The forth crusade. Ashgate, London 2008.*
15. Kazhdan, A. (Editor). : The Oxford Dictionary of Byzantium III. *Oxford – New York 1991.*
16. Kean, Roger Michael: Ιστορικός Άτλας της Βυζαντινής Αυτοκρατορίας. *Μετάφραση Δημ. Κατσικερός. Εκδόσεις Σαβάλλας, Αθήνα 2006.*

17. Laskaratos, J. Dalla-Vorgia, P.: The penalty of mutilation for crimes in the Byzantine era (324–1453 AD). *International Journal of Risk & Safety in Medicine. 1997, 10: 51–56.*
18. Laskaratos, J. Cohen, M. Voros, D.: Plastic surgery of the face in Byzantium in the fourth century. *Plastic and Reconstructive Surgery 1998, 102: 1274–1280.*
19. Marketos, S.G, Laskaratos, J. Malakates, S.: The first record of lithotripsy in the early Byzantine era. *British Journal of Urology 1994, 74: 405–408.*
20. Meriç, T. Öztürk T.: The provincial aristocracy in Byzantine Asia Minor (1081–1261). *Master of Arts. Institute for Graduate Studies in the Social Sciences. Boğaziçi Universitesi, Istanbul 2013*
21. Miller, T.S.: Η γέννησις του νοσοκομείου στην Βυζαντινή Αυτοκρατορία. *Μετάφραση Ι. Κελέρμενος. Εκδόσεις ΒΗΤΑ Αθήνα 1998.*
22. Miller, T.S.: The Orphans of Byzantium. Child Welfare in the Christian Empire. *Catholic University of America., Washincton D.C. 2003.*
23. Nicol, Donald M: Βυζάντιο και Βενετία. Μελέτη των διπλωματικών και πολιτιστικών σχέσεων. *Μετάφραση Χριστίνα Μουτσοπούλου. Εκδόσεις Παπαδήμας, Αθήνα 2002.*
24. Ostrogorsky, Georg : Ιστορία Του Βυζαντινού Κράτους. *Εκδόσεις Σ. Βασιλόπουλου, Αθήνα 1978.*
25. Ouspensky, Léonide: La théologie de l'icône dans l'Église orthodoxe. *Editions Le Cerf, Paris 1960, 2001.*
26. Patlagean, E. : Pauvreté économique et pauvreté sociale à Byzance aux 4ème–7ème siècles. *Editions La Haye, Paris 1977.*
27. Pentogalos, G., Lascaratos, J.: A surgical operation performed on siamese twins during the tenth century in Byzantium. *Bulletin of the History of Medicine 1984, 58: 99–102.*
28. Pollak, Kurt: Η Ιατρική στην Αρχαιότητα: Ελλάδα– Ρώμη– Βυζάντιο. *Εκδόσεις Παπαδήμας, Αθήνα 2005.*
29. Raeder, J.: Oribasii Collectionum Medicarum Reliquiae. *Στο Teubner BG, Lipsiae et Berolini 1931.*
30. Remesnyder, JP, Bigelow, ME, Goldwyn, RM.: Justinian II and Carmagnola: A Byzantine rhinoplasty? *Plastic &. Reconstructive Surgery 1979, 63: 19–25.*
31. Runciman. Steven: Βυζαντινός Πολιτισμός. *Μετάφραση Δ. Καμπάνη-Δετζώρτζη. Εκδόσεις Ερμείας, Αθήνα 1993.*
32. Runciman, Steven: Η τελευταία βυζαντινή αναγέννηση. *Μετάφραση Λάμπρος Καμπερίδης, Εκδόσεις Δόμος, Αθήνα 2005.*
33. Singer, A.C. Underwood, E.A.: A Short History of Medicine. *Εκδόσεις Blekiston, Philadelphia 1958.*
34. Vasiliev, A.A.: Ιστορία της Βυζαντινής Αυτοκρατορίας. *Εκδόσεις Πελεκάνος, Αθήνα 2006.*
35. Villehardouin, Geoffroy de: La Conquète de Constantinople. *Traduction et Presentation Jean Dufournet : Editions Flammarion, Paris 2004.*

36. Walter, Gérard: Η καθημερινή ζωή στο Βυζάντιο στον αιώνα των Κομνηνών 1081–1180 . *Μετάφραση Κ. Παναγιώτου, Εκδόσεις Ωκεανίς, Αθήνα 1970.*
37. Αγγελίδη, Χριστίνα: Αρχαιότητα-Βυζάντιο, μια δύσκολη σχέση. *Στο Βυζαντινοί και Αρχαιότητα, (ed. Δ. Δαμάσκος). Καθημερινή*, 12 Ιανουαρίου 2003.
38. Αγγελίδη, Χριστίνα: *Καταγώγια, νοσοκομεία και ξενώνες. Η διαδρομή της περίθαλψης στο Βυζάντιο.* Ινστιτούτο Βυζαντινών Ερευνών. Αρχαιολογία και τέχνες, 2007, 103: 16–19
39. Ακομινάτος Χωνιάτης Νικήτας: Χρονική Διήγησις του Χωνιάτου κυρ Νικήτα αρχομένη από της βασιλείας Ιωάννου του Κομνηνού και λήγουσα μέχρι της αλώσεως της Κωνσταντινουπόλεως. *https://byzantium.gr/keimena/choniatis.php.*
40. Ακροπολίτης Γεώργιος: Χρονική συγγραφή. *Μετάφραση και σχόλια Σπύρος Σπυρόπουλος.* Εκδόσεις Ζήτρος. Αθήνα 2004.
41. Γιαννακόπουλος, *Κωνσταντίνος: Ο αυτοκράτωρ Μιχαήλ Παλαιολόγος και η Δύση.* Έκδοση, Κουλτούρα-Καραβίας. Αθήνα 1969.
42. Γιαρένης, Ηλίας: *Η Δ΄ Σταυροφορία, η άλωση της Κωνσταντινουπόλεως και η συγκρότηση των κρατών.* Academia edu. ! Giarenis. PDF.
43. Γιαρένης, Ηλίας: *Η συγκρότηση και η εδραίωση της αυτοκρατορίας της Νίκαιας. Ο αυτοκράτορας Θεόδωρος Α΄ Κομνηνός Λάσκαρις.* Έκδοση Εθνικό Ίδρυμα Ερευνών, Ινστιτούτο Βυζαντινών Ερευνών, Αθήνα 2008.
44. Ευτυχιάδης, Αριστοτέλης: *Αρχές Φιλοσοφίας και Ιστορίας της Ιατρικής,* Εκδόσεις Βήτα, Αθήνα 2001.
45. Ζακυθηνός Διονύσιος: Βυζάντιον. *Λήμμα από την Μεγάλη Ελληνική Εγκυκλοπαίδεια. Συμπλήρωμα Παύλου Δρανδάκη, τόμος Β. Εκδόσεις Ο Φοίνιξ, Αθήνα 1956.*
46. Θεοδοσίου Σ., Δανέζης Μ. : Στα χρόνια του Βυζαντίου. Οι θετικοί επιστήμονες, ιατροί, χρονολόγοι και αστρονόμοι. *Εκδόσεις Δίαυλος, Αθήνα 2010.*
47. *Ιστορία του Ελληνικού Έθνους.* Επιμέλεια Γ. Χριστόπουλος, Ι. Μπαστιάς. Τόμος Θ΄. Εκδοτική Αθηνών, Αθήνα 1979.
48. Ιωάννου Σιναΐτου: Λόγος προς ποιμένα. *«Κλίμαξ Ιωάννου του Σιναΐτου».* Εκδόσεις Αστήρ, Αθήνα 1979.
49. Καλαντζής Γ., Τσιάμης Κ., Πουλάκου Ρεμπελάκου Ε.: «Ορειβάσιος και Παύλος Αιγινήτης, δύο Βυζαντινοί ιατροί, πρωτοπόροι στην πλαστική χειρουργική», *Αρχεία Ελληνικής Ιατρικής 2006, 23: 536–540*
50. Καραμπερόπουλος, Δημήτριος: *Παύλος Αιγινήτης (625–690).* Ελευθεροτυπία 2004, Ιστορικά, αρ. 277.
51. Καραμπερόπουλος, Δημήτριος.: *Βυζαντινή θεραπευτική. Πρακτικά Συνεδρίου «Βυζάντιο-Βενετία-Νεότερος Ελληνισμός.* Εθνικό Ίδρυμα Ερευνών, 2003.
52. Κέκης, Βασίλειος.: «Μέγας Βασίλειος ο Ιατρός». *Σύγχρονη Ιατρική Ενημέρωση.* Αθήνα, Δεκέμβριος 2001.

53. Κουρκουτά, Λαμπρινή: *Η Νοσηλευτική στο Βυζάντιο*. Διδακτορική διατριβή. ΕΚΠΑ, Αθήνα 1993.
54. Κουτσούκος, Γρηγόριος: *Ιστορία της χειρουργικής αναισθησίας κατά την Βυζαντινή περίοδο*. Διδακτορική διατριβή. ΕΚΠΑ, Αθήνα 2005.
55. Κρουμβάχερ, Κ.: *Ιστορία της Βυζαντινής Λογοτεχνίας*. Έκδοση Βιβλιοθήκης Μαρασλή. Αθήνα 1900.
56. Κωνσταντέλος, Δημήτριος: *Πενία, Κοινωνία και Φιλανθρωπία στον μεταγενέστερο μεσαιωνικό Ελληνικό κόσμο*. Εκδόσεις Βάνιας, Θεσσαλονίκη 1994.
57. Λασκαράτος, Ιωάννης: *Κύλικες ζωής κατευνάστριαι. Ιστορική και ιατρική προσέγγιση στις δηλητηριάσεις της Βυζαντινής περιόδου*. Ιδιωτική έκδοση, Αθήνα 1994.
58. Λασκαράτος, Ιωάννης: *Ιστορία της Ιατρικής*, τόμος Ι. Ιατρικές Εκδόσεις Πασχαλίδης, Αθήνα 2003.
59. Λεονάρδος, Γιώργος: *Μιχαήλ Η΄ Παλαιολόγος, ο Ελευθερωτής*. Εκδόσεις Λιβάνης, Αθήνα 2005.
60. Λούβη-Κίζη, Ασπασία: *Η εκπαίδευση στο Βυζάντιο*. https://www.archaiologia.gr/wp-content.
61. Λυμπέρης, Λεωνίδας Ν: *Η εκπαίδευση στα Βυζαντινά χρόνια. Ο συνδετικός κρίκος του αρχαίου με το νεότερο Ελληνισμό. Τα Εκπαιδευτικά*, τ. 107–108: 131–143, Αθήνα 2013.
62. Μανιός Α., Παπαδάκης Μ., Φραγκάκης Μ., Σχορετσανίτης Γ., Τσιφτσής Δ.: «Η θυρεοειδεκτομή για βρογχοκήλη στην Βυζαντινή περίοδο», *Archives of Hellenic Medicine* 2008, 25(3): 384–388.
63. Μαρκέτος, Σπύρος: *Λήμματα από το Παγκόσμιο Βιογραφικό Λεξικό*. Εκδοτική Αθηνών, Αθήνα 1984.
64. Ματσάγγας, Αριστομένης: *Η οργάνωση και η λειτουργία των Βυζαντινών Νοσοκομείων και ιδιαίτερα του Νοσοκομείου της Μονής του Παντοκράτορος*. Διδακτορική Διατριβή. ΕΚΠΑ, Αθήνα 1984.
65. Μεντής, Α.Φ., Καραρίζου, Ε: *Η διαλεκτική μεταξύ Ιατρικής και θαυμάτων στην Ανατολική Χριστιανική Ρωμαϊκή Αυτοκρατορία*. Archives of Hellenic Medicine, 2011, 28(4):561–568.
66. Μεργιαλή-Σαχά, Σοφία: *Πειρατές και ασκητές: Το φαινόμενο της πειρατείας μέσα από τα αγιολογικά κείμενα της Παλαιολόγειας εποχής*. Ιόνιος Λόγος, τ. 2, Κέρκυρα 2010.
67. Μεργιαλή-Σαχά, Σοφία: «Αμφίδρομες πολιτισμικές διαδρομές ανάμεσα στο Βυζάντιο και την αναγεννησιακή Ιταλία», *Βυζαντινά* (2012), 32: 227–244.
68. Μεργιαλή-Σαχά, Σοφία: *Γράφοντας ιστορία με τους αγίους: από την κοινωνία των αγίων στην κοινωνία τον Παλαιολόγων (1261–1453)*, Εκδόσεις Ηρόδοτος 2014.
69. Μοσχονάς, Ν.Γ. (επιμελητής εκδόσεως): Η Τετάρτη Σταυροφορία και ο Ελληνικός κόσμος. *Το Βυζάντιο σήμερα*. Εθνικό Ίδρυμα Ερευνών, Ινστιτούτο Βυζαντινών ερευνών, Αθήνα 2008.

70. Μουντζάλη, Αφέντρα: «Περίθαλψη ασθενών στο Βυζάντιο», *Αρχαιολογία και Τέχνες*, 2007, 103: 10–13.
71. Μυλωνάς, Αναστάσιος: *Η στοματική και γναθοπροσωπική χειρουργική στο Βυζάντιο*. Διδακτορική διατριβή. ΕΚΠΑ. Αθήνα 2011.
72. Παπαγεωργίου, Γεώργιος: *Ο Άγιος Λουκάς της Κριμαίας και ο Αλβέρτος Σβάιτσερ. Παράθεση δύο μεγάλων*. Εκδόσεις Επιστροφή 2016.
73. Παπαγεωργίου Γεώργιος: «Η χειρουργική και τα νοσοκομεία στο Βυζάντιο», In *Η Χειρουργική των Ελλήνων δια μέσου των αιώνων*. (ed. Ιωάννης Μπράμης), τόμος Α'. Εκδόσεις Μίλητος, Αθήνα 2019.
74. Παπαδάκης, Μάριος: *Η μελέτη της εξέλιξης των χειρουργικών επεμβάσεων και εργαλείων της πλαστικής χειρουργικής κατά την Ελληνική Αρχαιότητα και το Βυζάντιο*. Διδακτορική διατριβή. Πανεπιστήμιο Κρήτης. Ηράκλειο 2011.
75. Παπαρρηγόπουλος, Κωνσταντίνος: *Ιστορία του Ελληνικού Έθνους*. Επιμέλεια Παύλου Καρολίδου. Τόμος Δ' Μέρος Β' και Τόμος Ε' Μέρος Α'. Εκδόσεις Ελευθερουδάκης, Αθήνα 1932.
76. Πολίτη, Ειρήνη: *Η μόρφωση της γυναίκας την εποχή των Παλαιολόγων μέσα από την επιστολογραφία της Χούμναινας (1290–1360). Πρόσβαση στη γνώση και μαθητεία την εποχή των Παλαιολόγων (1261–1453.)* Μεταπτυχιακή εργασία. ΕΚΠΑ, 2013.
77. Σταυρακάκης, Ν.: «Το γηροκομείο, λεπροκομείο και το μοναστικό θεραπευτήριο της αυτοκρατορικής μονής του Παντοκράτορος Σωτήρος Χριστού στην Κωνσταντινούπολη (15/10/1136 έως 29/5/1453)», *Αρχεία Ελληνικής Ιατρικής*, 2017, 34(6): 824–829
78. Σπανδάγος, Β., Σπανδάγου Ρ., Τραυλού Δ.: *Οι θετικοί Επιστήμονες της Βυζαντινής Εποχής*. Εκδόσεις Αίθρα, Αθήνα 1996.
79. Στεφανίδης, Μάνος: *Μια ιστορία της ζωγραφικής. Από το Βυζάντιο στην Αναγέννηση και από τους Ιμπρεσιονιστές στον Πικάσο*. Εκδόσεις Καστανιώτης, Αθήνα 1997.
80. Τουλιάτος, Δ.Π.: *Η Ελληνική Ιατρική δια μέσου των Αιώνων. Ιατρική και Θρησκεία – Επιστήμη και Θαύμα. Η πίστις ως βασικός θεραπευτικός παράγων*. Εκδόσεις Φρίξου Μπουκούρη, Αθήνα 1954.
81. Τουλιάτος, Δ.Π.: *Αρρώστιες – Ιατροί και Φάρμακα ανά τον κόσμον και τους Αιώνας*. Εκδόσεις Φρίξου Μπουκούρη, Αθήνα 1958.
82. Τράκα, Ντιάνα.: *Η Βυζαντινή Ιατρική. Αρχαιολογία και Τέχνες*, 2007, τ. 103 Αθήνα.
83. Τσιόπας, Ζ.: *Ένα βυζαντινό νοσοκομείο του 12ου αιώνα*. https://vizantinonistorika.blogspot.com/2013.
84. Τσιπούρας, Στυλιανός: *Αγωγή και εκπαίδευση στο Βυζάντιο. Σπουδή στην κανονική και πατερική γραμματεία*. Διπλωματική εργασία. Αριστοτέλειο Πανεπιστήμιο Θεσσαλονίκης 2027.

Abbreviations - Image Sources

Zonaras: Ιωάννης Ζωναράς, *Επιτομή Ιστοριών, Codex Mutinensis graecus 122,* Biblioteca Estense in Modena, Italy

Skylitzes: Skylitzes, John. *Synopsis of Histories. Codex Matritensis gr.* Vitr. 26-2 (the "Madrid Skylitzes"), 12th century. National Library of Spain, Madrid Nacional de España.

Aubert David (1449–79) *Croniques abregies commençans au temps de Herode Antipas, persecuteur de la chrestienté, et finissant l'an de grace mil IIc et LXXVI* edited by Danielle Quéruel, *Cultures et civilisations médiévales,* Paris 1999

Biedermann Hans, *Medicina magica, metaphysische Heilmethoden in spatantiken und mittelalterlichen Handschriften,* Graz 1978

Delacoux Alois, *Biographies des sages-femmes célèbres anciennes, modernes et contemporaines,* ed. Trinquart, Paris 1834

Dölger Franz, *Facsimiles byzantinischer Kaiserurkunden. Mittel- und neugriechisches Seminar der Universität München,* Munich 1931

Dovaston Margaret (1884–1954), in *History of the Nations,* ed. Hutchinson, Λονδίνο 1915

Fossati Gaspard, *Aya Sofia Constantinople, A recently restored by Order of H.M. the Sultan Abdul Medjid,* ed. P. & C. Colhaghi, London 1852

Guillaume de Tyr, Histoire d' outremer, avec continuation jusqu'en 1275. National Library of France, Paris

Janin R., *Constantinople Byzantine. Developpement urbain et repertoire topographique,* Paris 1950

Köhler's medizinal-Pflanzen in naturgetreuen Abbildungen mit kurz erläuterndrem Text, Atlas zur Pharmacopoea germanica, austriaca, belgica, danica, helvetica, 1887

Michaud Joseph-Francois, *Histoire des Croisades, illustrée de 100 grandes compositions par Gustave Doré,* ed. Hachette, Paris 1877

Salzenberg Wilhelm, *Alt-Christliche Baudenkmale von Constantinopel vom V. bis XII. Jahrhundert,* ed. Von Ernst & Korn, Berlin 1854

African Journals Online: p. 90
Ancientmedicine.org: pp. 64, 89 (bottom)
Anglo norman dictionary: pp.179 (top–left), 208
https://www.antoine-helbert.com: 31, 51 (top), 52, 55, 58, 59, 60, 67, 859 (bottom), 94, 101 (top), 124, 141, 157, 159 (top), 175
Bridgeman images: p. 182
byzantineempire: p. 19 (top)
Flickr: p. 95 (top), 117
garouphalis.gr: p. 143 (left–right), 144 (left–right)
Getty images: p. 33, 130, 152, 164, 176, 1959
Google Books: p. 120
iKivotos: p. 16
ime (Ίδρυμα Μείζονος Ελληνισμού): pp. 18, 107 (top)
jwstudybibles: p. 22 (top left)
Médecine des Arts: p. 115
medieval ware: p. 174
Open Culture: Antoine Helbert
Orthodox Christianity then and now: pp. 32, 136 ()
pastorjasonelder.com: p. 98
Pinterest: p. 43
Reddit: p. 28
research gate: p. 191, 200 (right)
Romano Impero: p. 112
runivers.ru/book4: p. 190
Teacher Curator: p. 82 (top)
The Byzantium Blogger: p. 116 (top)
University of Virginia: p. 86 (left)
Wikimedia Commons: 8, 14, 15, 19 (bottom left), 26 (bottom), 29, 33, 36, 38, 46, 51, 54, 62, 68, 69, 71 (left), 71 (right), 72, 74, 75 (right), 76, 771, 78, 80, 83 (top), 83 (bottom), 85 (top), 86 (left), 89 (top), 92, 99, 100, 102, 105 (top), 107 (bottom), 109 (bottom), 110, 113, 114 (bottom), 125, 127, 128 (top–bottom), 136 (left), 150 (top–bottom), 150 (top), 153, 156, 162, 163, 168, 173 (top–bottom), 178, 185, 189, 199, 200 (left), 201, 202 (2 photos left), 204 (left), 205 (right), 209 (top–bottom), 212, 213
Wikipedia: pp. 20, 22 (top), 27, 50, 56, 61, 62, 66, 73, 75 (left), 84 (bottom), 87, 95, 96, 103, 105 (bottom), 108, 118, 119, 121 (top–bottom), 122, 123, 138 (bottom), 139 (top), 140, 145, 147, 148, 150 (bottom), 154 (top–bottom), 158, 159 (bottom), 160, 167, 177, 180, 181, 183, 184, 186 (left–right), 198, 202 (middle), 203 (bottom), 204 (right), 205 (left), 207, 210, 215
wordpress: p. 155
World History Encyclopedia: p. 109 (top)
Αρχαιολογία online: pp. 192, 216
Διακόνημα: p. 211

Εθνικό Μουσείο της Ελβετίας, Ζυρίχη (Schweizerisches Landesmuseum): p. 53
Πεμπτουσία: pp. 97, 138 (top)
Ταμείο Αρχαιολογικών Πόρων (ΤΑΠ): p. 101
Υπουργείο Πολιτισμού: p. 70

Textual Quotations

Παπαγεωργίου Γεώργιος Κ., *Ο Άγιος Λουκάς της Κριμαίας και ο Αλβέρτος Σβάιτσερ*, ed. Επιστροφή 2016, p. 105

Καραμπερόπουλος Δ., *Παύλος Αιγινήτης* 1 (625–690 μ. Χ.), Ιστορικά Ελευθεροτυπίας, No. 277, p. 38–41

Κ .Π. Καβάφης, *Ποιήματα Α'*, επιμ. Γ. Π. Σαββίδη, ed. Ίκαρος 1965, p. 47

Sheila Dillon et Sharon L. James, *A companion to Women in the Ancient World*, Wiley-Blackwell 2012

Κουκουλές Φαίδων, *Βυζαντινών Βίος και Πολιτισμός*, vol. 6, ed. Παπαζήση 1949, p. 24

Το Χρονικόν του Μωρέως, ed. Εκάτη χ.χ., pp. 4075–4092

Brief Biographical Note

Georgios C. Papageorgiou was born in Patras in 1945. He studied at the Medical School of the University of Athens and specialized in Surgery at Evangelismos Hospital.

He pursued further training in Endocrine Surgery in England and France.

He served for many years at Evangelismos as Registrar and, in his last ten years there, as Coordinating Director. Since 1998 he has collaborated with the KEDAS Association in the work of Medical Mission in Africa, in Kampala (Uganda) and in Bukoba (Tanzania).

In addition to his medical publications and treatises, he has authored five books: 1) *Saint Luke of Crimea and Albert Schweitzer* (in Greek and English), 2) *Demos of Dreams* (in Greek), 3) *Saint-Exupéry, the Last Knight of the Sky* (in Greek and English), 4) *Those Who Dared* (the history of physicians in Africa during the colonial period) (in Greek), and 5) *Oscar's Fantastic Journey to the Sky* (in Greek and German).

He holds a Doctorate from the University of Athens and the title of Emeritus (Assoc.) Professor of Surgery.

For this Edition Collaborated

Author
Dr. Georgios C. Papageorgiou

General Editing
Dr. Olga Mentzafou-Polyzou

Artistic Editing & Image Processing
Vana Roussioti

Technical Editing
Giannis Chrysanthopoulos

Publication Supervision & Coordination
Nikos Komn. Chatzigeorgiou

Greek ISBN: 978-960-89349-6-2

© Text Copyright
Georgios C. Papageorgiou

© Worldwide Edition Copyright
Athens 2024
Hellenic Facsimile Editions (Ελληνικές Ομοιογραφικές Εκδόσεις)

HELLENIC
FACSIMILE
EDITIONS

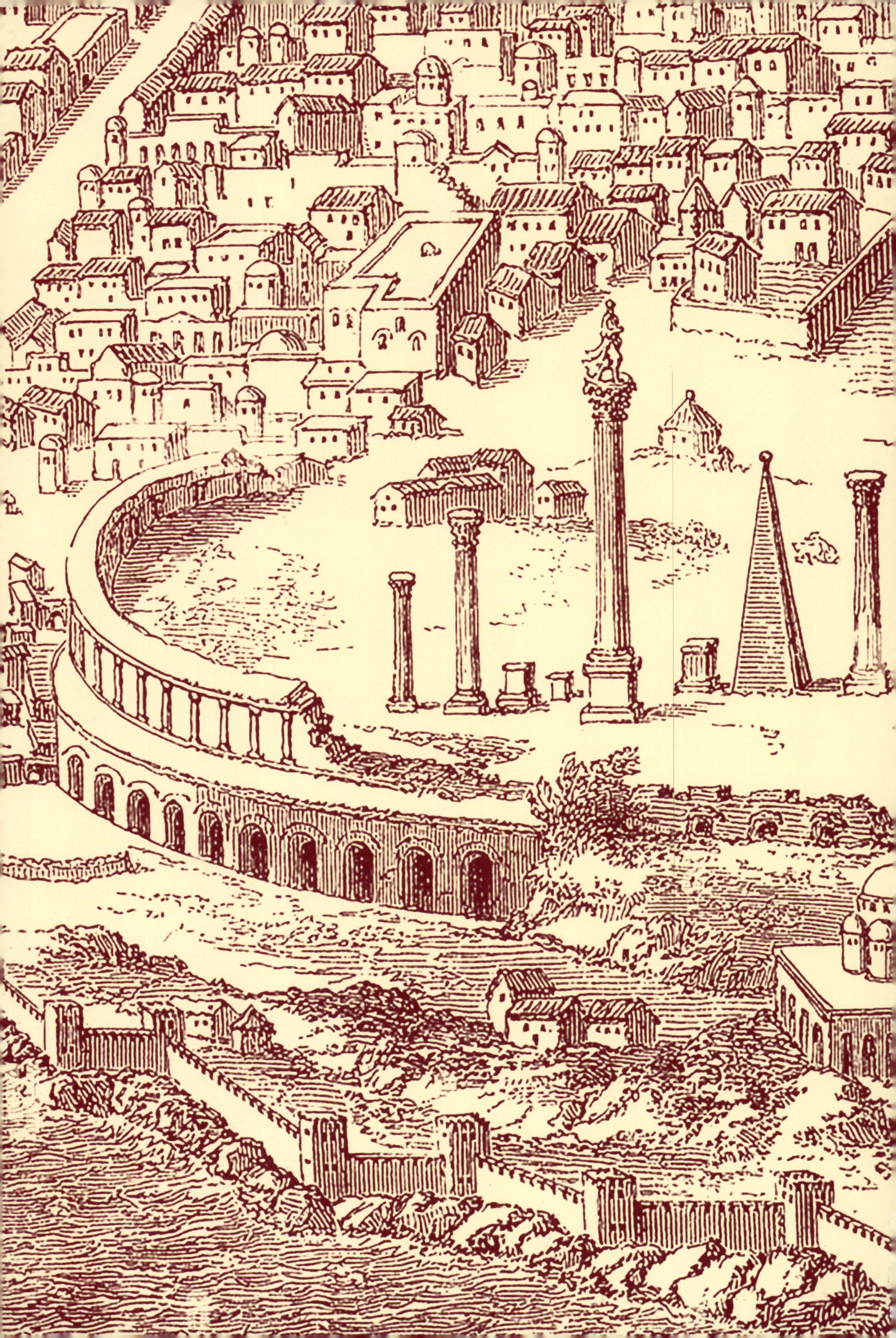